Muscle Energy Techniques

For Churchill Livingstone:

Editorial Director, Health Professions: Mary Law
Head of Project Management: Ewan Halley
Project Development Manager: Katrina Mather
Design Direction: George Ajayi

Muscle Energy Techniques

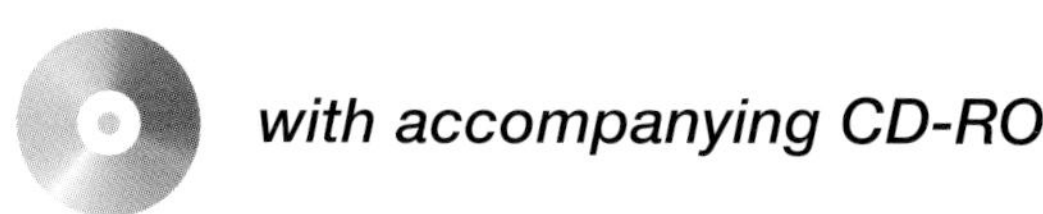

Leon Chaitow ND DO
Registered Osteopathic Practitioner and Senior Lecturer, University of Westminster, London, UK

with contribution from

Craig Liebenson DC (Chapter 5: Manual resistance techniques in rehabilitation)
Private Practitioner, Los Angeles, CA, USA

Foreword by

Donald R Murphy DC DACAN
Clinical Director, Rhode Island Spine Center,
Clinical Teaching Associate, Brown University
School of Medicine, Providence, RI, USA

Illustrated by

Graeme Chambers BA (Hons)
Medical Artist

SECOND EDITION

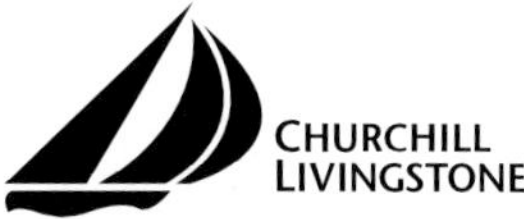

EDINBURGH LONDON NEW YORK PHILADELPHIA ST LOUIS SYDNEY TORONTO 2001

CHURCHILL LIVINGSTONE
An imprint of Harcourt Publishers Limited

First edition 1996
Second edition 2001

ISBN 0 443 06496 2

British Library Cataloguing in Publication Data
A catalogue record for this book is available from the British Library

Library of Congress Cataloging in Publication Data
A catalog record for this book is available from the Library of Congress

Note
Medical knowledge is constantly changing. As new information becomes available, changes in treatment, procedures, equipment and the use of drugs become necessary. The author and the publishers have taken care to ensure that the information given in this text is accurate and up to date. However, readers are strongly advised to confirm that the information, especially with regard to drug usage, complies with the latest legislation and standards of practice.

Neither the publishers nor the author will be liable for any loss or damage of any nature occasioned to or suffered by any person acting or refraining from acting as a result of reliance on the material contained in this publication.

The publisher's policy is to use **paper manufactured from sustainable forests**

Printed in China

Contents

The CD-ROM accompanying this text includes video sequences of all the techniques indicated in the text by the icon. To look at the video for a given technique, click on the relevant icon on the CD-ROM. The CD-ROM is designed to be used in conjunction with the text and not as a stand-alone product.

Glossary and abbreviations

Active Muscular Relaxation Techniques
MET - Muscle Energy Techniques = PIR = Post Isometric Relaxation
+RI = Reciprocal Inhibition

PNF: Proprioceptive Neuromuscular Facilitation
Manual Resistance Techniques = Post Contraction Relaxation

Agonist: prime mover (e.g. biceps during elbow flexion)
AIS: active isolated stretching
Antagonist: muscle which has the opposite action to the agonist (e.g. triceps during elbow flexion)
ASIS: anterior superior iliac spine
ATP: adenosine triphosphate
Barrier phenomenon: restriction of mobility either physiological, pathological or anatomical
CCP: common compensatory pattern
CNS: central nervous system
Concentric: muscle contraction involving shortening of the length of the muscle
CP: cerebral palsy
CR: contract–relax – a proprioceptive neuromuscular facilitation (PNF) technique used to relax and stretch tight muscles. Particularly good for large muscles
CRAC: contract–relax, antagonist contract – a PNF technique used to relax and stretch tight muscles. Involves use of agonist and antagonist muscles
CT: cervicothoracic
Eccentric: muscle contraction involving lengthening of the muscle
EMG: electromyogram
Facilitation: spontaneous activation of a specific muscle's contractile ability, often via reflex means
FMS: fibromyalgia syndrome
Functional (neutral) range: the painless range used for exercise training where proper form and proximal stability are maintained
HCP: health care provider
HR: hold–relax – a PNF technique used to relax and stretch tight muscles, especially when there is pain present
HVT: high velocity/low amplitude thrusts
INIT: integrated neuromuscular inhibition technique
Isometric: muscle contraction involving no change in the muscle's length (c.f. concentric and eccentric)
Isotonic: muscle contraction involving a change in muscle length (c.f. concentric and eccentric)
Joint centration: neutral position of a joint which achieves both maximum congruence of joint surfaces and normalises length/tension relationships of antagonist muscles
LDJ: lumbodorsal junction
LS: lumbosacral
MEP: muscle energy procedure
MET: muscle energy technique
MPI: myofascial pain index
MPS: myofascial pain syndrome
MRT: manual resistance technique
MTPJ: metatarsophalangeal joint
MVC: maximum voluntary contraction
NMT: neuromuscular technique
OA: occipitoatlantal
OMT: osteopathic manipulative therapy
PFS: postfacilitation stretch – used for stretching muscle or fascia
PIR: postisometric relaxation – like HR except that forces are gentler. Can be used to relax tense muscle, mobilise joint or aid in traction
PNF: proprioceptive neuromuscular facilitation

PSIS: posterior superior iliac spine
QL: quadratus lumborum
Release phenomenon: viscous or inhibitory release of pathological barrier in soft tissues which occurs with manipulation (thrust, PIR, oscillation, myofascial release, etc.)
RI: reciprocal inhibition – Sherrington's law states that when an agonist contracts, its antagonist will be inhibited (due to inhibitory neurotransmitter release at the antagonist site)
SCM: sternocleidomastoid
SCS: strain/counterstrain
SIJ: sacroiliac joint
SLR: straight leg raised
Synergist: a muscle which assists an agonist during a movement, but which has other primary actions
TFL: tensor fascia lata
TL: thoracolumbar
TMJ: temporomandibular joint

same Side inhibition by "Shortening of Shortened/Tight Muscle.

Foreword

As the art and science of neuromusculoskeletal care evolve, it is becoming increasingly clear that manual techniques are essential in the proper management of patients with problems in this area. What is less easily measured, however, is the impact of the degree of skill with which these techniques are applied on the outcome of management. Most clinicians who use manual techniques in the treatment of dysfunction in the locomotor system would agree, however, that the level of skill with which a practitioner applies a certain technique is of the utmost importance in the success of any management strategy. Intuition would tell us that a clinician with limited skill and a limited variety of methods in his or her armamentarium would be less effective, especially for a difficult case, than one who possesses wide-ranging knowledge and ability.

It has been said that you can't learn manual skills from a book. However, you can build upon an existing body of knowledge, skill and experience with a written source that introduces new methodology and instructs in the scientific basis and proper application of one's current methodology. In addition, a written source of high-quality, clinically applicable information can be an excellent source of support material when one is taking an undergraduate or postgraduate course in manual therapy. Leon Chaitow has produced such a book.

One of the unique aspects of manual therapy that one discovers early in practice is that no two patients are alike and no two locomotor systems are alike. As a result, each patient requires a highly individualized approach that addresses his or her unique circumstances. This means that one must be meticulous about identifying those specific dysfunctions, be they joint, muscle or otherwise, that are most important in producing the disorder from which the patient suffers, and choosing those specific treatment approaches that are most likely to correct the identified dysfunctions. Muscle energy techniques (METs) are among the most valuable tools that any manual clinician can have in his or her tool box. There are many reasons for this.

First, METs have a wide application. They can be applied to muscle hypertonicity and muscle tightness, but can be equally effectively applied to joint dysfunction and joint capsule adhesions. Important modifications must be made for each application, as demonstrated in this book. But because the method is as flexible as it is, the clinician is provided with a tool that he or she can modify for a variety of types of dysfunction. In addition, METs can be used as an important aspect of an overall rehabilitation strategy, as brought out by Craig Liebenson in his chapter.

Second, METs can be applied in a gentle manner. In manual therapy, we always want to be as gentle as possible, in a way that still provides effective correction of dysfunction. MET, particularly when applied to muscle hypertonicity and to joint dysfunction, is both gentle and effective. For those of us who use thrust techniques, METs also represent a different method of applying joint manipulation that is well tolerated by the apprehensive patient, or the acute situation. And, MET has been shown to be equally effective as thrust techniques.

Third, METs actively involve the patient in the process. One of the essential ingredients in a successful management strategy involves empowering the patient to take charge of his or her own recovery. This means that the patient must not be a passive recipient of treatment, but rather an active participant. Unlike many manual procedures, with METs, the patient must be involved in every step, contracting at the appropriate time, relaxing at the appropriate time, engaging in eye movements, breathing, etc. METs allow the clinician to apply corrective measures while at the same time beginning the process of transferring responsibility to the patient.

Finally, METs are effective. This has been demonstrated both experimentally and in the clinical experience of the many clinicians who use this method. I can say for myself that I could not imagine how I would attempt to manage the majority of patients that I see without this all-important tool at my disposal.

But, to realize all these benefits of METs, one must apply them with skill and precision. And they must be applied in the context of a management strategy that takes into consideration the entire person. This book represents an important step in this direction.

Providence, RI, USA Donald R. Murphy

Preface

Muscle energy techniques (MET) evolved in osteopathic medicine from a variety of roots, including the pioneering work of TJ Ruddy DO (1961). Ruddy's approach ('rapid resistive duction') was just one stimulus that inspired the work of Fred Mitchell Sr DO, who is generally credited with the formulation of the basis of MET, to refine and modify an approach that he described as 'muscular energy technique'. Other sources that guided Mitchell include the founder of osteopathic medicine, Andrew Taylor Still, whom Mitchell (1958) quotes as saying, 'The attempt to restore joint integrity before soothingly restoring muscle and ligamentous normality [is] putting the cart before the horse.' Over the years since 1958, when Mitchell first published details of MET, many others both within the osteopathic profession (such as Kuchera & Kuchera 1994), as well as from manual medicine (most notably Karel Lewit MD 1999 and Vladimir Janda MD 1993), physiotherapy (for example Jull & Janda 1987) and chiropractic (for example Craig Liebenson DC 1996 - see chapter 5) have all devised enhancements and modifications to MET's original model of use.

The basic concepts of MET involve using the intrinsic power of muscles to achieve a variety of effects, involving isometric and isotonic contraction variations, and this volume aims to offer insights into, and practical applications of, most of these.

There are no contraindications to the use of MET if it is applied thoughtfully, taking account of the patient's particular and specific needs. It is perfectly appropriate to utilise MET in an acute and extremely painful situation, working with minute contractions, sometimes involving no more than eye movement as the instigator of muscular toning. Alternatively, MET may involve robust stretching following an isometric contraction (of agonist or antagonist), or it might be deemed appropriate to apply a passive stretch during the contraction, or there may be no stretching at all - merely a repetitive facilitation of tone in inhibited structures (echoing in many particulars Ruddy's original pulsing approach).

The permutations in methodology that can be applied to the basic concepts of MET are as numerous and as varied as the conditions they are being applied to, ranging from acute to chronic, with objectives as disparate as relaxing a muscle, stretching a muscle, strengthening a muscle, retraining appropriate function in a muscle, deactivating trigger points, freeing a restricted joint, preparing supporting tissues for manipulation of a joint, enhancing local circulation ... and more.

MET methods may at times be usefully employed in isolation, but are more commonly found to be useful when combined with appropriate associated modalities and methods, including manipulation of joints (adjustments), positional release techniques, myofascial release, soft tissue manipulation, neuromuscular techniques, massage therapy, physical therapy and chiropractic rehabilitation. MET methods are sometimes used before and sometimes following application of other modalities, and sometimes in intricate sequences such as integrated neuromuscular inhibition (see chapter 7).

Whichever aspect of MET is employed it is important to appreciate the context in which it is being used, and the objectives it is being asked to encourage. In health care in general, and bodywork in particular, objectives can usually be seen to have one of three goals (with an overlap of several at a time in some instances), all of which encourage the self-regulating mechanisms of the body to perform more efficiently. The initial objective may be to lessen the adaptive demands on an area, or on the body as a whole (releasing tight structures, mobilising restricted joints, toning inhibited structures, improving function, etc.); or to encourage more efficient handling by the body of the adaptive demands it is facing (by creating more resilient and stable structures); and/or to treat symptoms (e.g. easing pain). Whichever of these is the therapeutic objective, MET is capable of playing a role, if utilised appropriately, without imposing further adaptive demands. The thinking practitioner's goals are to understand the modus operandi of the available therapeutic choices, to acquire the skills to utilise them, and to apply them appropriately and safely. The multiple application potentials of muscle energy technique offer an invaluable set of such choices.

Corfu 2001 LC

REFERENCES

Janda V 1993 Assessment and treatment of impaired movement patterns and motor recruitment. Presentation to Physical Medicine Research Foundation Montreal, 9-11 October 1993

Jull G, Janda V 1987 Muscles and motor control in low back pain. In: Twomey L, Taylor J (eds) Physical therapy for the low back. Churchill Livingstone, New York, NY

Kuchera W, Kuchera M 1994 Osteopathic principles in practice, 2nd edn. Greyden Press, Columbus, OH

Lewit K 1999 Manipulation in rehabilitation of the locomotor system, 3rd edn. Butterworth, London

Liebenson C 1996 Rehabilitation of the spine Williams & Wilkins, Baltimore, MD

Mitchell FL Sr 1958 Structural pelvic function. In: Barnes M (ed) Yearbook of the Academy of Applied Osteopathy, Indianapolis, IN 1958:79

Ruddy TJ 1961 Osteopathic rhythmic resistive duction therapy. In: Barnes M (ed) Yearbook of the Academy of Applied Osteopathy, Indianapolis, IN 1961:58

Acknowledgements

The acknowledgements given in the first edition of this book are repeated since without the pioneering work of Drs Korr, Stiles, Mitchell, Ruddy and Patterson in the osteopathic profession and medical researchers and clinicians such as Karel Lewit and Vladimir Janda, MET would not have developed to its present refined state. Particular thanks go to Dr Craig Liebenson, who has brought these methods into mainstream chiropractic rehabilitation methodology. His excellent compilation of information is found in Chapter 5. Additionally numerous physiotherapists, massage therapists and basic science researchers have contributed to the methods distilled into this book, and my thanks go to all of them. I wish also to thank my colleagues at the University of Westminster School of Integrated Health, where a module of MET, based on this text, is taught – particularly Mark Gray, who has so enthusiastically assisted me in its teaching.

CHAPTER CONTENTS

1

An introduction to muscle energy techniques

MUSCLE ENERGY TECHNIQUES (MET)

A revolution has taken place in manipulative therapy involving a movement away from high velocity/low amplitude thrusts (HVT – now commonly known as 'mobilisation with impulse' and characteristic of most chiropractic and, until recently, much osteopathic manipulation) towards gentler methods which take far more account of the soft tissue component (DiGiovanna 1991, Lewit 1999, Travell & Simons 1992).

Greenman (1996) states that: 'Early [osteopathic] techniques did speak of muscle relaxation with soft tissue procedures, but specific manipulative approaches to muscle appear to be 20th century phenomena.' One such approach – which targets the soft tissues primarily, although it also makes a major contribution towards joint mobilisation – has been termed muscle energy technique (MET) in osteopathic medicine. There are a variety of other terms used to describe this approach, the most general (and descriptively accurate) of which was that used by chiropractor Craig Liebenson (1989, 1990) when he described 'muscle energy' techniques as 'active muscular relaxation techniques'. MET evolved out of osteopathic procedures developed by pioneer practitioners such as T. J. Ruddy (1961), who termed his approach 'resistive duction', and Fred Mitchell Snr (1967). As will become clear in this chapter, there also exists a commonality between MET and various procedures used in orthopaedic and physiotherapy methodology, such as proprioceptive neuromuscular facilitation (PNF).

Largely due to the work of experts in physical medicine such as Karel Lewit (1999), MET has evolved and been refined, and now crosses all interdisciplinary boundaries.

MET has as one of its objectives the induced relaxation of hypertonic musculature and, where appropriate (see below), the subsequent stretching of the muscle. This objective is shared with a number of 'stretching' systems, and it is necessary to examine and to compare the potential benefits and drawbacks of these various methods (see Box 1.1).

MET, as presented in this book, owes most of its development to osteopathic clinicians such as T. J. Ruddy (1961) and Fred Mitchell Snr (1967), with more recent refinements deriving from the work of people such as Karel Lewit (1986, 1999) and Vladimir Janda (1989) of the former Czechoslovakia, both of whose work will be referred to many times in this text.

T. J. Ruddy (1961)

In the 1940s and 50s, osteopathic physician T. J. Ruddy developed a treatment method involving patient-induced, rapid, pulsating contractions against resistance which he termed 'rapid resistive duction'. It was in part this work which Fred Mitchell Snr used as the basis for the evolution of MET (along with PNF methodology, see Box 1.1). Ruddy's method called for a series of rapid, low amplitude muscle contractions against resistance, at a rate a little faster than the pulse rate. This approach is now known as pulsed MET, rather than the tongue-twisting 'Ruddy's rapid resistive duction'.

As a rule, at least initially, these patient-directed pulsating contractions involve an effort towards the barrier, using antagonists to shortened structures. This approach can be applied in all areas where sustained contraction muscle energy technique procedures are appropriate, and is particularly useful for self-treatment, following instruction from a skilled practitioner. Ruddy suggests that the effects include improved local oxygenation, venous and lymphatic circulation, as well as a positive influence on both static and kinetic posture, because of the effects on proprioceptive and interoceptive afferent pathways.

Ruddy's work formed part of the base on which Mitchell Snr and others constructed MET and aspects of its clinical application are described in Chapter 3.

Fred Mitchell Snr

No single individual was alone responsible for MET, but its inception into osteopathic work must be credited to F. L. Mitchell Snr, in 1958. Since then his son F. Mitchell Jnr (Mitchell et al 1979) and many others have evolved a highly sophisticated system of manipulative methods (F. Mitchell Jnr, tutorial on biomechanical procedures, American Academy of Osteopathy, 1976) in which the patient 'uses his/her muscles, on request, from a precisely controlled position in a specific direction, against a distinctly executed counterforce'.

Philip Greenman

Professor of biomechanics Philip Greenman (1996) states that:

> The function of any articulation of the body which can be moved by voluntary muscle action, either directly or indirectly, can be influenced by muscle energy procedures … . Muscle energy techniques can be used to lengthen a shortened, contractured or spastic muscle; to strengthen a physiologically weakened muscle or group of muscles; to reduce localized edema, to relieve passive congestion, and to mobilize an articulation with restricted mobility.

Sandra Yale

Osteopathic physician Sandra Yale (in DiGiovanna 1991) extols MET's potential in even fragile and severely ill patients:

> Muscle energy techniques are particularly effective in patients who have severe pain from acute somatic dysfunction, such as those with a whiplash injury from a car accident, or a patient with severe muscle spasm from a fall. MET methods are also an excellent treatment modality for hospitalized or bedridden patients. They can be used in older patients who may have severely restricted motion from arthritis, or who have brittle osteoporotic bones.

Box 1.1 Stretching variations

Facilitated stretching
This active stretching approach represents a refinement of PNF (see below), and is largely the work of Robert McAtee (McAtee & Charland 1999). This approach uses strong isometric contractions of the muscle to be treated, followed by active stretching by the patient. An acronym, CRAC, is used to describe what is done (contract–relax, antagonist contract). The main difference between this and MET lies in the strength of the contraction and the use of spiral, diagonal patterns, although these concepts (spiral activities) have also been used in MET in recent years (consider scalene MET treatment in Ch. 4, for example). The debate as to how much strength should be used is unresolved. MET prefers lighter contractions than facilitated stretching and PNF because:

- It is considered that once a greater degree of strength than 25% of available force is used, recruitment is occurring of phasic muscle fibres, rather than the postural fibres which will have shortened and require stretching (Liebenson 1996). (The importance of variations in response between phasic and postural muscles is discussed in detail in Ch. 2).
- It is far easier for the practitioner to control light contractions than it is strong ones, making MET a less arduous experience.
- There is far less likelihood of provoking cramp, tissue damage or pain when light contractions rather than strong ones are used, making MET safer and gentler.
- Physicians and researchers such as Karel Lewit (1999) have demonstrated that *extremely* light isometric contractions, utilising breathing and eye movements alone, are often sufficient to produce postisometric relaxation, and in this way to facilitate subsequent stretching.

Proprioceptive neuromuscular facilitation (PNF) variations (including hold–relax and contract–relax) (Voss et al 1985, Surburg 1981)
Most PNF variations involve stretching which is either passive or passive-assisted, following a strong contraction. The same reservations listed above (in the facilitated stretching discussion) apply to these methods. There are excellent aspects to their use, however, the author considers MET, as detailed in this text, to have distinct advantages, and no drawbacks.

Active isolated stretching (AIS) (Mattes 1995)
Flexibility is encouraged in AIS, which uses active stretching by the patient and reciprocal inhibition (RI) mechanisms. AIS, unlike MET (which combines RI and PIR as well as active patient participation), does not utilise the benefits of postisometric relaxation (PIR). In AIS:

1. The muscle needing stretching is identified.
2. Precise localisation should be used to ensure that the muscle receives specific stretching.
3. Use should be made of a contractile effort to produce relaxation of the muscles involved.
4. Repetitive, fairly short duration, isotonic muscle contractions are used to increase local blood flow and oxygenation.
5. A synchronised breathing rhythm is established, using inhalation as the part returns to the starting position (the 'rest' phase) and exhalation as the muscle is taken to, and through, its resistance barrier (the 'work' phase).
6. The muscle to be stretched is taken into stretch just beyond a point of light irritation – with the patient's assistance – and held for 1–2 seconds before being returned to the starting position.
7. Repetitions continue until adequate gain has been achieved.

Mattes uses patient participation in moving the part through the barrier of resistance in order to prevent activation of the myotatic stretch reflex, and this component of his specialised stretching approach has been incorporated into MET methodology by many practitioners.

As noted, a key feature of AIS is the rapid rate of stretching, and the deliberately induced irritation of the stretched tissues. The undoubted ability of AIS to lengthen muscles rapidly is therefore achieved at the expense of some degree of microtrauma, which is not always an acceptable exchange. AIS may be more suited to athletic settings than to use on more vulnerable individuals.

Yoga stretching (and static stretching)
Adopting specific postures based on traditional yoga and maintaining these for some minutes at a time (combined, as a rule, with deep relaxation breathing) allows a slow release of contracted and tense tissues to take place. A form of self-induced viscoelastic myofascial release (see discussion of 'creep' in Ch. 2) seems to be taking place as tissues are held, unforced, at their resistance barrier. Yoga stretching, applied carefully, after appropriate instruction, represents an excellent means of home care. There are superficial similarities between yoga stretching and static stretching as described by Anderson (1984). Anderson, however, maintains stretching at the barrier for short periods (usually no more than 30 seconds) before moving to a new barrier. In some settings the stretching aspect of this method is assisted by the practitioner.

Ballistic stretching (Beaulieu 1981)
A series of rapid, 'bouncing', stretching movements are the key feature of ballistic stretching. Despite claims that it is an effective means of lengthening short musculature rapidly, in the view of the author the risk of irritation, or frank injury, makes this method undesirable.

Edward Stiles

Among the key MET clinicians is Edward Stiles, who elaborates on the theme of the wide range of MET application (Stiles 1984a, 1984b). He states that:

> Basic science data suggests the musculoskeletal system plays an important role in the function of other systems. Research indicates that segmentally related somatic and visceral structures may affect one another directly, via viscerosomatic and somaticovisceral reflex pathways. Somatic dysfunction may increase energy demands, and it can affect a wide variety of bodily processes; vasomotor control, nerve impulse patterns (in facilitation), axionic flow of neurotrophic proteins, venous and lymphatic circulation and ventilation. The impact of somatic dysfunction on various combinations of these functions may be associated with myriad symptoms and signs. A possibility which could account for some of the observed clinical effects of manipulation.

As to the methods of manipulation he now uses clinically, Stiles states that he employs muscle energy methods on about 80% of his patients, and functional techniques (such as strain/counterstrain) on 15–20%. He uses high velocity thrusts on very few cases. The most useful manipulative tool available is, he maintains, muscle energy technique.

J. Goodridge and W. Kuchera

Modern osteopathic refinements of MET – for example the emphasis on very light contractions which has strongly influenced this text – owe much to physicians such as John Goodridge and William Kuchera, who consider that (Goodridge & Kuchera 1997):

> Localization of force is more important than intensity. Localization depends on palpatory proprioceptive perception of movement (or resistance to movement) at or about a specific articulation … . Monitoring and confining forces to the muscle group or level of somatic dysfunction involved are important for achieving desirable changes. *Poor results are most often due to improperly localized forces, often with excessive patient effort.* [italics added]

Early sources of MET

MET emerged squarely out of osteopathic tradition, although a synchronous evolution of treatment methods, involving isometric contraction and stretching, was taking place independently in physical therapy, called PNF (see Box 1.1).

Fred Mitchell Snr (1958) quoted the words of the developer of osteopathy, Andrew Taylor Still: 'The attempt to restore joint integrity before soothingly restoring muscle and ligamentous normality was putting the cart before the horse.' As stated earlier, Mitchell's work drew on the methods developed by Ruddy; however, it is unclear whether Mitchell Snr, when he was refining MET methodology in the early 1950s, had any awareness of proprioceptive neuromuscular facilitation (PNF), a method which had been developed a few years earlier, in the late 1940s, in a physical therapy context (Knott & Voss 1968).

PNF method tended to stress the importance of rotational components in the function of joints and muscles, and employed these using resisted (isometric) forces, usually involving extremely strong contractions. Initially, the focus of PNF related to the strengthening of neurologically weakened muscles, with attention to the release of muscle spasticity following on from this, as well as to improving range of motion at intervertebral levels (Kabat 1959, Levine et al 1954) (see Box 1.1).

Postisometric relaxation and reciprocal inhibition: two forms of MET (Box 1.2)

A term much used in more recent developments of muscle energy techniques is postisometric relaxation (PIR), especially in relation to the work of Karel Lewit (1999). The term postisometric relaxation refers to the effect of the subsequent reduction in tone experienced by a muscle, or group of muscles, after brief periods during which an isometric contraction has been performed.

The terms proprioceptive neuromuscular facilitation (PNF) and postisometric relaxation (PIR) (the latent hypotonic state of a muscle following isometric activity) therefore represent variations on the same theme. A further variation involves the physiological response of the antagonists of a muscle which has been isometrically contracted – reciprocal inhibition (RI).

Box 1.2 Defining the terms used in MET

The terms used in MET require clear definition and emphasis:

1. An isometric contraction is one in which a muscle, or group of muscles, or a joint, or region of the body, is called upon to contract, or move in a specified direction, and in which that effort is matched by the operator's effort, so that no movement is allowed to take place.
2. An isotonic contraction is one in which movement does take place, in that the counterforce offered by the operator is either less than that of the patient, or is greater.
   In the first isotonic example there would be an approximation of the origin and insertion of the muscle(s) involved, as the effort exerted by the patient more than matches that of the operator. This has a tonic effect on the muscle(s) and is called a concentric isotonic contraction. This method is useful in toning weakened musculature.
3. The other form of isotonic contraction involves an eccentric movement in which the muscle, while contracting, is stretched. The effect of the operator offering greater counterforce than the patient's muscular effort is to lengthen a muscle which is trying to shorten. This is also called an isolytic contraction. This manoeuvre is useful in cases where there exists a marked degree of fibrotic change. The effect is to stretch and alter these tissues – inducing controlled microtrauma – thus allowing an improvement in elasticity and circulation.

When a muscle is isometrically contracted, its antagonist will be inhibited, and will demonstrate reduced tone immediately following this. Thus the antagonist of a shortened muscle, or group of muscles, may be isometrically contracted in order to achieve a degree of ease and additional movement potential in the shortened tissues.

Sandra Yale (in DiGiovanna 1991) acknowledges that, apart from the well understood processes of reciprocal inhibition, the precise reasons for the effectiveness of MET remain unclear – although in achieving PIR the effect of a sustained contraction on the Golgi tendon organs seems pivotal, since their response to such a contraction seems to be to set the tendon and the muscle to a new length by inhibiting it (Moritan 1987). Other variations on this same theme include 'hold–relax' and 'contract–relax' techniques (see Box 1.1).

Lewit & Simons (1984) agree that while reciprocal inhibition is a factor in some forms of therapy related to postisometric relaxation techniques, it is not a factor in PIR itself, which is a phenomenon resulting from a neurological loop, probably involving the Golgi tendon organs (see Figs 1.1 and 1.2).

Liebenson (1996) discusses both the benefits of, and the mechanisms involved in, use of muscle

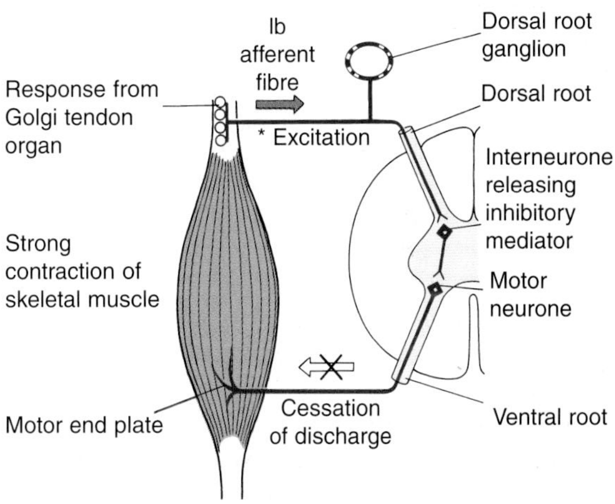

Figure 1.1 Schematic representation of the neurological effects of the loading of the Golgi tendon organs of a skeletal muscle by means of an isometric contraction, which produces a postisometric relaxation effect in that muscle.

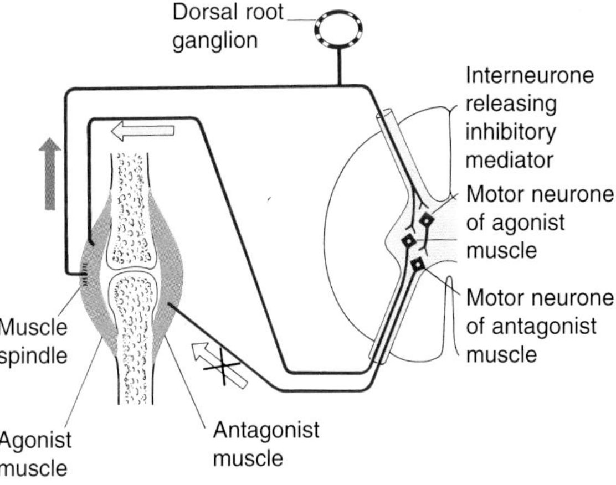

Figure 1.2 Schematic representation of the reciprocal effect of an isometric contraction of a skeletal muscle, resulting in an inhibitory influence on its antagonist.

energy technique (which he terms 'manual resistance techniques', or MRT):

> Two aspects to MRT [i.e. MET by another name] are their ability to relax an overactive muscle ... and their ability to enhance stretch of a shortened muscle or its associated fascia when connective tissue or viscoelastic changes have occurred.
>
> Two fundamental neurophysiological principles account for the neuromuscular inhibition that occurs during application of these techniques. The first is postcontraction inhibition [also known as postisometric relaxation, or PIR], which states that after a muscle is contracted, it is automatically in a relaxed state for a brief, latent, period. The second is reciprocal inhibition (RI) which states that when one muscle is contracted, its antagonist is automatically inhibited.

Liebenson suggests that there is evidence that the receptors responsible for PIR lie within the muscle and not in the skin or associated joints (Robinson 1982).

Where pain of an acute or chronic nature makes controlled contraction of the muscles involved difficult, the therapeutic use of the antagonists can patently be of value. Thus modern MET incorporates both postisometric relaxation and reciprocal inhibition methods, as well as aspects unique to itself, such as isokinetic techniques, described later (see p. 11).

A number of researchers, including Karel Lewit of Prague (Lewit 1999), have reported on the usefulness of aspects of MET in the treatment of trigger points, and this is seen by many to be an excellent method of treating these myofascial states, and of achieving the restoration of a situation where the muscle in which the trigger lies is once more capable of achieving its full resting length, with no evidence of shortening.

Travell & Simons (1992) mistakenly credited Lewit with developing MET, stating that 'The concept of applying post-isometric relaxation in the treatment of myofascial pain was presented for the first time in a North American journal in 1984 [by Lewit]'. In fact Mitchell Snr had described the method some 25 years previously, a fact acknowledged by Lewit (Lewit & Simons 1984).

KEY POINTS ABOUT MODERN MET

MET methods all employ variations on a basic theme. This primarily involves the use of the patient's own muscular efforts in one of a number of ways, usually in association with the efforts of the therapist:

1. The operator's force may exactly match the effort of the patient (so producing an isometric contraction) allowing no movement to occur – and producing as a result a physiological neurological response (via the Golgi tendon organs) involving a combination of:
   - reciprocal inhibition of the antagonist(s) of the muscle(s) being contracted, as well as
   - postisometric relaxation of the muscle(s) which are being contracted.
2. The operator's force may overcome the effort of the patient, thus moving the area or joint in the direction opposite to that in which the patient is attempting to move it (this is an isotonic eccentric contraction, also known as an isolytic contraction).
3. The operator may partially match the effort of the patient, thus allowing, although slightly retarding, the patient's effort (and so producing an isotonic concentric, isokinetic, contraction).

Other variables may be also introduced, for example involving:

- Whether the contraction should commence with the muscle or joint held at the resistance barrier or short of it – a factor decided largely on the basis of the degree of chronicity or acuteness of the tissues involved
- How much effort the patient uses – say, 20% of strength, or more, or less
- The length of time the effort is held – 7–10 seconds, or more, or less (Lewit (1999) favours 7–10 seconds; Greenman (1989), Goodridge & Kuchera (1997) all favour 3–5 seconds)
- Whether, instead of a single maintained contraction, to use a series of rapid, low amplitude contractions (Ruddy's rhythmic resisted duction method, also known as pulsed muscle energy technique)
- The number of times the isometric contraction (or its variant) is repeated – three repetitions are thought to be optimal (Goodridge & Kuchera 1997)
- The direction in which the effort is made – towards the resistance barrier or away from it,

thus involving either the antagonists to the muscles or the actual muscles (agonists) which require 'release' and subsequent stretching (these variations are also known as 'direct' and 'indirect' approaches, see p. 8)

- Whether to incorporate a held breath and/or specific eye movements to enhance the effects of the contraction – desirable if possible, it is suggested (Goodridge & Kuchera 1997, Lewit 1999)
- What sort of resistance is offered (for example by the operator, by gravity, by the patient, or by an immovable object)
- Whether the patient's effort is matched, overcome or not quite matched – a decision based on the precise needs of the tissues – to achieve relaxation, reduction in fibrosis or tonifying/ re-education
- Whether to take the muscle or joint to its new barrier following the contraction, or whether or not to stretch the area/muscle(s) beyond the barrier – this decision is based on the nature of the problem being addressed (does it involve shortening? fibrosis?) and its degree of chronicity
- Whether any subsequent (to a contraction) stretch is totally passive, or whether the patient should participate in the movement, the latter being thought by many to be desirable in order to reduce danger of stretch reflex activation (Mattes 1995)
- Whether to utilise MET alone, or in a sequence with other modalities such as the positional release methods of strain/counterstrain, or the ischaemic compression/inhibitory pressure techniques of neuromuscular technique (NMT) – such decisions will depend upon the type of problem being addressed, with myofascial trigger point treatment frequently benefiting from such combinations (see description of integrated neuromuscular inhibition (INIT), p. 197 (Chaitow 1993)).

Greenman summarises the requirements for the successful use of MET in osteopathic situations as 'control, balance and localisation'. His suggested basic elements of MET include the following:

- A patient/active muscle contraction, which
  — commences from a controlled position
  — is in a specific direction (towards or away from a restriction barrier)
- The operator applies distinct counterforce (to meet, not meet, or to overcome the patient's force)
- The degree of effort is controlled (sufficient to obtain an effect but not great enough to induce trauma or difficulty in controlling the effort).

What is done subsequent to the contraction may involve any of a number of variables, as will be explained.

The essence of MET then is that it uses the energy of the patient, and that it may be employed in one or other of the manners described above with any combination of variables depending upon the particular needs of the case. Goodridge (one of the first osteopaths to train with Mitchell Snr in 1970) summarises as follows: 'Good results [with MET] depend on accurate diagnosis, appropriate levels of force, and sufficient localization. Poor results are most often caused by inaccurate diagnosis, improperly localized forces, or forces that are too strong' (Goodridge & Kuchera 1997) (see also Box 1.3).

Using agonist or antagonist? (Box 1.4)

As mentioned, a critical consideration in MET, apart from degree of effort, duration and

Box 1.3 Muscle energy sources (Jacobs & Walls 1997, Lederman 1998, Liebenson 1996, Schafer 1987)

- Muscles are the body's force generators. In order to achieve this function, they require a source of power, which they derive from their ability to produce mechanical energy from chemically bound energy (in the form of adenosine triphosphate – ATP).
- Some of the energy so produced is stored in contractile tissues for subsequent use when activity occurs. The force which skeletal muscles generate is used to either produce or prevent movement, to induce motion or to ensure stability.
- Muscular contractions can be described in relation to what has been termed a *strength continuum*, varying from a small degree of force, capable of lengthy maintenance, to a full-strength contraction, which can be sustained for very short periods only.
- When a contraction involves more than 70% of available strength, blood flow is reduced and oxygen availability diminishes.

Box 1.4 Direct and indirect action

It is sometimes easier to describe the variations used in MET in terms of whether the operator's force is the same as, less than, or greater than that of the patient.

In any given case there is going to exist a degree of limitation in movement, in one direction or another, which may involve purely soft tissue components of the area, or actual joint restriction (and even in such cases there is bound to be some involvement of soft tissues).

The operator establishes, by palpation and by mobility assessments (motion palpation), the direction of maximum 'bind' or restriction.

This is felt as a definite point of limitation in one or more directions. In many instances the muscle(s) will be shortened and incapable of stretching and relaxing. Should the isometric, or isotonic, contraction which the patient is asked to perform, be one in which the contraction of the muscles or movement of the joint is *away from the barrier* or point of bind, while the operator is using force in the direction which goes towards, or through that barrier, then this form of treatment involves what is called a *direct* action.

Should the opposite apply, with the patient attempting to take the area/joint/muscle towards the barrier, while the operator is resisting, then this is an *indirect* manoeuvre.

Experts differ

As with so much in manipulative terminology, there is disagreement even in this apparently simple matter of which method should be termed 'direct' and which 'indirect'. Grieve (1985) describes the variations thus: 'Direct action techniques in which the patient attempts to produce movement towards, into or across a motion barrier; and indirect techniques, in which the patient attempts to produce motion away from the motion barrier, i.e. the movement limitation is attacked indirectly.'

On the other hand, Goodridge (1981), having previously illustrated and described a technique where the patient's effort was directed away from the barrier of restriction, states: 'The aforementioned illustration used the direct method. With the indirect method the component is moved by the operator away from the restrictive barrier.'

Thus:

- If the operator is moving away from the barrier, then the patient is moving towards it, and in Goodridge's terminology (i.e. osteopathic) this is an indirect approach.
- In Grieve's terminology (physiotherapy) this is a direct approach.

Plainly these views are contradictory.

Since muscle energy techniques always involve two opposing forces (the patient's and the operator's), it is more logical to indicate which force is being used in order to characterise a given technique. Thus an operator-direct method can also equally accurately be described as a patient-indirect method.

Operator-direct methods (in which the patient is utilising muscles – the agonists – already in a shortened state) may be more appropriate to managing chronic conditions, rather than acute ones, for example during rehabilitation, where muscle shortening has occurred.

When acute, shortened muscles could have sustained fibre damage, or may be oedematous, and could be painful and/or go into spasm were they asked to contract. It would therefore seem both more logical, and safer, to contract their antagonists.

frequency of use, involves the direction in which the effort is made. This may be varied, so that the operator's force is directed towards overcoming the restrictive barrier (created by a shortened muscle, restricted joint, etc.); or indeed opposite forces may be used, in which the operator's counter-effort is directed away from the barrier.

There is general consensus among the various osteopathic experts already quoted that the use of postisometric relaxation is more useful than reciprocal inhibition in normalising hypertonic musculature. This, however, is not generally held to be the case by experts such as Lewit and Janda, who see specific roles for the reciprocal inhibition variation.

Osteopathic clinicians such as Stiles and Greenman believe that the muscle which requires stretching (the agonist) should be the main source of 'energy' for the isometric contraction, and suggest that this achieves a more significant degree of relaxation, and so a more useful ability to subsequently stretch the muscle, than would be the case were the relaxation effect being achieved via use of the antagonist (i.e. using reciprocal inhibition).

Following on from an isometric contraction – whether agonist or antagonist is being used – there is a refractory, or latency, period of approximately 15 seconds during which there can be an easier (due to reduced tone) movement towards the new position (new resistance barrier) of a joint or muscle.

Variations on the MET theme

Liebenson (1989, 1990) describes three basic variations which are used by Lewit and Janda as well as by himself in a chiropractic rehabilitation setting.

Lewit's (1999) modification of MET, which he calls postisometric relaxation, is directed towards relaxation of hypertonic muscle, especially if this relates to reflex contraction or the involvement of myofascial trigger points. Liebenson (1996) notes that 'this is also a suitable method for joint mobilisation when a thrust is not desirable'.

Lewit's postisometric relaxation method

(Lewit 1999)

1. The hypertonic muscle is taken, without force or 'bounce', to a length just short of pain, or to the point where resistance to movement is first noted (Fig. 1.3).
2. The patient gently contracts the affected hypertonic muscle away from the barrier (i.e. the agonist is used) for between 5 and 10 seconds, while the effort is resisted with an exactly equal counterforce. Lewit usually has the patient inhale during this effort.
3. This resistance involves the operator holding the contracting muscle in a direction which would stretch it, were resistance not being offered.
4. The degree of effort, in Lewit's method, is minimal. The patient may be instructed to think in terms of using only 10 or 20% of his available strength, so that the manoeuvre is never allowed to develop into a contest of strength between the operator and the patient.
5. After the effort, the patient is asked to exhale and to let go completely, and only when this is achieved is the muscle taken to a new barrier with all slack removed but no stretch – to the extent that the relaxation of the hypertonic muscles will now allow.
6. Starting from this new barrier, the procedure is repeated two or three times.
7. In order to facilitate the process, especially where trunk and spinal muscles are involved, Lewit usually asks the patient to assist by looking with his eyes in the direction of the contraction during the contracting phase, and in the direction of stretch during the stretching phase of the procedure.

The key elements in this approach, as in most MET, involve precise positioning, as well as taking out slack and using the barrier as the starting and ending points of each contraction.

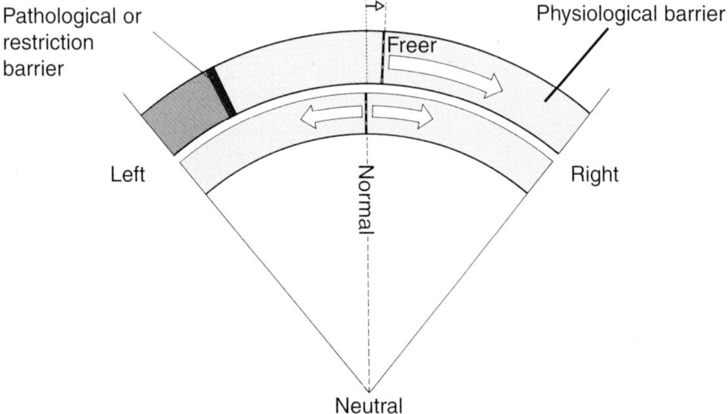

Figure 1.3 A schematic representation of the directions in which a muscle or joint can move – towards a restriction barrier (at which point MET could be usefully applied) or towards a position of relative ease.

What is happening?

Karel Lewit, discussing MET methods (Lewit 1999), states that medullary inhibition is not capable of explaining their effectiveness. He considers that the predictable results obtained may relate to the following facts:

- During resistance using minimal force (isometric contraction) only a very few fibres are active, the others being inhibited
- During relaxation (in which the shortened musculature is taken gently to its new limit without stretching) the stretch reflex is avoided – a reflex which may be brought about even by passive and non-painful stretch (see Mattes' views p. 3).

He concludes that this method demonstrates the close connection between tension and pain, and between relaxation and analgesia.

The use of eye movements as part of the methodology is based on research by Gaymans (1980) which indicates, for example, that flexion is enhanced by the patient looking downwards, and extension by the patient looking upwards. Similarly, sidebending is facilitated by looking towards the side involved. These ideas are easily proved by self-experiment: an attempt to flex the spine while maintaining the eyes in an upwards (towards the forehead) looking direction will be found to be less successful than an attempt made to flex while looking downwards. These eye-direction aids are also useful in manipulation of the joints.

Effects of MET

Lewit (1999) discusses the element of passive muscular stretch in MET and maintains that this factor does not always seem to be essential. In some areas, self-treatment, using gravity as the resistance factor, is effective, and such cases sometimes involve no element of stretch of the muscles in question. Stretching of muscles during MET, according to Lewit (1999), is only required when contracture due to fibrotic change has occurred, and is not necessary if there is simply a disturbance in function. He quotes results in one series of patients in his own clinic in which 351 painful muscle groups, or muscle attachments, were treated by MET (using post-isometric relaxation) in 244 patients. Analgesia was immediately achieved in 330 cases and there was no effect in only 21 cases. These are remarkable results by any standards.

Lewit suggests, as do many others, that trigger points and 'fibrositic' changes in muscle will often disappear after MET contraction methods. He further suggests that referred local pain points, resulting from problems elsewhere, will also disappear more effectively than where local anaesthesia or needling (acupuncture) methods are employed.

Janda's postfacilitation stretch method

Janda's variation on this approach (Janda 1993), known as 'postfacilitation stretch', uses a different starting position for the contraction and also a far stronger isometric contraction than that suggested by Lewit and most osteopathic users of MET:

1. The shortened muscle is placed in a mid-range position about halfway between a fully stretched and a fully relaxed state.
2. The patient contracts the muscle isometrically, using a maximum degree of effort for 5–10 seconds while the effort is resisted completely.
3. On release of the effort, a rapid stretch is made to a new barrier, without any 'bounce', and this is held for at least 10 seconds.
4. The patient relaxes for approximately 20 seconds and the procedure is repeated between three and five times more.

Some sensations of warmth and weakness may be anticipated for a short while following this more vigorous approach.

Reciprocal inhibition variation

This method, which forms a component of PNF methodology (see Box 1.1) and MET, is mainly used in acute settings, where tissue damage or pain precludes the use of the more usual agonist contraction, and also commonly as an addition to such methods, often to conclude a series of stretches whatever other forms of MET have been used (Evjenth & Hamberg 1984):

1. The affected muscle is placed in a mid-range position.
2. The patient is asked to push firmly towards the restriction barrier and the operator either completely resists this effort (isometric) or allows a movement towards it (isotonic). Some degree of rotational or diagonal movement may be incorporated into the procedure.
3. On ceasing the effort, the patient inhales and exhales fully, at which time the muscle is passively lengthened.

Liebenson notes that 'a resisted isotonic effort towards the barrier is an excellent way in which to facilitate afferent pathways at the conclusion of treatment with active muscular relaxation techniques or an adjustment (joint). This can help reprogram muscle and joint proprioceptors and thus re-educate movement patterns.' (See Box 1.2.)

Strengthening variation

Another major muscle energy variation is to use what has been called isokinetic contraction (also known as progressive resisted exercise). In this the patient starts with a weak effort but rapidly progresses to a maximal contraction of the affected muscle(s), introducing a degree of resistance to the operator's effort to put the joint, or area, through a full range of motion. The use of isokinetic contraction is reported to be a most effective method of building strength, and to be superior to high repetition, lower resistance exercises (Blood 1980). It is also felt that a limited range of motion, with good muscle tone, is preferable (to the patient) to having a normal range with limited power. Thus the strengthening of weak musculature in areas of permanent limitation of mobility is seen as an important contribution in which isokinetic contractions may assist.

Isokinetic contractions not only strengthen the fibres which are involved, but also have a training effect which enables them to operate in a more coordinated manner. There is often a very rapid increase in strength. Because of neuromuscular recruitment, there is a progressively stronger muscular effort as this method is repeated. Isokinetic contractions, and accompanying mobilisation of the region, should take no more than 4 seconds at each contraction in order to achieve maximum benefit with as little fatiguing as possible, either of the patient or the operator. Prolonged contractions should be avoided. The simplest, safest, and easiest-to-handle use of isokinetic methods involves small joints, such as those in the extremities. Spinal joints may be more difficult to mobilise while muscular resistance is being fully applied.

The options available in achieving increased strength via these methods therefore involve a choice between either a partially resisted isotonic contraction, or the overcoming of such a contraction, at the same time as the full range of movement is being introduced (note that both isotonic concentric and eccentric contractions will take place during the isokinetic movement of a joint). Both of these options should involve maximum contraction of the muscles by the patient. Home treatment of such conditions is possible, via self-treatment, as in other MET methods.

Isolytic MET

Another application of the use of isotonic contraction occurs when a direct contraction is resisted and overcome by the operator (Fig. 1.4). This has been termed isolytic contraction, in that it involves the stretching, and sometimes the breaking down, of fibrotic tissue present in the affected muscles. Adhesions of this type are reduced by the application of force by the operator which is just greater than that being exerted by the patient. This procedure can be uncomfortable, and the patient should be advised of this. Limited degrees of effort are therefore called for at the outset of isolytic contractions. This is an isotonic eccentric contraction, in that the origins and insertions of the muscles involved will become further separated, despite the patient's effort to approximate them. In order to achieve the greatest degree of stretch (in the condition of myofascial fibrosis, for example), it is necessary for the largest number of fibres possible to be involved in the isotonic contraction. Thus

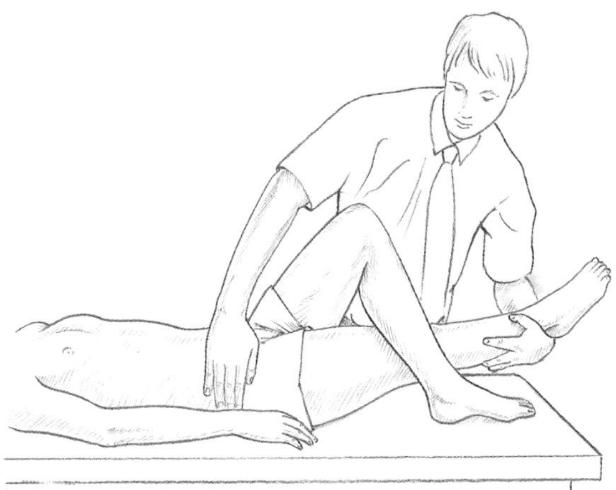

Figure 1.4 Example of an isolytic contraction in which the patient is attempting to move the right leg into abduction towards the right at exactly the same time as the operator is overriding this effort. This stretches the muscles which are contracting (TFL shown in example) thereby inducing a degree of controlled microtrauma, with the aim of increasing the elastic potential of shortened or fibrosed tissues.

there is a contradiction in that, in order to achieve this large involvement, the degree of contraction should be a maximal one, and yet this is likely to produce pain, which is contraindicated. It may also, in many instances, be impossible for the operator to overcome.

The patient should be instructed to use about 20% of possible strength on the first contraction, which is resisted and overcome by the operator, in a contraction lasting 3–4 seconds. This is then repeated, but with an increased degree of effort on the part of the patient (assuming the first effort was relatively painless). This continuing increase in the amount of force employed in the contracting musculature may be continued until, hopefully, a maximum contraction effort is possible, again to be overcome by the operator. In some muscles, of course, this may require a heroic degree of effort on the part of the operator, and alternative methods are therefore desirable. Deep tissue techniques, such as neuromuscular technique, would seem to offer such an alternative. The isolytic manoeuvre should have as its ultimate aim a fully relaxed muscle, although this will not always be possible.

Why fibrosis occurs naturally

An article in the *Journal of the Royal Society of Medicine* (Royal Society of Medicine 1983) discusses connective tissue changes:

> Aging affects the function of connective tissue more obviously than almost any organ system. Collagen fibrils thicken, and the amounts of soluble polymer decrease. The connective tissue cells tend to decline in number, and die off. Cartilages become less elastic, and their complement of proteoglycans changes both quantitatively and qualitatively. The interesting question is how many of these processes are normal, that contribute blindly and automatically, beyond the point at which they are useful? Does prevention of aging, in connective tissues, simply imply inhibition of crosslinking in collagen fibrils, and a slight stimulation of the production of chondroitin sulphate proteoglycan?

The effects of various soft tissue approaches such as NMT and MET will impact directly on these tissues as well as on the circulation and drainage of the affected structures, which suggests that the ageing process can be influenced. Destruction of collagen fibrils, however, is a serious matter (for example when using isolytic stretches), and although the fibrous tissue may be replaced in the process of healing, scar-tissue formation is possible, and this makes repair inferior to the original tissues, both in functional and structural terms. An isolytic contraction has the ability to break down tight, shortened tissues and the replacement of these with superior material will depend, to a large extent, on the subsequent use of the area (exercise, etc.), as well as the nutritive status of the individual. Collagen formation is dependent on adequate vitamin C, and a plentiful supply of amino acids such as proline, hydroxyproline and arginine. Manipulation, aimed at the restoration of a degree of normality in connective tissues, should therefore take careful account of nutritional requirements.

The range of choices in stretching, irrespective of the form of prelude to this – strong or mild isometric contraction, starting at or short of the barrier – therefore covers the spectrum from all-passive to all-active, with many variables in between.

PUTTING IT TOGETHER

Many may prefer to use the variations, as described above, within individual settings. The recommendation of this text, however, is that they should be 'mixed and matched' so that elements of all of them may be used in any given setting, as appropriate. Lewit's (1999) approach seems ideal for more acute and less chronic conditions, while Janda's (1989) more vigorous methods seem ideal for hardy patients with chronic muscle shortening.

MET offers a spectrum of approaches which range from those involving hardly any active contraction at all, relying on the extreme gentleness of mild isometric contractions induced by breath-holding and eye movements only, all the way to the other extreme of full-blooded, total-strength contractions. Subsequent to isometric contractions – whether strong or mild – there is an equally sensitive range of choices, involving either energetic stretching or very gentle movement to a new restriction. We can see why Sandra Yale (in DiGiovanna 1991) speaks of the usefulness of MET in treating extremely ill patients.

Many patients present with a combination of recent dysfunction (acute in terms of time, if not in degree of pain or dysfunction) overlaid on chronic changes which have set the scene for their acute current problems. It seems perfectly appropriate to use methods which will deal gently with hypertonicity, and more vigorous methods which will help to resolve fibrotic change, in the same patient, at the same time, using different variations on the theme of MET. Other variables can be used which focus on joint restriction, or which utilise RI should conditions be too sensitive to allow PIR methods, or variations on Janda's more vigorous stretch methods (see Box 1.1).

Discussion of common errors in application of MET will help to clarify these thoughts.

Why MET might be ineffective at times

Poor results from use of MET may relate to an inability to localise muscular effort sufficiently, since unless local muscle tension is produced in the precise region of the soft tissue dysfunction, the method is likely to fail to achieve its objectives. Also, of course, underlying pathological changes may have taken place, in joints or elsewhere, which make such an approach of short-term value only, since such changes will ensure recurrence of muscular spasms, sometimes almost immediately.

MET will be ineffective, or cause irritation, if excessive force is used in either the contraction phase or the stretching phase.

The keys to successful application of MET therefore lie in a precise focusing of muscular activity, with an appropriate degree of effort used in the isometric contraction, for an adequate length of time, followed by a safe movement through the previous restriction barrier, usually with patient assistance.

Use of variations such as stretching chronic fibrotic conditions following an isometric contraction and use of the integrated approach (INIT) mentioned earlier in this chapter represent two examples of further adaptations of Lewit's basic approach which, as described above, is ideal for acute situations of spasm and pain.

To stretch or to strengthen?

Marvin Solit (1963), a former pupil of Ida Rolf, describes a common error in application of MET – treating the 'wrong' muscles the 'wrong' way:

> As one looks at a patient's protruding abdomen, one might think that the abdominal muscles are weak, and that treatment should be geared towards strengthening them. By palpating the abdomen, however, one would not feel flabby, atonic muscles which would be the evidence of weakness; rather, the muscles are tight, bunched and shortened. This should not be surprising because here is an example of muscle working overtime maintaining body equilibrium. In addition these muscles are supporting the sagging viscera, which normally would be supported by their individual ligaments. As the abdominal muscles are freed and lengthened, there is a general elevation of the rib cage, which in turn elevates the head and neck.

Attention to tightening and hardening these supposedly weak muscles via exercise, observes

Solit, results in no improvement in posture, and no reduction in the 'pot-bellied' appearance. Rather, the effect is to further depress the thoracic structures, since the attachments of the abdominal muscles, superiorly, are largely onto the relatively mobile, and unstable, bones of the rib cage. Shortening these muscles simply achieves a degree of pull on these structures towards the stable pelvic attachments below.

The approach to this problem adopted by Rolfers is to free and loosen these overworked and only apparently weakened tissues. This allows for a return to some degree of normality, freeing the tethered thoracic structures, and thus correcting the postural imbalance. Attention to the shortened, tight musculature, which will also be inhibiting their antagonist muscles, should be the primary aim. Exercise is not suitable at the outset, before this primary goal is achieved.

The common tendency in some schools of therapy to encourage the strengthening of weakened muscle groups in order to normalise postural and functional problems is also discussed by Vladimir Janda (1978). He expresses the reasons why this approach is 'putting the cart before the horse': 'In pathogenesis, as well as in treatment of muscle imbalance and back problems, tight muscles play a more important, and perhaps even primary, role in comparison to weak muscles' (Fig. 1.5). He continues with the following observation:

> Clinical experience, and especially therapeutic results, support the assumption that (according to Sherrington's law of reciprocal innervation) tight muscles act in an inhibitory way on their antagonists. Therefore, it does not seem reasonable to start with strengthening of the weakened muscles, as most exercise programmes do. It has been clinically proved that it is better to stretch tight muscles first. It is not exceptional that, after stretching of the tight muscles, the strength of the weakened antagonists improves spontaneously, sometimes immediately, sometimes within a few days, without any additional treatment.

This sound, well-reasoned, clinical and scientific observation, which directs our attention and efforts towards the stretching and normalising of those tissues which have shortened and tightened, seems irrefutable, and this theme will be pursued further in Chapter 2.

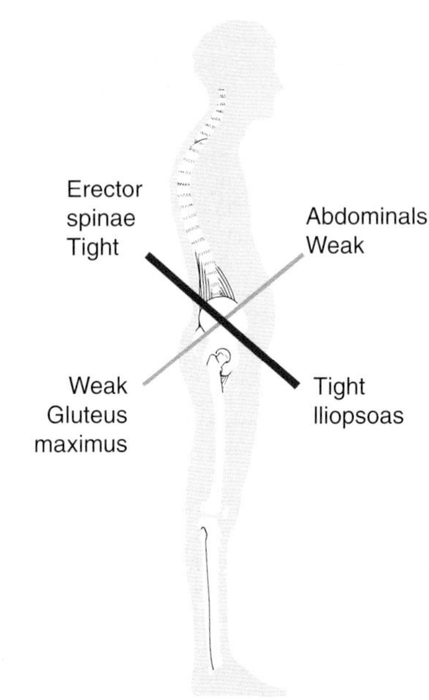

Figure 1.5 Lower crossed syndrome. An example of a common postural imbalance pattern, involving a chain reaction of hypertonia and hypotonia in which excessively tight and short muscles are inhibiting their antagonists.

MET is designed to assist in this endeavour and, as discussed above, also provides an excellent method for assisting in the toning of weak musculature, should this still be required, after the stretching of the shortened antagonists, by use of isotonic methods.

Tendons

Aspects of the physiology of muscles and tendons are worthy of a degree of review, in so far as MET and its effects are concerned (see also Box 1.5). The tone of muscle is largely the job of the Golgi tendon organs. These detect the load applied to the tendon, via muscular contraction. Reflex effects, in the appropriate muscles, are the result of this information being passed from the Golgi tendon organ back along the cord. The reflex is an inhibitory one, and thus differs from the muscle spindle stretch reflex. Sandler (1983) describes some of the processes involved:

> When the tension on the muscles, and hence the tendon, becomes extreme, the inhibitory effect from

Box 1.5 Muscle tone and contraction

- Muscles display excitability – the ability to respond to stimuli, and, by means of a stimulus, to be able to *actively contract, extend* (lengthen), or to *elastically recoil* from a distended position, as well as to be able to *passively relax* when stimulus ceases.
- Lederman (1998) suggests that *muscle tone* in a resting muscle relates to biomechanical elements – a mix of fascial and connective tissue tension together with intramuscular fluid pressure, with no neurological input (therefore, not measurable by electromyogram (EMG)).
- If a muscle has altered morphologically (due to chronic shortening, for example, or compartment syndrome), then muscle tone even at rest will be altered and palpable.
- Lederman (1998) differentiates this from *motor tone* which is measurable by means of EMG, and which is present in a resting muscle only under abnormal circumstances – for example when psychological stress or protective activity is involved.
- Motor tone is either *phasic* or *tonic*, depending upon the nature of the activity being demanded of the muscle – to move something (phasic) or to stabilise it (tonic). In normal muscles, both activities vanish when gravitational and activity demands are absent.
- Contraction occurs in response to a motor nerve impulse acting on muscle fibres.
- A motor nerve fibre will always activate more than one muscle fibre, and the collection of fibres it innervates is the *motor unit.*
- The greater the degree of fine control a muscle is required to produce, the fewer the number of muscle fibres a nerve fibre will innervate in that muscle. This can range from between 6 and 12 muscle fibres being innervated by a single motor neuron in the extrinsic eye muscles, to one motor neuron innervating 2000 fibres in major limb muscles (Gray 1973).
- Because there is a diffuse spread of influence from a single motor neuron throughout a muscle (i.e. neural influence does not necessarily correspond to fascicular divisions), only a few need to be active to influence the entire muscle.
- The functional contractile unit of a muscle fibre is its sarcomere, which contains filaments of actin and myosin. These myofilaments (actin and myosin) interact in order to shorten the muscle fibre.
- When a muscle is idle some of its extrafusal fibres (innervated by motor neurons) will contract to maintain normal tone while others rest.
- The muscle spindles (intrafusal fibres innervated by gamma fibres) monitor both the tone and length of the muscle. When the spindles are stretched they report to the cord both the fact of changing length and also the rate at which this is taking place.
- The Golgi tendon organs report on muscle tension so that, as this increases, fine tuning of tone occurs via the cord. As Greenman (1996) reports: 'The control of muscle tone is highly complex and includes afferent information coming from mechanoreceptors of the articulations, periarticular structures, and from the muscle spindle and Golgi tendon apparatus. This information is processed at the cord level with many muscle functions being preprogrammed … through local reflexes and propriospinal tracts. *The cord has the capacity to learn both normal and abnormal programs* [italics added].'

the tendon organ can be so great that there is sudden relaxation of the entire muscle under stretch. This effect is called the lengthening reaction, and is probably a protective reaction to the force which, if unprotected, can tear the tendon from its bony attachments. Since the Golgi tendon organs, unlike the [muscle] spindles, are in series with the muscle fibres, they are stimulated by both passive and active contractions of the muscles.

Pointing out that muscles can either contract with constant length and varied tone (isometrically), or with constant tone and varied length (isotonically), he continues: 'In the same way as the gamma efferent system operates as a feedback to control the length of muscle fibres, the tendon reflex serves as a reflex to control the muscle tone'.

The relevance of this to soft tissue techniques is explained as follows:

In terms of longitudinal soft tissue massage, these organs are very interesting indeed, and it is perhaps the reason why articulation of a joint, passively, to stretch the tendons that pass over the joint, is often as effective in relaxing the soft tissues as direct massage of the muscles themselves. Indeed, in some cases, where the muscle is actively in spasm, and is likely to object to being pummelled directly, articulation, muscle energy technique, or functional balance techniques, that make use of the tendon organ reflexes, can be most effective.

The use of this knowledge in therapy is obvious and Sandler explains part of the effect of massage on muscle: 'The [muscle] spindle and its reflex connections constitute a feedback device which can operate to maintain constant muscle length, as in posture; if the muscle is stretched the spindle discharges increase, but if the muscle is shortened, without a change in the rate of gamma discharge, then the spindle discharge will decrease, and the muscle will relax.'

Sandler believes that massage techniques cause a decrease in the sensitivity of the gamma efferent, and thus increase the length of the muscle fibres rather than a further shortening of them; this produces the desired relaxation of the muscle. MET provides for the ability to influence both the muscle spindles and also the Golgi tendon organs.

Joints and MET

Bourdillon (1982) tells us that shortening of muscle seems to be a self-perpetuating phenomenon which results from an over-reaction of the gamma-neuron system. It seems that the muscle is incapable of returning to a normal resting length as long as this continues. While the effective length of the muscle is thus shortened, it is nevertheless capable of shortening further. The pain factor seems related to the muscle's inability thereafter to be restored to its anatomically desirable length. The conclusion is that much joint restriction is a result of muscular tightness and shortening. The opposite may also apply where damage to the soft or hard tissues of a joint is a factor. In such cases the periarticular and osteophytic changes, all too apparent in degenerative conditions, are the major limiting factor in joint restrictions. In both situations, however, MET may be useful, although more useful where muscle shortening is the primary factor.

The restriction which takes place as a result of tight, shortened muscles is usually accompanied by some degree of lengthening and weakening of the antagonists. A wide variety of possible permutations exists in any given condition involving muscular shortening which may be initiating, or be secondary to, joint dysfunction combined with weakness of antagonists. A combination of isometric and isotonic methods can effectively be employed to lengthen and stretch the shortened groups, and to strengthen and shorten the weak, overlong muscles.

Paul Williams (1965) stated a basic truth which is often neglected by the professions which deal with musculoskeletal dysfunction:

> The health of any joint is dependent upon a balance in the strength of its opposing muscles. If for any reason a flexor group loses part, or all of its function, its opposing tensor group will draw the joint into a hyperextended position, with abnormal stress on the joint margins. This situation exists in the lumbar spine of modern man.

Lack of attention to the muscular component of joints in general, and spinal joints in particular, results in frequent inappropriate treatment of the joints thus affected. Correct understanding of the role of the supporting musculature would frequently lead to normalisation of these tissues, without the need for heroic manipulative efforts. MET and other soft tissue approaches focus attention on these structures and offer the opportunity to correct both the weakened musculature and the shortened, often fibrotic, antagonists.

More recently, Norris (1999) has pointed out that:

> The mixture of tightness and weakness seen in the muscle imbalance process alters body segment alignment and changes the equilibrium point of a joint. Normally the equal resting tone of the agonist and antagonist muscles allows the joint to take up a balanced position where the joint surfaces are evenly loaded and the inert tissues of the joint are not excessively stressed. However if the muscles on one side of a joint are tight and the opposing muscles relax, the joint will be pulled out of alignment towards the tight muscle(s).

Such alignment changes produce weight-bearing stresses on joint surfaces, and result also in shortened soft tissues chronically contracting over time. Additionally such imbalances result in reduced segmental control with chain reactions of compensation emerging (see Ch. 2).

Several studies will be detailed (Chs 5 and 8) showing the effectiveness of MET application in diverse population groups, including a Polish study on the benefits of MET in joints damaged by haemophilia, and a Swedish study on the effects of MET in treating lumbar spine dysfunction, as well as an American/Czech study involving myofascial pain problems. In the main, the results indicate a universal role in providing resolution or relief of such problems by means of the application of safe and effective muscle energy techniques.

REFERENCES

Anderson B 1984 Stretching. Shelter Publishing, Nolinas, California

Beaulieu J 1981 Developing a stretching program. Physician and Sports Medicine 9(11): 59–69

Blood S 1980 Treatment of the sprained ankle. Journal of the American Osteopathic Association 79(11): 689

Bourdillon J 1982 Spinal manipulation, 3rd edn. Heinemann, London

Chaitow L 1993 Integrated neuromuscular inhibition technique (INIT) in treatment of pain and trigger points. British Journal of Osteopathy 13: 17–21

DiGiovanna E 1991 Osteopathic approach to diagnosis and treatment. Lippincott, Philadelphia

Evjenth O, Hamberg J 1984 Muscle stretching in manual therapy. Alfta, Sweden

Gaymans F 1980 Die Bedeuting der atemtypen fur mobilisation der werbelsaule maanuelle. Medizin 18: 96

Goodridge J P 1981 Muscle energy technique: definition, explanation, methods of procedure. Journal of the American Osteopathic Association 81(4): 249–254

Goodridge J, Kuchera W 1997 Muscle energy treatment techniques. In: Ward R (ed) Foundations of osteopathic medicine. Williams and Wilkins, Baltimore

Gray's Anatomy 1973 Churchill Livingstone, Edinburgh

Greenman P 1989 Manual therapy. Williams and Wilkins, Baltimore

Greenman P 1996 Principles of manual medicine, 2nd edn. Williams and Wilkins, Baltimore

Grieve G P 1985 Mobilisation of the spine. Churchill Livingstone, Edinburgh, p 190

Jacobs A, Walls W 1997 Anatomy. In: Ward R (ed) Foundations of osteopathic medicine. Williams and Wilkins, Baltimore

Janda V 1978 Muscles, central nervous regulation and back problems. In: Korr I (ed) Neurobiological mechanisms in manipulative therapy. Plenum Press, New York

Janda V 1989 Muscle function testing. Butterworths, London

Janda V 1993 Presentation to Physical Medicine Research Foundation, Montreal, Oct 9–11

Kabat H 1959 Studies of neuromuscular dysfunction. Kaiser Permanente Foundation Medical Bulletin 8: 121–143

Knott M, Voss D 1968 Proprioceptive neuromuscular facilitation, 2nd edn. Harper and Row, New York

Lederman E 1998 Fundamentals of manual therapy. Churchill Livingstone, Edinburgh

Levine M et al 1954 Relaxation of spasticity by physiological techniques. Archives of Physical Medicine 35: 214–223

Lewit K 1986 Muscular patterns in thoraco-lumbar lesions. Manual Medicine 2: 105

Lewit K 1999 Manipulative therapy in rehabilitation of the motor system, 3rd edn. Butterworths, London

Lewit K, Simons D 1984 Myofascial pain: relief by post isometric relaxation. Archives of Physical Medical Rehabilitation 65: 452–456

Liebenson C 1989 Active muscular relaxation techniques (part 1). Journal of Manipulative and Physiological Therapeutics 12(6): 446–451

Liebenson C 1990 Active muscular relaxation techniques (part 2). Journal of Manipulative and Physiological Therapeutics 13(1): 2–6

Liebenson C (ed) 1996 Rehabilitation of the spine. Williams and Wilkins, Baltimore

McAtee R, Charland J 1999 Facilitated stretching, 2nd edn. Human Kinetics, Champaign, Illinois

Mattes A 1995 Flexibility – active and assisted stretching. Mattes, Sarasota

Mitchell F L Snr 1958 Structural pelvic function. Yearbook of the Academy of Osteopathy 1958, Carmel, p 71 (expanded in references in 1967 yearbook)

Mitchell F L Snr 1967 Motion discordance. Yearbook of the Academy of Applied Osteopathy 1967, Carmel, pp 1–5

Mitchell F Jnr, Moran P S, Pruzzo N 1979 An evaluation and treatment manual of osteopathic muscle energy procedures. Valley Park, Illinois

Moritan T 1987 Activity of the motor unit during concentric and eccentric contractions. American Journal of Physiology 66: 338–350

Norris C 1999 Functional load abdominal training (part 1). Journal of Bodywork and Movement Therapies 3(3): 150–158

Robinson K 1982 Control of soleus motoneuron excitability during muscle stretch in man. Journal of Neurology and Neurosurgical Psychiatry 45: 699

Royal Society of Medicine 1983 Connective tissues: the natural fibre reinforced composite material. Journal of the Royal Society of Medicine 76

Ruddy T 1961 Osteopathic rhythmic resistive duction therapy. Yearbook of Academy of Applied Osteopathy 1961, Indianapolis, p 58

Sandler S 1983 Physiology of soft tissue massage. British Osteopathic Journal 15: 1–6

Schafer R 1987 Clinical biomechanics, 2nd edn. Williams and Wilkins, Baltimore

Solit M 1963 A study in structural dynamics. Yearbook of Academy of Applied Osteopathy 1963

Stiles E 1984a Patient Care May 15: 16–97

Stiles E 1984b Patient Care August 15: 117–164

Surburg P 1981 Neuromuscular facilitation techniques in sports medicine. Physician and Sports Medicine 9(9): 115–127

Travell J, Simons D 1992 Myofascial pain and dysfunction, vol. 2, Williams and Wilkins, Baltimore

Voss D, Ionta M, Myers B 1985 Proprioceptive neuromuscular facilitation, 3rd edn. Harper and Row, Philadelphia

Williams P 1965 The lumbo-sacral spine. McGraw Hill, New York

CHAPTER CONTENTS

2

Patterns of function and dysfunction

Why do soft tissues change from their normal elastic, pliable, adequately toned functional status to become short, contracted, fibrosed, weak, lengthened and/or painful? The reasons are many and varied, and usually compound, and may be summarised under broad headings such as biomechanical, biochemical and psychosocial – or under more pointed headings such as 'overuse, abuse, misuse, disuse', and usually with some sort of status distinction (acute, subacute or chronic) which may be time-related.

Most musculoskeletal dysfunction can be shown to emerge out of adaptive processes, as the body – or part of it – compensates for what is being demanded of it in its daily activities. As a rule these adaptive demands relate to a combination of processes, repetitive use patterns, postural habits, emotional turmoil, chronic changes (e.g. arthritic) and so on. Onto such evolving patterns sudden blows and strains are all too often superimposed, adding new demands and directions to the adaptive efforts of the body.

Our bodies compensate (often without obvious symptoms) until the adaptive capacities of tissues are exhausted, at which time *decompensation* begins, and symptoms become apparent: pain, restriction, limitation of range of movement, etc. The processes of decompensation then progress towards chronic dysfunction and possibly disability.

Grieve (1986) explains how a patient presenting with pain, loss of functional movement or altered patterns of strength, power or endurance will probably either have suffered a major trauma which has overwhelmed the physiological limits of relatively healthy tissues, or will be displaying 'gradual decompensation, demonstrating slow exhaustion of the tissue's adaptive potential, with or without trauma'. As this process continues, progressive postural adaptation, influenced by time factors and possibly by trauma, leads to exhaustion of the body's adaptive potential and results in dysfunction and, ultimately, symptoms.

Grieve reminds us of Hooke's law, which states that within the elastic limits of any substance, the ratio of the stress applied to the strain produced is constant (Bennet 1952). Hooke's law is expressed as follows: 'The stress applied to stretch or compress a body is proportional to the strain, or change in length thus produced, so long as the limit of elasticity of the body is not exceeded' (Stedman 1998).

In simple terms, this means that tissue capable of deformation will absorb or adapt to forces applied to it within its elastic limits, beyond which it will break down or fail to compensate (leading to decompensation). Grieve rightly reminds us that while attention to specific tissues incriminated in producing symptoms often gives excellent short-term results, 'unless treatment is also focused towards restoring function in asymptomatic tissues responsible for the original postural adaptation and subsequent decompensation, the symptoms will recur.'

CONSTRUCTING A CREDIBLE STORY

In order to make sense of what is happening when a patient presents with symptoms, it is necessary to be able to extract information, to construct a story – or possibly several stories – based on what the patient says, what the history suggests, and what can be palpated and tested. These 'stories' should ideally tally, and offer direction as to where therapeutic efforts should be concentrated.

Out of this should emerge a rationale for treatment, involving objectives which might reasonably be achievable. Reasonable objectives might sometimes involve complete recovery, or, in other circumstances, no more than a partial degree of improvement in the present condition. In other settings, ensuring that for the time being matters do not worsen may be the best possible scenario. Whatever the plan of action involves, it should be discussed and agreed with the patient, and should ideally involve active patient participation in the process.

Maps and grids

In order to make sense of the patient's history and perspective on what is happening, and of the many pieces of information made available via observation, palpation and examination, a series of 'grids' or maps may be created. This collection of maps and grids might, for example, include (in no particular order of importance):

- Postural (structural) evaluation grid: including an anteroposterior perspective showing the relative positions of the major landmarks (ankles, knees, pelvis, spinal curves, head) as well as a bilateral comparison of the relative heights of ears, shoulders, scapulae, pelvic crest, hips and knees. This offers a structural framework onto which the soft tissues are attached.
- Motion (functional) restriction grid: in which joints are evaluated for their functional ranges, compared side with side, and with established norms. This would include spinal joints.
- Individual characteristics map: demonstrating restrictions or dysfunctional patterns specific to the patient, possibly including loss of range of movement, or hypermobility and/or inappropriate firing patterns in muscles when activated, and/or neurological signs.
- Postural muscle grid: including evidence of relative shortness of the postural muscles of the body. (See later in this chapter for discussion of different ways of catagorising muscles, as *stabilisers* or *mobilisers*, or as *global* or *local*.)
- Muscular weakness grid: including evaluation of relative strength/weakness of muscles associated with the patient's problem.
- Fascial patterns (for example those described by Zink & Lawson (1979) and Myers (1998) – see later this chapter). This is associated with what can be termed 'loose–tight' (or ease–bind) evaluations, involving a general or specific comparison

of the freedom of movement of tissues on one side compared with the other (see below).

- Local dysfunction maps: including detailed evidence of, for example, the presence of active myofascial trigger points.
- Breathing function (and dysfunction) grid: in which aspects of breathing function are evaluated.

Space does not allow for a full discussion of all these possibilities, however, some will be explored and described.

More questions to ask

It is useful to examine the viewpoints of different experts if we are to come to an understanding of soft tissue dysfunction in particular, and of its place in the larger scheme of things in relation to musculoskeletal and general dysfunction. A commonality will be noted in many of the views which will be presented, as well as distinctive differences in emphasis. It is not the position of the author to be dogmatic, but to present evidence from which the reader can make choices.

Most models include a progression, a sequence of events, a chain reaction, and a process of adaptation, modification, attempted homeostatic accommodation to whatever is taking place.

In order adequately to deal with soft tissue or joint dysfunction, it is axiomatic that what is dysfunctional should first be accurately assessed and identified. Based on such verifiable data as are available, a treatment plan with a realistic prognosis can be formulated, irrespective of the methods of treatment chosen. The assessment findings are then capable of being used as a yardstick against which results can be assessed and evaluated. If progress is not forthcoming, a reassessment is required.

Among the many pertinent questions which need answering are:

1. Which muscle groups have shortened and contracted?
2. Is the evident restriction in a specific soft tissue structure related to neuromuscular influence (which could be recorded on an EMG reading of the muscle), or tightness due to connective tissue fibrosis (which would not show on an EMG reading), or both?
3. Which muscles have become significantly weaker, and is this through inhibition or through atrophy?
4. What 'chain reactions' of functional imbalance have occurred as one muscle group (because of its excessive hypertonicity) has inhibited and weakened its antagonists?
5. What joint restrictions are associated with these soft tissue changes – either as a result, or as a cause of these?
6. Is a restriction primarily of soft tissue or of joint origin, or a mixture of both?
7. How does the obvious dysfunction relate to the nervous system and to the rest of the musculoskeletal system of this patient?
8. What patterns of compensating postural stress have such changes produced (or have produced them) and how is this further stressing the body as a whole, affecting its energy levels and function?
9. Within particular muscle areas that are stressed, what local soft tissue changes (fascial, etc.) have occurred leading, for example, to myofascial trigger point development?
10. What symptoms, whether of pain or other forms of dysfunction, are the result of reflexogenic activity such as trigger points?

In other words, what palpable, measurable, identifiable evidence is there which connects what we can observe, test and palpate to the symptoms (pain, restriction, fatigue, etc.) of this patient?

And further:

11. What, if anything, can be done to remedy or modify the situation, safely and effectively?
12. Is this a self-limiting condition which treatment can make more tolerable as it normalises?
13. Is this a condition which can be helped towards normalisation by therapeutic intervention?
14. Is this a condition which cannot normalise but which can be modified to some extent, so making function easier or reducing pain?
15. What mobilisation, relaxation and/or strengthening strategies are most likely to be of

assistance, and how can this patient learn to use herself less stressfully following treatment?

16. To what degree can the patient participate in the process of recovery, normalisation, rehabilitation?

Fortunately, as a part of such therapeutic intervention, a vast range of muscle energy techniques exist which can be taught as self-treatment, thus involving and empowering the patient.

VIEWING SYMPTOMS IN CONTEXT

Clearly the answers to this range of questions will vary enormously from person to person, even if symptoms appear similar at the outset. The context within which symptoms appear and exist will largely determine the opportunities available for successful therapeutic intervention.

Pain is probably the single most common symptom experienced by humans and, along with fatigue, is the most frequent reason for anyone consulting a doctor in industrialised societies – indeed the World Health Organization (1981) has suggested that pain is 'the primary problem' for developed countries.

Within that vast area of pain, musculoskeletal dysfunction in general, and back pain in particular, feature large. If symptoms of pain and restriction are viewed in isolation, with inadequate attention being paid to the degree of acuteness or chronicity, their relationship with the whole body and its systems (including the musculoskeletal and nervous systems) – as well as, for example, the emotional and nutritional status of the individual and of the multiple environmental, occupational, social and other factors which impinge upon them – then it is quite possible that they will be treated inappropriately.

A patient with major social, economic and emotional stressors current in her life and who presents with muscular pain and backache is unlikely to respond – other than in the short term – to manual approaches which ignore the enormous and multiple coping strains she is handling. In many instances, the provision of a job, a new home, a new spouse (or removal of the present one) would be the most appropriate treatment in terms of addressing the real causes of such pain or backache. However, the practitioner must utilise those skills available so that suitable treatment will, if nothing else, minimise the patient's mechanical and functional strains – even if they do not always deal with what is really wrong!

Suitable treatment for pain and dysfunction which has evolved out of the somatisation by the patient of emotional distress might well be helped more through application of deep relaxation methods, non-specific 'wellness' bodywork methods and/or counselling and enhancement of stress-coping abilities, rather than specific musculoskeletal interventions which impose yet another adaptation demand on an already overextended system. The art of successfully applied manual approaches to healing lies, at least in part, in recognising when intervention should be specific and when it needs to be more general.

The role of the emotions in musculoskeletal dysfunction

Sandman has analysed the interaction between mind influences on those neurological and metabolic functions which regulate physiological responses, and concludes that there is a synergistic relationship which results in a need to address both the psychological and the physiological aspects of stress which have emerged from the effects of (among others) familial, relationship, career, social, health, traumatic and financial stressors (Sandman 1984, Selye 1976). Unless both aspects (mind and body) are addressed, 'no permanent reduction of the negative feedback loop is possible'.

Sandman reviews the process by means of which stress and secondary stress influence muscles:

1. Stress causes biochemical changes in the brain – partly involving neurotransmitter production which increases neural excitability.

2. Postural changes follow in muscles, commonly involving increased tone which retards circulatory efficiency and increases calcium, lactic acid and hyaluronic acid accumulation.

3. Local contractile activity in muscle is increased because of the interaction between

calcium and adenosine triphosphate (ATP), leading to physiological contractions which shorten and tense muscle bundles.

4. Sustained metabolic activity in such muscles increases neural hyper-reactivity which may stimulate reflex vasoconstriction, leading to local tenderness and referred pain.

5. Relative oxygen lack and reduced energy supply result from decreased blood flow leading to an energy-deficient muscle contraction in which the sarcoplasmic reticulum becomes damaged.

6. The energy-sensitive calcium pump responds by increasing muscle contraction due to the lack of energy supply, leading to ever greater depletion.

7. Pain is a feature of this process, possibly due to accumulation locally of chemicals, which might include bradykinin, substance P, inflammatory exudates, histamine and others.

8. Local pressure build-up involving these chemicals and local metabolic wastes, and/or local ischaemia, are sufficient causes to produce local spasm which might involve local and/or referred pain.

9. If at this time the muscle is stretched, the locked actin and myosin filaments will release the contraction and sufficient ATP can then accumulate to allow a more normal sarcoplasmic reticulum, which would allow for removal of the build-up of metabolites.

10. The degree of damage which the muscle sustains due to this sequence depends entirely upon the length of time during which these conditions are allowed to continue: 'At this point physiological aspects as well as psychological should be addressed ... to stop the debilitating cycle.'

Sandman's method of relieving the physical aspects of the condition involves active and passive stretching alongside pressure and vibratory techniques.

Latey's perspective

Australian-based British osteopath Philip Latey (1996) has found a useful metaphor for describing observable and palpable patterns of distortion which coincide with particular clinical problems. He uses the analogy of 'clenched fists' because, he says, the unclenching of a fist correlates with physiological relaxation while the clenched fist indicates fixity, rigidity, overcontracted muscles, emotional turmoil, withdrawal from communication and so on. Failure to express emotion results in suppression of activity and, ultimately, chronic contraction of the muscles which would have been used were these emotions (e.g. rage, fear, anger, joy, frustration, sorrow) expressed. Latey points out that all areas of the body producing sensations which arouse emotional excitement may have their blood supply reduced by muscular contraction. When considering the causes of hypertonicity and muscle shortening, emotional factors should be one of the areas investigated. Failure to do so will almost certainly lead to unsatisfactory results.

Korr's 'orchestrated movement' concept

It is necessary to conceptualise muscular function and dysfunction as being something other than a local event. Irwin Korr (1976) stated the position elegantly and eloquently:

> The spinal cord is the keyboard on which the brain plays when it calls for activity. But each 'key' in the console sounds not an individual 'tone' such as the contraction of a particular group of muscle fibres, but a whole 'symphony' of motion. In other words, built into the cord is a large repertoire of patterns of activity, each involving the complex, harmonious, delicately balanced orchestration of the contractions and relaxation of many muscles. The brain thinks in terms of whole motions, not individual muscles. It calls, selectively, for the preprogrammed patterns in the cord and brain stem, modifying them in countless ways and combining them in an infinite variety in still more complex patterns. Each activity is subject to further modulation refinement, and adjustment by the feedback continually streaming in from the participating muscles, tendons and joints.

We must never forget the complex interrelationships between the soft tissues, the muscles, fascia and tendons and their armies of neural reporting stations, as we attempt to understand the nature of dysfunction and of what is required to achieve normalisation.

A proprioceptive model of dysfunction

Let us visualise an area at relative ease, in which there is some degree of difference between antagonist muscles, one group comfortably stretched, the other short of their normal resting length and equally comfortable, such as might exist in someone comfortably bending forwards to lift something. Imagine a sudden demand for stability in this setting. As this happened, the annulospiral receptors in the short (flexor) muscles would respond to the sudden demand (the person or whatever they are lifting unaccountably slips for example) by contracting even more (Mathews 1981).

The neural reporting stations in these shortened muscles (which would be rapidly changing length to provide stability) would be firing impulses as if the muscles were being stretched, even when the muscle remained well short of its normal resting length. At the same time the stretched extensor muscles would rapidly shorten in order to stabilise the situation. Once stability has been achieved, they are likely to still be somewhat longer than their normal resting length.

Korr (1947, 1975) has described what happens in the abdominal muscles (flexors) in such a situation. He says that because of their relaxed status, short of their resting length, there occurs a silencing of the spindles. However, due to the demand for information from the higher centres, gamma gain is increased reflexively and as the muscle contracts rapidly to stabilise the alarm demands, the central nervous system would receive information that the muscle, which is actually short of its neutral resting length, was being stretched. In effect, the muscles would have adopted a position of somatic dysfunction as a result of 'garbled' or inappropriate proprioceptive reporting. As DiGiovanna (1991) explains:

> With trauma or muscle effort against a sudden change in resistance, or with muscle strain incurred by resisting the effects of gravity for a period of time, one muscle at a joint is strained and its antagonist is hyper-shortened. When the shortened muscle is suddenly stretched the annulospiral receptors in that muscle are stimulated causing a reflex contraction of the already shortened muscle. The proprioceptors in the short muscle now fire impulses as if the shortened muscle were being stretched. Since this inappropriate proprioceptor response can be maintained indefinitely a somatic dysfunction has been created.

In effect, the two opposing sets of muscles would have adopted a stabilising posture to protect the threatened structures, and in doing so would have become locked into positions of imbalance in relation to their normal function. One would be shorter and one longer than their normal resting length. At this time any attempt to extend the area/joint(s) would be strongly resisted by the tonically shortened flexor group. The individual would be locked into a forward-bending distortion (in our example). The joint(s) involved would not have been taken beyond their normal physiological range and yet the normal range would be unavailable due to the shortened status of the flexor group (in this particular example). Going further into flexion, however, would present no problems or pain.

Walther (1988) summarises the situation as follows (Fig. 2.1A–C):

> When proprioceptors send conflicting information there may be simultaneous contraction of the antagonists ... without antagonist muscle inhibition, joint and other strain results ... a reflex pattern develops which causes muscle or other tissue to maintain this continuing strain. It [strain dysfunction] often relates to the inappropriate signaling from muscle proprioceptors that have been strained from rapid change that does not allow proper adaptation.

We can recognise this 'strain' situation in an acute setting in torticollis in whiplash, as well as in acute 'lumbago'. It is also recognisable as a feature of many types of chronic somatic dysfunction in which joints remain restricted due to muscular imbalances of this type.

Van Buskirk's nociceptive model

A variation on the theme of a progression of dysfunctional changes has been proposed by Van Buskirk (1990), who suggests the following sequence:

1. Nociceptors (peripheral pain receptors) in a muscle are activated by minor trauma from a chemical, mechanical, thermal or other damag-

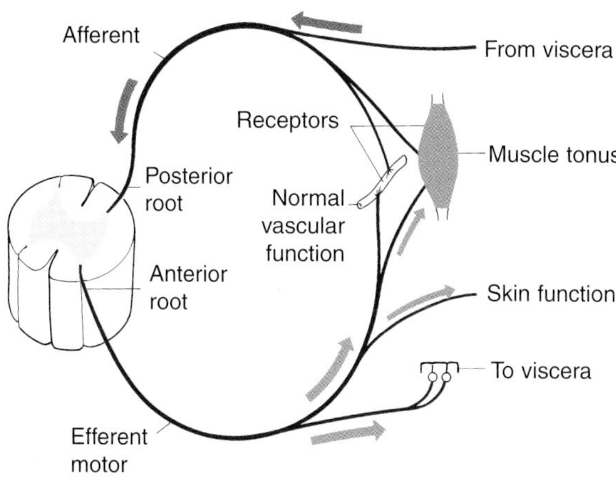

Figure 2.1A Schematic representation of normal afferent influences deriving from visceral, muscular and venous sources, on the efferent supply to those same structures.

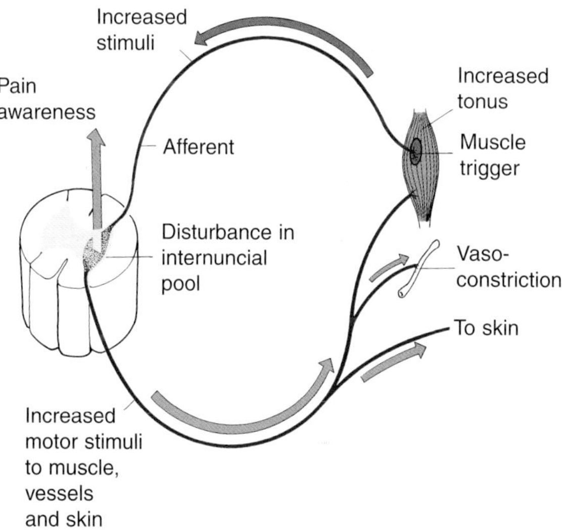

Figure 2.1B Schematic representation of normal afferent influences deriving from a muscle which displays excessively increased tonus and/or trigger point activity, both in pain awareness and on the efferent motor supply to associated muscular, venous and skin areas.

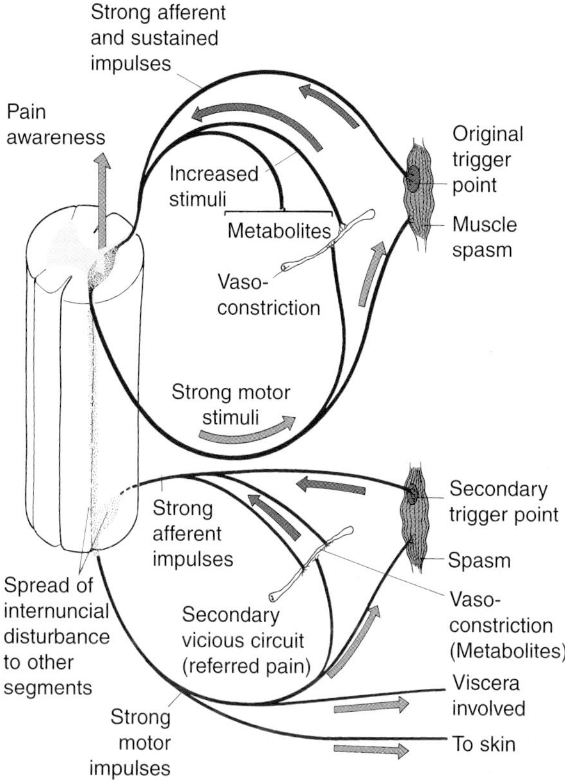

Figure 2.1C Schematic representation of the secondary spread of neurologically induced influences deriving from acute or chronic soft tissue dysfunction, and involving trigger point activity and/or spasm.

ing stimuli source (any disease or trauma in any somatic or visceral structure produces nociceptive activation).

2. Nociceptive activation transmits impulses to other axons in the same nociceptor as well as to the spinal cord.

3. Various peptide transmitters in the axon branches are released resulting in vasodilatation and the gathering of immune cells around and in the trauma site.

4. These in turn release chemicals, which enhance the vasodilatation and extravasation while also lowering the nociceptive threshold.

5. Organs at a distance may display axon reflex effects; for example, skeletal muscles and the heart may be simultaneously affected.

6. Spinal neurons will be stimulated by impulses entering the cord synaptically, which influences aspects of the higher CNS which registers pain; or the impulses might stimulate preganglionic autonomic neurons or even the spinal skeletal muscle motor pool, producing nocifensive reflexes.

7. There may be poor localisation of pain at this stage, if it is perceived at all, due to the many sources influencing the same spinal neurons, as well as the divergence of signals along neighbouring spinal segments. Pain will, however, be most noticeable in the originating segment.

8. Any sympathetic response to this chain of events will depend upon the effects of sympathetic stimulus to the target organ, and could (among others) involve cardiopressor, gastrointestinal stasis, bronchodilatation, vasopressor or vasodilator or negative immune function effects.

9. Muscular responses could involve local or multisegmental changes, including shortening of the injured muscle itself via synergistic or self-generated action from non-injured fibres; or overlying muscle might attempt to guard underlying tissues, or some other defensive action might ensue.

10. Direct mechanical restriction of the affected muscles derives from vasodilatation which, along with chemicals associated with tissue injury (bradykinin, histamine, serotonin, etc.) causes stimulation of local nociceptors in the muscle associated with the original trauma, or those reflexively influenced.

11. A new defensive muscular arrangement will develop which will cause imbalance and a shortening of the muscles involved. These will not be held at their maximal degree of shortening nor in their previously neutral position.

12. This continued contraction results in additional nociceptive action as well as fatigue, which tends to cause recruitment of additional muscular tissues to maintain the abnormal situation.

13. After a matter of hours or days the abnormal joint positions which result from this defensive muscular activity become chronic as connective tissue reorganisation involving tissue fibrocytes commences.

14. Connective tissues will be randomly orientated in the shortened muscles and less capable of handling stress along normal lines of force.

Van Buskirk (1990) describes the progression as follows: 'In the lengthened muscles, creep will elongate the connective tissue, producing slack without stressing the lengthened muscles. Now maintenance of the joint in the non-neutral position dictated by both the nocifensive reflexes and the connective tissue changes no longer requires continuous muscle activity.' Now:

- Active contraction only occurs when the area is stressed which would reactivate the nociceptors.
- At the same time the joint is neither 'gravitationally, posturally, nor functionally balanced', making it far more likely to be stressed and to produce yet more nociceptive activation.
- There would exist a situation of restricted motion deriving from the original shortening, chronic nociceptive activation, as well as autonomic activation.

In effect, there is now neurologically-derived restriction as well as structural modifications and fibrotic connective tissue changes, both of which require normalising in order to restore normal function. Both the original tissues which were stressed as well as others which have modified in a protective manner are influencing the unbalanced, unphysiological situation.

An example of nociceptive modulated dysfunction. Let us consider someone involved in a simple neck stress as their car came to an unexpected halt. The neck would be thrown backwards into hyperextension, stressing the flexor group of muscles. The extensor group would be rapidly shortened and various proprioceptive changes leading to strain and reflexive shortening would operate (as described above in relation to a bending strain), inducing them to remain in a shortened state. At the time of the sudden hyperextension, the flexors of the neck would be violently stretched, inducing actual tissue damage.

Nociceptive responses (which are more powerful than proprioceptive influences) would occur, and these multisegmental reflexes would produce a flexor withdrawal – increasing tone in the flexor muscles.

The neck would now have hypertonicity of both the extensors and the flexors – pain, guarding and stiffness would be apparent and the role of clinician would be to remove these restricting influences layer by layer.

Where pain is a factor in strain this has to be considered as producing an overriding influence over whatever other more 'normal' (proprioceptive) reflexes might be operating. In the example of neck strain described, it is obvious that in real life matters are likely to be even more complicated, since a true whiplash would introduce both rapid hyperextension and hyperflexion, so producing a multitude of conflicting layers of dysfunction.

The proprioceptive and nociceptive reflexes which might be involved in the production of strain are likely to also involve other factors. As Bailey (Bailey & Dick 1992) explains: 'Probably few dysfunctional states result from a purely proprioceptive or nociceptive response. Additional factors such as autonomic responses, other reflexive activities, joint receptor responses, or emotional states must also be accounted for.'

However, it is at the level of our basic neurological awareness that understanding of the complexity of these problems commences and we need to be aware of the choices which are available for resolving such dysfunction.

How would MET be able to influence this situation? Various approaches are likely to be helpful, including a variety of techniques derived from positional release methods, such as strain/counterstrain (SCS) (Jones 1964), facilitated positional release (DiGiovanna 1991), functional technique (Greenman 1989), etc., as well as various modifications of muscle energy technique.

Van Buskirk (1990) states it thus:

> In indirect 'muscle energy' the skeletal muscles in the shortened area are initially stretched to the maximum extent allowed by the somatic dysfunction [to the barrier]. With the tissues held in this position the patient is instructed to contract the affected muscle voluntarily. This isometric activation of the muscle will stretch the internal connective tissues. Voluntary activation of the motor neurons to the same muscles also blocks transmission in spinal nociceptive pathways. Immediately following the isometric phase, passive extrinsic stretch is imposed, further lengthening the tissues towards the normal easy neutral position.

It is as well to emphasise that these models of the possible chain reaction of events taking place in acute and chronic musculoskeletal dysfunction are included in order to help us to understand what *might* be happening in the complex series of events which surround, and which flow from, such problems. These elegant attempts at interpreting our understanding of stress and strain are not definitive; there are other models, and some of them will be touched on as we progress through our exploration of the patterns of dysfunction which confront us clinically.

Janda's 'primary and secondary' responses

It has become a truism that we need to consider the body as a whole. However, local focus still seems to be the dominant clinical approach. Janda (1988) gives examples of why this is shortsighted in the extreme.

He discusses the events which follow on from the presence of a short leg – which might well include an altered pelvic position, scoliosis, altered head position, changes at the cervicocranial junction, compensatory activity of the small cervico-occipital muscles, later compensation of neck musculature, increased muscle tone, muscle spasm, probable joint dysfunction, particularly at cervicocranial junction ... and a sequence of events which would then include compensation and adaptation responses in many muscles, followed by the evolution of a variety of possible syndromes involving head/neck, TMJ, shoulder/arm or others (see discussion of upper and lower 'crossed' syndromes later in this chapter, pp. 50–52).

Janda's point is that at such a time, after all the adaptation that has taken place, treatment of the most obvious cervical restrictions, where the patient might be aware of pain and restriction, would offer limited benefit.

He points to the existence of oculopelvic and pelviocular reflexes which indicate that any change in pelvic orientation alters the position of the eyes and vice versa, and to the fact that eye position modifies muscle tone, particularly the suboccipital muscles (look up and extensors tighten, look down and flexors prepare for activity, etc.). The implications of modified eye position due to altered pelvic position therefore becomes yet another factor to be considered as we try to unravel chain reactions of interacting elements (Komendatov 1945).'These examples,' Janda says, 'serve to emphasise that one should not limit consideration to local clinical symptomatology ... but [that we] should always maintain a general view.'

Prior's 'foot dysfunction' example

Consultant podiatrist Trevor Prior (1999) reminds us of the ways in which body-wide dysfunctional patterns can evolve from a very simple foot dysfunction. He points out that normal flexibility of the first metatarsophalangeal joints (MTPJ) is essential to normal gait. Dysfunction of this joint might occur in a condition known as functional halux limitus ('stiff big toe'). He states that:

> 1st MPTJ dorsiflexion is essential to allow the metatarsal rocker phase to occur ... . 1st MTPJ dorsiflexion is accompanied by ankle plantarflexion. A failure of this to occur results in early knee joint flexion (prior to heel strike of the [other] swing limb) and thus reduced hip joint extension. Insufficient hip joint extension prevents the hip flexors gaining mechanical advantage and thus removes their ability to initiate motion via a swing of the limb. As a result, the gluteals and quadratus lumborum on the contralateral side become active in order to help pull the weightbearing leg into swing. This will destabilize the contralateral lower back and sacroiliac joint and may predispose to piriformis overactivity. Furthermore the position of the hip at the time of hip flexor activity means that the leg effectively acts as a dead weight. As the hip flexors are unable to accelerate the leg forwards, they effectively pull the leg downwards, exacerbating the effect of the dead weight. This results in lateral rotation on the spine and trauma to the intervertebral disks. Whilst this abnormal function is of low magnitude, it is its repetitive nature that causes the problem over a sustained period of time. The average person takes 5000 steps per day, or 2500 per foot, thus subtle imbalances are repeated thousands of times per day.

It is easy to translate the picture drawn by Prior, and to move the dysfunctional stresses upwards towards the upper back, neck and shoulders.

The lesson that we can learn from this excellent example of 'chain reactions of dysfunction' is that all efforts to normalise postural stresses should commence with attention to the foundations of the body, the feet.

Isaacson's 'functional unit'

Isaacson (1980) helps us to understand the interaction of associated parts in terms of spinal motion. He describes spinal muscles as being divided into two groups, with one set being prime movers (extrinsic) and the others stabilisers (intrinsic) including the erector spinae muscle mass. Although the component parts of the erector spinae muscle group are often referred to individually as discrete entities (multifidus, intertransverse, interspinal, etc.), this is basically inaccurate. He states that, 'various functions have been assigned to these intrinsic muscles, on the assumption that they actually move vertebrae; however, the arrangement and position of the muscle bundles making up this group would seem to make it improbable that they have much to do in this regard.' They are, instead, stabilisers and proprioceptive sensory receptors which facilitate the coordinated activity of the vertebral complex (as in Korr's 'whole motions').

The force required to move the vertebral column comes from the large, extrinsic, muscles. Analysis of the multifidus group, which is particularly thick in the lumbar region, indicates that its component fascicles could not be prime movers, and that they serve effectively as maintainers of the position, normal or abnormal, in which the prime movers place the vertebrae. The same finding is made in relation to the semispinal group of muscles. These are responsible for compensatory lesions, derived from the vertebra above and below, by virtue of the arrangement of groups of pairs of stabilising fascicles. These groups of muscles are, Isaacson maintains, responsible in large part for the coordinated, synchronous, function of the spinal column which is a complex of the two functions of the different types of muscles in the region; those that stabilise, and those that move. Isaacson goes so far as to suggest that the evidence points to the spinal region being a vast network of information gathering tissues: 'Arranged as they are in a variety of positions some of the individual muscle bundles are placed on a stretch by any change of position in the vertebral column, and the tension so produced is translated into terms of proprioceptive sensation and reported to the CNS.'

Thus the vertebral column and the body must be viewed as a functional unit, and not as a collection of parts and organs which function independently of each other. This is a concept which, while obvious, is often neglected in practice.

As we will discover later in this chapter, extrinsic prime movers and intrinsic stabilisers behave differently not only in their normal function but also, most importantly, in their dysfunction (see notes on *stabilisers* and *mobilisers* later in this chapter).

Fascial considerations

If we are to have anything like a clear overview of soft tissue dysfunction it is necessary to add into the equation the influence of fascia, which invests, supports, divides, enwraps, gives cohesion to and is an integral part of every aspect of soft tissue structure and function throughout the body and which represents a single structural entity, from the inside of the skull to the soles of the feet.

Rolf (1962) puts fascia and its importance into perspective when she discusses its properties:

> Our ignorance of the role of fascia is profound. Therefore even in theory it is easy to overlook the possibility that far-reaching changes may be made not only in structural contour, but also in functional manifestation, through better organisation of the layer of superficial fascia which enwraps the body. Experiment demonstrates that drastic changes may be made in the body, solely by stretching, separating and relaxing superficial fascia in an appropriate manner. Osteopathic manipulators have observed and recorded the extent to which all degenerative changes in the body, be they muscular, nervous, circulatory or organic, reflect in superficial fascia. Any degree of degeneration, however minor, changes the bulk of the fascia, modifies its thickness and draws it into ridges in areas overlying deeper tensions and rigidities. Conversely, as this elastic envelope is stretched, manipulative mechanical energy is added to it, and the fascial colloid becomes more 'sol' and less 'gel'. As a result of the added energy, as well as of a directional contribution in applying it, the underlying structures, including muscles which determine the placement of the body parts in space, and also their relations to each other, come a little closer to the normal.

Muscle energy techniques, which involve passive and active stretching of shortened and often fibrosed structures, have marked effects on fascial changes such as those hinted at by Rolf, and which have universal involvement in total body function, as indicated by osteopathic physician Angus Cathie's list of the properties of fascia (Cathie 1974). Fascia, he tells us:

- Is richly endowed with nerve endings
- Has the ability to contract and relax elastically
- Provides extensive muscular attachments
- Supports and stabilises all structures, so enhancing postural balance
- Is vitally involved in all aspects of movement
- Assists in circulatory economy, especially of venous and lymphatic fluids
- Will demonstrate changes preceding many chronic degenerative diseases
- Will frequently be associated with chronic passive tissue congestion when such changes occur
- Will respond to tissue congestion by formation of fibrous tissue, followed by increased hydrogen ion concentration in articular and periarticular structures
- Will form specialised 'stress bands' in response to the load demanded of it
- Commonly produces a pain of a burning nature in response to sudden stress-trauma
- Is a major arena of many inflammatory processes
- Is the medium along the fascial planes of which many fluids and infectious processes pass
- Is the tissue which surrounds the CNS.

Cathie also points out that many 'trigger' spots correspond to sites where nerves pierce fascial investments. Stress on the fascia can be seen to result from faulty muscular patterns of use, altered bony relationships, altered visceral position and postural imbalance, whether of a sustained nature or violently induced by trauma.

It is safe to say that there are no musculoskeletal problems which do not involve fascia and, since it is a continuous structure throughout the body, any alterations in its structural integrity, by virtue of tensions, shortening, thickening or calcification, are bound to impact on areas at a distance from the site of the stress.

Fascia and posture

The specialised fascial structures – plantar, iliotibial, lumbodorsal, cervical and cranial – stabilise the body and permit an easier maintenance of the upright position, and these are among the first to show signs of change in response to postural defects.

Korr (1986) once again, as in so much of his writing, sums up what we know in a manner which enlightens further:

> While biomechanical dysfunction is usually viewed as a causative or contributing factor in the patient's problem, it is itself a consequence of the imperfections in that person's total adaptation to the relentless force of gravity … . It is no semantic accident that 'posture' and 'attitude' apply to both the physical and psychological domains. Given the unity of the body and mind, posture reflects the history and status of both and helps in determining where and how the body framework is vulnerable.

What causes abnormal fascial tension?

Cisler (1994) summarises the commonest factors which produce fascial stress as:

- Faulty muscular activity
- Altered position of fascia in response to osseous changes
- Changes in visceral position (ptosis)
- Sudden or gradual alterations in vertebral mechanics.

He also tells us that, 'In specific regions, where fascial tension is great due to associated muscular attachments, or closely related articulations, skeletal disorders are likely to be the site of a marked, burning type of pain in localised fascia.' Changes in the fascia can result from passive congestion which results in fibrous infiltration. Under healthy conditions, ground substance follows the laws of fluid mechanics. Clearly the more resistive drag there is in a colloidal substance, the greater will be the difficulty in normalising this.

Scariati (1991) points out that colloids are not rigid: they conform to the shape of their container, and respond to pressure even though they are not compressible. The amount of resistance they offer increases proportionally to the velocity of motion applied to them, which makes a gentle touch a fundamental requirement if viscous drag and resistance are to be avoided when attempting to produce a release.

When stressful forces (either undesirable or therapeutic) are applied to fascia, there is a first reaction in which a degree of slack is allowed to be taken up, followed by what is colloquially referred to as 'creep' – a variable degree of resistance (depending upon the state of the tissues). 'Creep' is an honest term which accurately describes the slow, delayed yet continuous stretch which occurs in response to a continuously applied load, as long as this is gentle enough to not provoke the resistance of colloidal 'drag'. This highlights the absolute need in applying MET (as will be described in later chapters) for stretching to be slow and gentle, involving 'taking out of slack', followed by stretch at the pace the tissues allow, unforced, if a defensive response is to be avoided.

Since the fascia comprises a single structure, the implications for body-wide repercussions of distortions in that structure are clear. An example of one possible negative influence of this sort is to be found in the fascial divisions within the cranium, the tentorium cerebelli and falx cerebri which are commonly warped during birthing difficulties (too long or too short a time in the birth canal, forceps delivery, etc.) and which are noted in craniosacral therapy as affecting total body mechanics via their influence on fascia (and therefore the musculature) throughout the body (Brookes 1984).

Cantu (Cantu & Grodin 1992) describes what he sees as the 'unique' feature of connective tissue as its 'deformation characteristics'. This refers to a combined viscous (permanent) deformation characteristic, as well as an elastic (temporary) deformation characteristic. This leads to the clinically important manner in which connective tissue responds to applied mechanical force by first changing in length, followed by some of this change being lost while some remains. The implications of this phenomenon can be seen in the application of stretching techniques to such tissues as well as in the way they respond to postural and other repetitive insults.

Such changes are not, however, permanent since collagen (the raw material of fascia/connective tissue) has a limited (300–500 day) half-life and, just as bone adapts to stresses imposed upon it, so will fascia. If, therefore, negative stresses (posture, use, etc.) are modified for the better and/or positive 'stresses' are imposed – manipulation and/or exercise for example – dysfunctional connective tissue can usually be improved over time (Neuberger et al 1953).

Cantu and Grodin, in their evaluation of the myofascial complex, conclude that therapeutic approaches which sequence their treatment protocols to involve the superficial tissues (involving autonomic responses) as well as deeper tissues (influencing the mechanical components of the musculoskeletal system) and which also address the factor of mobility (movement), are in tune with the requirements of the body when dysfunctional. (See also Boxes 2.1 and 2.2, Figs 2.2–2.7.)

Box 2.1 Laws affecting tissues

The following summary of terms and basic laws affecting tissues has direct implications in relation to the application of stretching forces as used in MET:

Mechanical terms

Stress = force normalised over the area on which it acts

Strain = change in shape as a result of stress

Creep = continued deformation (increasing strain) of a viscoelastic material with time under constant load (traction, compression, twist)

All tissues exhibit stress/strain responses

Tissues comprise water absorbing collagen and ground substance (glycosaminoglycans, glycoproteins, etc.)

Biomechanical laws

- Wolff's law states that biological systems (including soft and hard tissues) deform in relation to the lines of force imposed on them
- Hooke's law states that deformation (resulting from strain) imposed on an elastic body is in proportion to the stress (force/load) placed on it
- Newton's third law states that when two bodies interact, the force exerted by the first on the second is equal in magnitude and opposite in direction to the force exerted by the second on the first

POSTURAL (FASCIAL) PATTERNS

(Zink & Lawson 1979)

Zink & Lawson (1979) have described patterns of postural patterning determined by fascial compensation and decompensation.

- Fascial *compensation* is seen to commonly involve useful, beneficial, and above all functional adaptations (i.e. no obvious symptoms emerge) on the part of the musculoskeletal system, for example in response to anomalies such as a short leg, or to overuse.
- *Decompensation* describes the same phenomenon, but only in relation to a situation in which adaptive changes are seen to be dysfunctional, to produce symptoms, evidencing a failure of homeostatic adaptation.

By testing the tissue 'preferences' in different areas it is possible to classify patterns in clinically useful ways:

- *Ideal* (minimal adaptive load transferred to other regions)
- *Compensated* patterns which alternate in directions, from area to area (e.g. atlanto-occipital–cervicothoracic–thoracolumbar–lumbosacral), and which represent positive adaptive modifications
- *Uncompensated* patterns which do not alternate, which are commonly the result of trauma, and which represent negative adaptive modifications.

FUNCTIONAL EVALUATION OF FASCIAL POSTURAL PATTERNS

Zink & Lawson (1979) have described methods for testing tissue preference:

There are four crossover sites where fascial tensions can be noted: occipitoatlantal (OA),

Box 2.2 Myers' fascial trains (Myers 1997, 2001) (Figs. 2.2–2.7)

Tom Myers, a distinguished Rolfer, has described a number of clinically useful sets of myofascial chains. The connections between different structures ('long functional continuities') which these insights allow should be kept in mind when consideration is given to the possibility of symptoms arising from distant causal sites. They are of particular importance in helping draw attention to (for example) dysfunctional patterns in the lower limb which impact directly (via these chains) on structures in the upper body.

The superficial back line (Figure 2.2) involves a chain which starts with:

- The plantar fascia, linking the plantar surface of the toes to the calcaneus
- Gastrocnemius, linking calcaneus to the femoral condyles
- Hamstrings, linking the femoral condyles to the ischial tuberosities
- Subcutaneous ligament, linking the ischial tuberosities to sacrum
- Lumbosacral fascia, erector spinae and nuchal ligament, linking the sacrum to the occiput
- Scalp fascia, linking the occiput to the brow ridge.

The superficial front line (Figure 2.3) involves a chain which starts with:

- The anterior compartment and the periosteum of the tibia, linking the dorsal surface of the toes to the tibial tuberosity
- Rectus femoris, linking the tibial tuberosity to the anterior inferior iliac spine and pubic tubercle
- Rectus abdominis as well as pectoralis and sternalis fascia, linking the pubic tubercle and the anterior inferior iliac spine with the manubrium
- Sternocleidomastoid, linking the manubrium with the mastoid process of the temporal bone.

The lateral line (Figure 2.4) involves a chain which starts with:

- Peroneal muscles, linking the 1st and 5th metatarsal bases with the fibular head
- Iliotibial tract, tensor fascia lata and gluteus maximus, linking the fibular head with the iliac crest
- External obliques, internal obliques and (deeper) quadratus lumborum, linking the iliac crest with the lower ribs
- External intercostals and internal intercostals, linking the lower ribs with the remaining ribs
- Splenius cervicis, iliocostalis cervicis, sternocleidomastoid and (deeper) scalenes, linking the ribs with the mastoid process of the temporal bone.

The spiral lines (Figure 2.5) involve a chain which starts with:

- Splenius capitis, which wraps across from one side to the other, linking the occipital ridge (say on the right) with the spinous processes of the lower cervical and upper thoracic spine on the left
- Continuing in this direction (see Fig. 2.5), the rhomboids (on the left) link via the medial border of the scapula with serratus anterior and the ribs (still on the left), wrapping around the trunk via the external obliques and the abdominal aponeurosis on the left, to connect with the internal obliques on the right and then to a strong anchor point on the anterior superior iliac spine (right side)
- From the ASIS, the tensor fascia lata and the iliotibial tract link to the lateral tibial condyle
- Tibialis anterior links the lateral tibial condyle with the 1st metatarsal and cuneiform
- From this apparent end point of the chain (1st metatarsal and cuneiform), peroneus longus rises to link with the fibular head
- Biceps femoris connects the fibular head to the ischial tuberosity
- The sacrotuberous ligament links the ischial tuberosity to the sacrum
- The sacral fascia and the erector spinae link the sacrum to the occipital ridge.

The deep front line describes several alternative chains involving the structures anterior to the spine (internally, for example):

- The anterior longitudinal ligament, diaphragm, pericardium, mediastinum, parietal pleura, fascia prevertebralis and the scalene fascia, which connect the lumbar spine (bodies and transverse processes) to the cervical transverse processes, and via longus capitis to the basilar portion of the occiput
- Other links in this chain might involve a connection between the posterior manubrium and the hyoid bone via the subhyoid muscles and
- The fascia pretrachealis between the hyoid and the cranium/mandible, involving suprahyoid muscles
- The muscles of the jaw linking the mandible to the face and cranium.

Myers includes in his chain description structures of the lower limbs which connect the tarsum of the foot to the lower lumbar spine, making the linkage complete. Additional smaller chains involving the arms are described as follows:

Back of the arm lines (Figure 2.6)

- The broad sweep of trapezius links the occipital ridge and the cervical spinous processes to the spine of the scapula and the clavicle
- The deltoid, together with the lateral intermuscular septum, connects the scapula and clavicle with the lateral epicondyle
- The lateral epicondyle is joined to the hand and fingers by the common extensor tendon
- Another track on the back of the arm can arise from the rhomboids, which link the thoracic transverse processes to the medial border of the scapula
- The scapula in turn is linked to the olecranon of the ulna by infraspinatus and the triceps

Box 2.2 Myers' fascial trains (Myers 1997, 2001) (Figs. 2.2–2.7) (*contd.*)

- The olecranon of the ulna connects to the small finger via the periosteum of the ulna
- A 'stabilisation' feature in the back of the arm involves latissimus dorsi and the thoracolumbar fascia, which connects the arm with the spinous processes, the contralateral sacral fascia and gluteus maximus, which in turn attaches to the shaft of the femur
- Vastus lateralis connects the femur shaft to the tibial tuberosity and (via this) to the periosteum of the tibia.

Front of the arm lines (Figure 2.7)

- Latissimus dorsi, teres major and pectoralis major attach to the humerus close to the medial intramuscular septum, connecting it to the back of the trunk
- The medial intramuscular septum connects the humerus to the medial epicondyle which connects with the palmar hand and fingers by means of the common flexor tendon
- An additional line on the front of the arm involves pectoralis minor, the costocoracoid ligament, the brachial neurovascular bundle and the fascia clavipectoralis, which attach to the coracoid process
- The coracoid process also provides the attachment for biceps brachii (or brachialis) linking this to the radius and the thumb via the flexor compartment of the forearm
- A 'stabilisation' line on the front of the arm involves pectoralis major attaching to the ribs, as do the external obliques, which then run to the pubic tubercle, where a connection is made to the contralateral adductor longus, gracilis, pes anserinus, and the tibial periosteum.

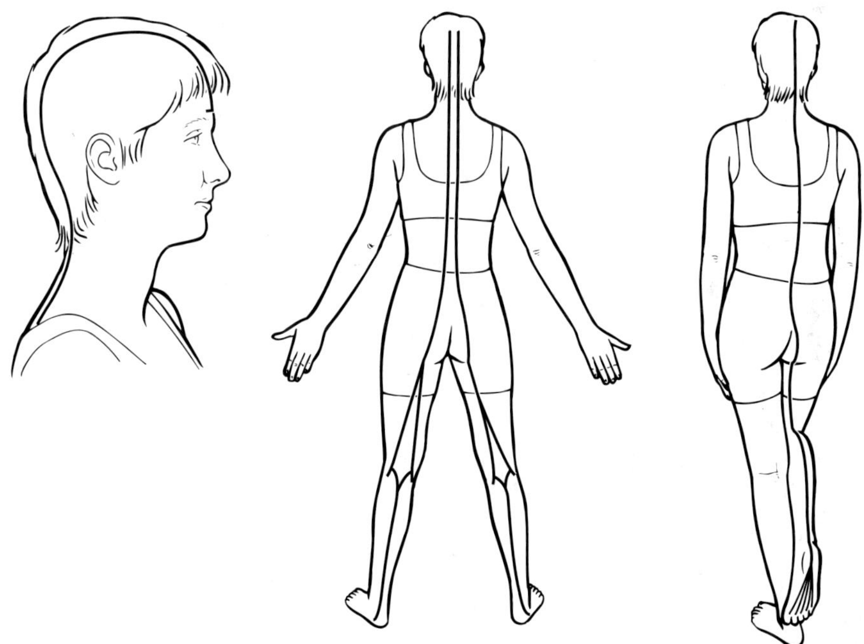

Figure 2.2 The superficial back line (SBL) (see Box 2.2).

cervicothoracic (CT), thoracolumbar (TL), lumbosacral (LS). These sites are tested for their rotation and sidebending preferences.

Zink & Lawson's research showed that most people display alternating patterns of rotatory preference, with about 80% of people showing a common pattern of left-right-left-right (termed the 'common compensatory pattern' or CCP) 'reading' from the occiptotatlantal region downwards. Zink & Lawson observed that the 20% of people whose compensatory pattern did not alternate commonly had poor health histories.

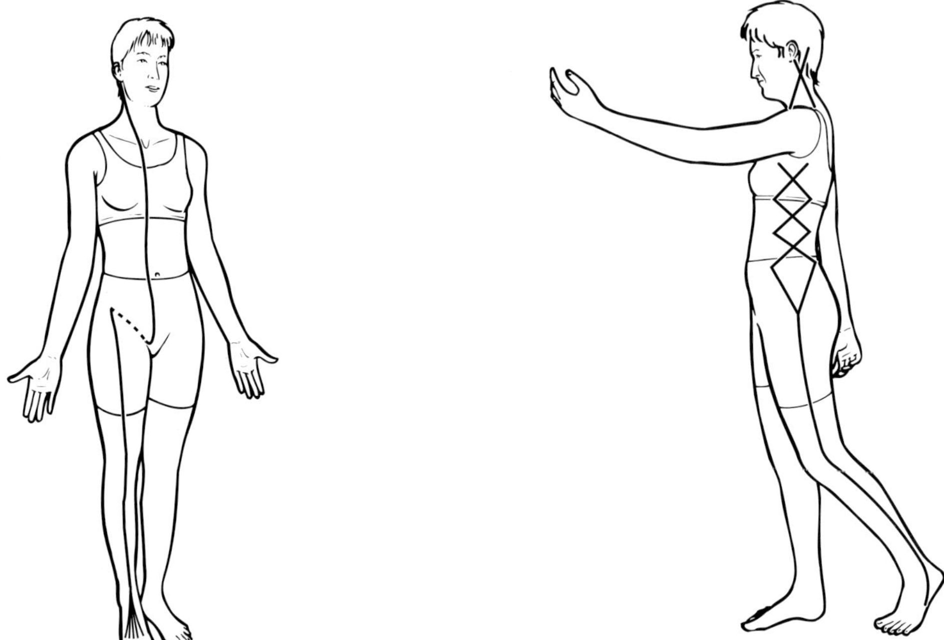

Figure 2.3 The superficial front line (SFL) (see Box 2.2).

Figure 2.4 The lateral line (see Box 2.2).

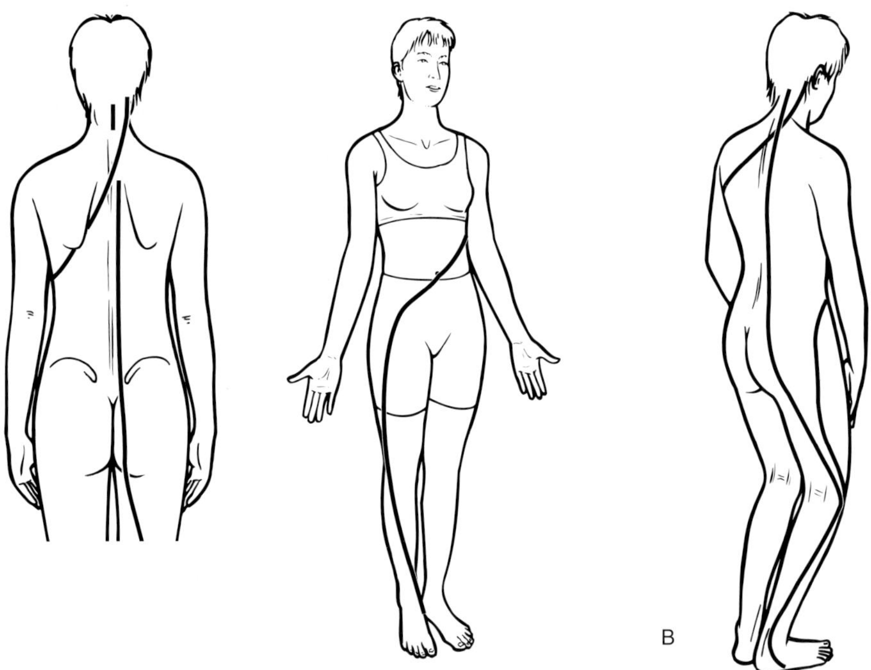

Figure 2.5 The spiral lines (see Box 2.2).

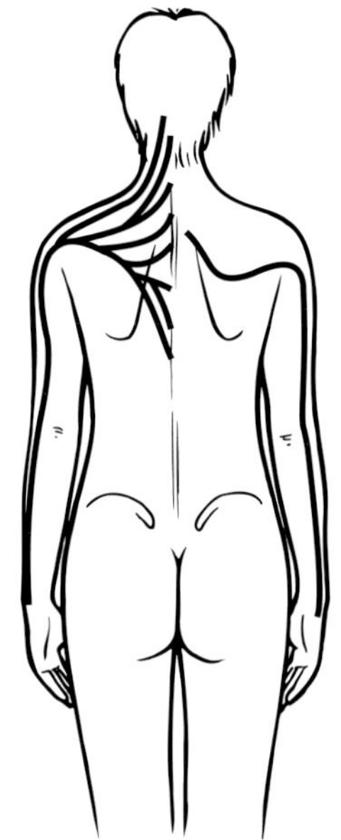

Figure 2.6 Back of arm lines (see Box 2.2).

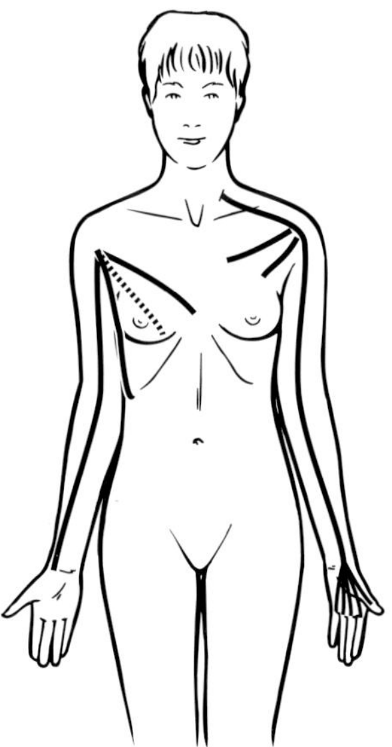

Figure 2.7 Front of arm lines (see Box 2.2).

Treatment of either CCP or uncompensated fascial patterns has the objective of trying as far as is possible to create a symmetrical degree of rotatory motion at the key crossover sites. The treatment methods used to achieve this range from direct muscle energy approaches to indirect positional release techniques. Restoration of an alternating compensatory pattern can be seen as evidence of successful therapeutic intervention.

Assessment of tissue preference

Occipitoatlantal (OA) area

The patient is supine. The practitioner sits at the patient's head, slightly to one side, and faces the corner of the table. One hand (caudal hand) cradles the occiput with opposed index finger and thumb palpating the atlas. The other hand is placed on the patient's forehead.

The hand palpating the occiptoatlantal joint evaluates the tissue preference (which way does it move most easily without force?) as the area is slowly rotated left and then right.

Cervicothoracic (CT) area

The patient is seated in a relaxed posture with the practitioner behind, with hands placed to cover the medial aspects of the upper trapezius so that his fingers rest over the clavicles and thumbs rest on the transverse processes of the T1/T2 area.

The hands assess the area being palpated for its 'tightness/looseness' preferences as a slight degree of rotation left and then right is introduced at the level of the cervicothoracic junction. If there was a preference for the OA area to rotate left, then there should ideally be a preference for right rotation at the CT junction.

Thoracolumbar (TL) area

The patient is supine or prone. The practitioner stands at waist level facing cephalad and places his hands over the lower thoracic structures, fingers along lower rib shafts laterally.

Treating the structure being palpated as a cylinder, the hands test the preference for the lower thorax to rotate around its central axis, one way and then the other. The preferred TL rotation direction should be compared with those of OA and CT test results. Alternation in these should be observed if a healthy adaptive process is occurring.

Lumbosacral (LS) area

The patient is supine. The practitioner stands below waist level facing cephalad and places his hands on the anterior pelvic structures, using the contact as a 'steering wheel' to evaluate tissue preference as the pelvis is rotated around its central axis, seeking information as to its 'tightness/looseness' preferences. Alternation with previously assessed preferences should be observed if a healthy adaptive process is occurring.

NOTE: By holding tissues in their 'tight' or bind positions and introducing an isometric contraction, changes can be encouraged.

Questions the practitioner should ask himself following the assessment exercise:

1. Was there an 'alternating' pattern to the tissue preferences?
2. Or was there a tendency for the tissue preference to be the same in all, or most of, the four areas assessed?
3. If the latter was the case, was this in an individual whose health is more compromised than average (in line with Zink & Lawson's observations)?
4. What therapeutic methods would produce a more balanced degree of tissue preference?

Example of sport-induced compensation

Kuchera and associates (Kuchera et al 1990) have shown that in healthy collegiate volunteers a significant correlation exists between a history of trauma and the type of athletic activity pursued, most notably in the golf team who displayed a rotation to the right around the right oblique sacral axis. The volunteers were subjected to a variety of assessments including palpatory structural analysis, anthropomorphic measurements, radiographic series as well as photographic centre of gravity analyses. Well-compensated patterns of fascia were noted in those who had a low incidence of back pain, whereas, conversely, a higher incidence of non-compensated patterning related to back pain within the previous year. Subjects reporting a significant history of psoas muscle problems were found to have a high incidence of non-compensated fascial patterning.

'Looseness and tightness' as part of the biomechanical model

Robert Ward DO (1997) discusses the 'loose–tight' concept as an image required to appreciate three-dimensionality as the body, or part of it, is palpated/assessed. This can involve large or small areas in which interactive asymmetry produces areas or structures which are 'tight and loose' relative to each other. Ward illustrates this with the following examples:

- A tight sacroiliac/hip on one side and loose on the other
- A tight SCM and loose scalenes on the same side
- One shoulder area tight and the other loose.

The terms 'ease' and 'bind' are also used to describe these phenomena. Assessment of the 'tethering' of tissues, and of the subtle qualities of 'end-feel' in soft tissues and joints, are prerequisites for appropriate treatment being applied, whether this is of a direct or indirect nature, or whether it is active or passive.

Indeed, the awareness of these features (end-feel, tight/loose, ease/bind) may be the determining factor as to which therapeutic approaches are introduced, and in what sequence.

These barriers (tight and loose) can also be seen to refer to the obstacles which are identified in preparation for direct methods such as muscle energy technique (where the barrier of restriction is engaged and movement is toward bind, tightness) and indirect methods such as strain/counterstrain (where movement is towards ease, looseness) (Jones 1982).

Is 'tight' always undesirable?

Clinically, it is always worth considering whether restriction barriers ought to be released, in case they are offering some protective benefit. As an example, van Wingerden (1997) reports that both intrinsic and extrinsic support for the sacroiliac joint derive in part from hamstring (biceps femoris) status. Intrinsically, the influence is via the close anatomical and physiological relationship between biceps femoris and the sacrotuberous ligament (they frequently attach via a strong tendinous link). He states that 'Force from the biceps femoris muscle can lead to increased tension of the sacrotuberous ligament in various ways. Since increased tension of the sacrotuberous ligament diminishes the range of sacroiliac joint motion, the biceps femoris can play a role in stabilization of the SIJ [sacroiliac joint]' (Vleeming et al 1989). Van Wingerden also notes that in low back patients forward flexion is often painful as the load on the spine increases. This happens whether flexion occurs in the spine or via the hip joints (tilting of the pelvis). If the hamstrings are tight and short they effectively prevent pelvic tilting. 'In this respect, an increase in hamstring tension might well be part of a defensive arthrokinematic reflex mechanism of the body to diminish spinal load.' If such a state of affairs is longstanding, the hamstrings (biceps femoris) will shorten (see discussion of the effects of stress on postural muscles in this and later chapters), possibly influencing sacroiliac and lumbar spine dysfunction. The decision to treat tight ('tethered') hamstring should therefore take account of why it is tight, and consider that in some circumstances it is offering beneficial support to the SIJ, or that it is reducing low back stress.

Lewit and 'tight–loose' thinking (Lewit 1996)

Lewit notes that pain is often noted on the 'loose' side when there is an imbalance in which a joint or muscle (group) on one side of the body differs from the other. 'A "tight and loose complex", i.e. one side is restricted and the other side is hypotonic, is frequently noted. Shifting [Lewit is referring to stretching of fascial structures] is examined and treated in a craniocaudal or caudocranial direction on the back, but it should be assessed and treated in a circular manner around the axis of the neck and the extremities.'

Pain and the tight–loose concept

Pain is more commonly associated with tight and bound/tethered structures, which may be due to local overuse/misuse/abuse factors, to scar tissue, to reflexively induced influences, or to centrally mediated neural control. When a tight tissue is then asked to either fully contract or fully lengthen, pain is often experienced.

Paradoxically, as pointed out by Lewit above, pain is also often noted in the loose rather than in the tight areas of the body, which may involve hypermobility and ligamentous laxity at the loose joint or site. These (lax, loose) areas are vulnerable to injury and prone to recurrent dysfunctional episodes (SI joint, TMJ, etc.). Myofascial trigger points may develop in either tight or loose structures, but usually appear more frequently and are more stressed in those which are tethered, restricted, tight. Myofascial trigger points will continue to evolve if the aetiological factors which created and/or sustained them are not corrected and, unless the trigger points are deactivated, they will help to sustain the dysfunctional postural patterns which subsequently emerge.

Three-dimensional patterns

Areas of dysfunction will usually involve vertical, horizontal and 'encircling' (also described as cross-over, or spiral, or 'wrap-around') patterns of involvement.

Ward (1997) offers a 'typical' wrap-around pattern associated with a tight left low back area (which ends up involving the entire trunk and cervical area) as tight areas evolve to compensate for loose, inhibited, areas (or vice versa):

- Tightness in the posterior left hip, SI joint, lumbar erector spinae and lower rib cage
- Looseness on the right low back
- Tightness in the lateral and anterior rib cage on the right
- Tight left thoracic inlet, posteriorly
- Tight left craniocervical attachments (involving jaw mechanics).

THE EVOLUTION OF MUSCULOSKELETAL DYSFUNCTION

(Guyton 1987, Janda 1985, Lewit 1974)

The normal response of muscle to any form of stress is to increase in tone (Barlow 1959, Selye 1976). Some of the stress factors which negatively influence musculoskeletal soft tissues structure or function, producing irritation, increased muscle tension and pain, are listed in Box 2.3 (see also Fig. 2.8).

Box 2.3 Stress factors leading to musculoskeletal dysfunction (Fig. 2.8)

- Acquired postural imbalances (Rolf 1977)
- 'Pattern of use' stress (occupational, recreational, etc.)
- Inborn imbalance (short leg, short upper extremity, small hemipelvis, fascial distortion via birth injury, etc.)
- The effects of hyper- or hypomobile joints, including arthritic changes
- Repetitive strain from hobby, recreation, sport, etc. (overuse)
- Emotional stress factors (Barlow 1959)
- Trauma (abuse), inflammation and subsequent fibrosis
- Disuse, immobilisation
- Reflexogenic influences (viscerosomatic, myofascial and other reflex inputs) (Beal 1983)
- Climatic stress such as chilling
- Nutritional imbalances (vitamin C deficiency reduces collagen efficiency for example) (Pauling 1976)
- Infection

A chain reaction will evolve as any one, or combination of, the stress factors listed in Box 2.3, or additional stress factors, cumulatively demand increased muscular tone in those structures obliged to compensate for, or adapt to them, resulting in the following events:

- The muscles antagonistic to the hypertonic muscles become weaker (inhibited) – as may the hypertonic muscles themselves.
- The stressed muscles develop areas of relative hypoxia and ultimately ischaemia while, simultaneously, there will be a reduction in the efficiency with which metabolic wastes are removed.
- The combined effect of toxic build-up (largely the by-products of the tissues themselves) (Cyriax 1962) and oxygen deprivation leads to irritation, sensitivity and pain, which feeds back into the loop, so creating more hypertonicity and pain. This feedback loop becomes self-perpetuating.
- Oedema may also be a part of the response of the soft tissues to stress.

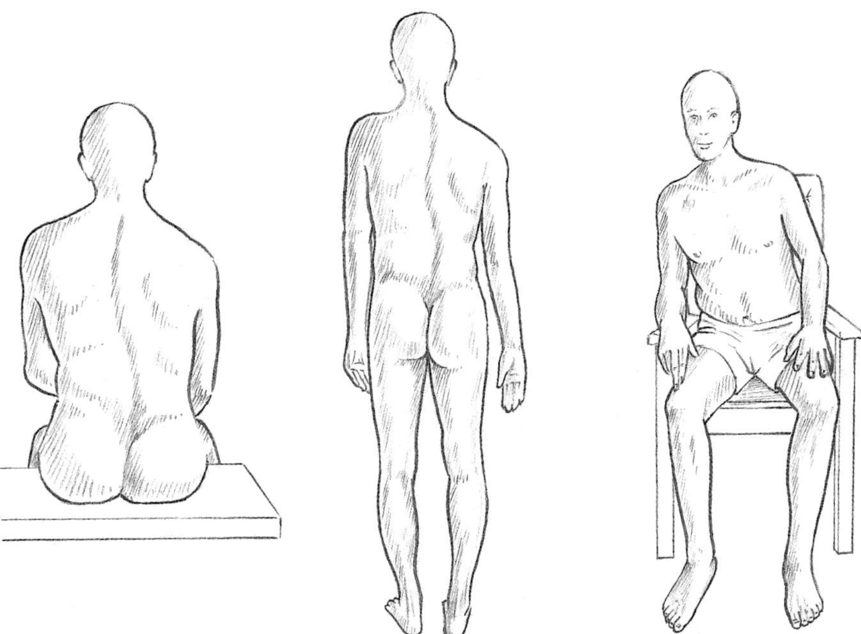

Figure 2.8 Examples of common congenital structural imbalances which result in sustained functional/postural stress – small hemipelvis, short leg and short upper extremity.

- If inflammation is part of the process, fibrotic changes in connective tissue may follow.
- Neural structures in the area may become facilitated, and therefore hyper-reactive to stimuli, further adding to the imbalance and dysfunction of the region (see discussion, later in this chapter, of myofascial trigger points and other areas of facilitation).
- Initially, the soft tissues involved will show a reflex resistance to stretch and after some weeks (some say less, see Van Buskirk's view earlier in this chapter, p. 26) a degree of fibrous infiltration may appear as the tissues under greatest stress mechanically, and via oxygen lack, adapt to the situation.
- The tendons and insertions of the hypertonic muscles will also become stressed and pain and localised changes will begin to manifest in these regions. Tendon pain and periosteal discomfort are noted (Lewit & Simons 1984).
- If any of the hypertonic structures cross joints, and many do, these become crowded and some degree of imbalance will manifest as abnormal movement patterns evolve (with antagonistic and synergistically related muscles being excessively hypertonic and/or hypotonic, for example), leading ultimately to joint dysfunction.
- Localised reflexively active structures (trigger points) will emerge in the highly stressed, most ischaemic, tissues, and these will themselves become responsible for the development of new dysfunction at distant target sites, typically inhibiting antagonist muscles (Travell & Simons 1983, Lewit & Simons 1984).
- Because of excessive hypertonic activity there will be energy wastage and a tendency to fatigue – both locally and generally (Gutstein 1955).
- Functional imbalances will occur, for example involving respiration, when chain reactions of hypertonicity and weakness impact on this vital function (Garland 1994, Lewit 1980).
- Muscles will become involved in 'chain reactions' of dysfunction. A process develops in which some muscles will be used inappropriately as they learn to compensate for other structures which are weak or restricted, leading to adaptive movements, and loss of the ability to act synergistically as in normal situations (see notes on crossed syndromes later in this chapter, and also Dr Liebenson's comments in Chapter 5, p. 150) (Janda 1985).
- Over time, the central nervous system learns to accept altered patterns of use as normal, adding further to the complication of recovery since rehabilitation will now demand a relearning process as well as the more obvious structural (shortness) and functional (inhibition/weakness) corrections (Knott & Voss 1968).

Fitness, weakness, strength and hypermobility influences

While much of the emphasis in the rationale of use of MET relates to hypertonic structures, it would be folly to neglect to mention the converse – hypotonia. In particular, Kraus (1970) presented evidence of the negative influence of relative lack of fitness on the evolution of low back pain.

Whether through acquired lack of fitness, reflex inhibition, or more seriously, inborn hypomobility, the fact is that lack of tone contributes enormously to musculoskeletal problems, imbalances and changes in functional sequence patterns, and generally causes a good deal of compensating overuse by synergistic or related muscles (Fahrni 1966, Janda 1960). Janda (1986a) describes weakness in muscles which relate to altered movement patterns, resulting from 'changed motor regulation and motor performance'. Structural and functional factors can be involved in a variety of complex ways: 'A motor defect [weakness] of a neurological origin can almost always be considered as a result of the combination of a direct structural (morphological) lesion of some motor neurons and of inhibition effects. Both causes may occur even in the same neuron'.

Deterioration of muscle function can be demonstrated by three syndromes, according to Janda:

- Hypotonia which can be determined by inspection and palpation
- Decrease in strength which can be determined by testing, (although, according

to Janda, evaluation of strength is 'difficult and inaccurate as it is often impossible to differentiate the function of individual muscles')

- Changed sequence of activation in principal movement patterns, which can be more easily observed and evaluated if they are well understood (see also Ch. 5).

Ligaments and muscles which are hypermobile do not adequately protect joints and therefore fail to prevent excessive ranges of motion from being explored. Without this stability, overuse and injury stresses evolve and muscular overuse is inevitable. Janda observes that in his experience, 'In races in which hypermobility is common there is a prevalence of muscular and tendon pain, whereas typical back pain or sciatica are rare.'

Logically, the excessive work rate of muscles which are adopting the role of 'pseudoligaments' leads to tendon stress and muscle dysfunction, increasing tone in the antagonists of whatever is already weakened and complicating an already complex set of imbalances, including altered patterns of movement (Beighton et al 1983, Janda 1984).

Characteristics of altered movement patterns

Among the key alterations which are demonstrable in patterns of altered muscle movement are:

- The start of a muscle's activation is delayed, resulting in an alteration in the order in which a sequence of muscles is activated.
- Non-inhibited synergists or stabilisers often activate earlier in the sequence than the inhibited, weak muscle.
- There is an overall decrease in activity in the affected muscle, which in extreme cases can result in EMG readings showing it to be almost completely silent. This can lead to a misinterpretation that muscle strength is totally lacking when in fact, after proper facilitation, it may be capable of being activated towards more normal function. (Janda calls these changes 'pseudoparesis'.)
- An anomalous response is possible from such muscles since, unlike the usually beneficial activation of motor units seen in isometric training, such work against resistance can actually decrease even further the activity of pseudoparetic muscles (similar to the effect seen in muscles which are antagonists of the muscles in spasm in poliomyelitis).
- Some muscles are more likely to be affected by hypotonia, loss of strength and the effects of altered movement patterns. Janda points to tibialis anticus, peronei, vasti, long thigh adductors, the glutei, the abdominal muscles, the lower stabilisers of the scapulae, the deep neck flexors.

Among the causes of such changes in mainly phasic muscles are the effects of reciprocal inhibition by tight muscles, and in such cases, Janda comments, 'Stretching and achievement of normal length of the tight muscles disinhibits the pseudoparetic muscles and improves their activity'.

The phenomenon of increased tone is the other side of the picture.

What does increased bind/tone actually represent? (Box 2.4)

Janda notes that the word 'spasm' is commonly used without attention to various functional causes of hypertonicity and he has divided this phenomenon into five variants (Janda 1989):

1. Hypertonicity of limbic system origin which may be accompanied by evidence of stress, and be associated with, for example, tension-type headaches.
2. Hypertonicity of a segmental origin, involving interneuron influence. The muscle is likely to be spontaneously painful, and will probably be painful to stretch and will certainly have weak (inhibited) antagonists.
3. Hypertonicity due to uncoordinated muscle contraction resulting from myofascial trigger point activity. The muscle will be painful spontaneously if triggers are active. There may only be increased tone in part of the muscle, which will be hyperirritable while neighbouring areas of the same muscle may be inhibited.
4. Hypertonicity resulting from direct pain irritation, such as might occur in torticollis. This muscle would be painful at rest, not only when

Box 2.4 Muscle spasm, tension, atrophy (Walsh 1992, Liebenson 1996)

- Muscles are often said to be short, tight, tense, or in spasm, however, these terms are used very loosely
- Muscles experience either neuromuscular, viscoelastic, or connective tissue alterations or combinations of these
- A tight muscle could have either increased neuromuscular tension or connective tissue modification (e.g. fibrosis)

Spasm (tension with EMG elevation)

- Muscle spasm is a neuromuscular phenomenon relating either to a upper motor neuron disease or an acute reaction to pain or tissue injury
- Electromyographic (EMG) activity is increased in these cases
- Examples include spinal cord injury, reflex spasm (such as in a case of appendicitis) or acute lumbar antalgia with loss of flexion relaxation response (Triano & Schultz 1987)
- Long-lasting noxious (pain) stimulation has been shown to activate the flexion withdrawal reflex (Dahl et al 1992)
- Using electromyographic evidence, Simons has shown that myofascial trigger points can 'cause reflex spasm and reflex inhibition in other muscles, and can cause motor incoordination in the muscle with the trigger point' (Simons 1994)

Contracture (tension of muscles without EMG elevation)

- Increased muscle tension can occur without a consistently elevated EMG (as, for example, in trigger points in which muscle fibres fail to relax properly)
- Muscle fibres housing trigger points have been shown to have different levels of EMG activity within the same functional muscle unit
- Hyperexcitability, as shown by EMG readings, has been demonstrated in the nidus of the trigger point, which is situated in a taut band (which shows no increased EMG activity) and has a characteristic pattern of reproducible referred pain (Hubbard & Berkoff 1993). When pressure is applied to an active trigger point, EMG activity is found to increase in the muscles to which sensations are being referred ('target area') (Simons 1994)

Increased stretch sensitivity

- Increased sensitivity to stretch can lead to increased muscle tension
- This can occur under conditions of local ischaemia, which have also been demonstrated in the nidus of trigger points, as part of the 'energy crisis' which, it is hypothesised (see Ch. 6), produces them (Mense 1993, Simons 1994)
- Liebenson (1996) confirms that 'local ischemia is a key factor involved in increased muscle tone. Under conditions of ischemia groups III and IV muscle afferents become more sensitive to stretch'
- These same afferents also become sensitised in response to a build-up of metabolites when sustained mild contractions occur, such as happens in prolonged, slumped sitting (Johansson 1991)
- Mense (1993) suggests that a range of dysfunctional events emerge from the production of local ischaemia which can occur as a result of venous congestion, local contracture and tonic activation of muscles by descending motor pathways
- Sensitisation (which is in all but name the same phenomenon as facilitation, discussed more fully in Ch. 6) involves a change in the stimulus–response profile of neurons, leading to a decreased threshold as well as increased spontaneous activity of types III and IV primary afferents
- Schiable & Grubb (1993) have implicated reflex discharges from (dysfunctional) joints in the production of such neuromuscular tension
- According to Janda (1991), neuromuscular tension can also be increased by central influences due to limbic dysfunction

palpated, and would demonstrate electromyographic evidence of increased activity even at rest. This could be described as reflex spasm due to nociceptive influence (see pp. 24–27 for more on nociceptive influences).

5. Overuse hypertonicity results in muscles becoming increasingly irritable, with reduced range of motion, tightness and painful only on palpation.

Thus increased tone of functional origin can result from pain sources, from trigger point activity, from higher centres or CNS influences and from overuse.

Liebenson (1990a) suggests that each type of hypertonicity requires different therapeutic approaches, ranging from adjustment (joint manipulation) through use of soft tissue and rehabilitation and facilitation approaches. The many different MET variations offer the opportunity to influence all stages of dysfunction, as listed above – the acute, the chronic and everything in between – as will become clear in our evaluation of the methods.

Clearly we all adapt and (de)compensate at our own rates, depending upon multiple variables ranging from our inherited tendencies, genetic make-up and nutritional status, to the degree, variety and intensity of the stressors confronting us, past and present.

Adding to the complexity of these responses is yet one more variable: the fact that there are predictable and palpable differences in the responses of the soft tissues to stress – some muscles becoming progressively weak while others become progressively hypertonic (Janda 1978) or actually lengthen (Norris 1999).

DIFFERENT STRESS RESPONSE OF MUSCLES

A debate is raging in academia and in clinical settings as to how best to tell the story of the way muscles respond to the stressful demands of overuse, misuse, abuse and disuse. A number of models have emerged in which respected clinicians and researchers take quite different standpoints in the way they interpret the functional characteristics of muscles. There are descriptions of the muscles of the body relating to whether they are 'postural or phasic', 'mobiliser or stabiliser', 'superficial or deep', 'polyarticular or monoarticular', and whether, as a result of their nature, they respond to 'stress' by shortening, weakening, lengthening, altering their firing patterns, atrophying or hypertrophying, or indeed whether some muscles are capable of a mixture of such responses.

It seems that in order to make sense of the complexities it is necessary, in biological science, to characterise and categorise the constituent parts of complicated organisations such as the musculoskeletal system. The problem emerges when there is no consensus as to how to perform the act of categorisation.

The author has worked with a particular model for many years, that promulgated by Janda (1978) and Lewit (1974) relating to 'postural' and 'phasic' muscles and their behaviour. This was the model used in the first edition of this text, and is described below as a part of an attempt to present readers with information in order that they should be able to investigate this conundrum further for themselves.

Postural and phasic muscles

The research and writings of prominent workers in physical medicine such as Lewit (1974), Korr (1980), Janda (1978), Basmajian (1978), Liebenson (1996), and others, suggest that muscles which have predominantly stabilising functions will shorten when stressed, while others which have more active 'moving', or phasic functions, will not shorten but will become weak (inhibited).

The muscles which shorten are said to be those which have a primarily postural rather than phasic (active, moving) role and it is possible to learn to conduct, in a short space of time (10 minutes or so) an assessment sequence in which the majority of these can be identified as being either short or relatively 'normal' (Chaitow 1991a).

Janda (1978) informs us that postural muscles have a tendency to shorten, not only under pathological conditions but also often under normal circumstances. He has noted, using electromyographic instrumentation, that 85% of the walking cycle is spent on one leg or the other, and that this is the most common postural position for man. Those muscles which enable this position to be satisfactorily adopted (one-legged standing) are genetically older; they have different physiological, and probably biochemical, qualities compared with phasic muscles which normally weaken and exhibit signs of inhibition in response to stress or pathology.

Later in this chapter other models in which muscles are grouped or characterised differently will be examined. Before that, orthopaedic surgeon Gordon Waddell's (1998) opinion is worth recording:

> Different muscles contain varying proportions of slow and fast muscle fibres. Slow fibres maintain posture; they activate more easily, are capable of more sustained contraction, and tend to become shortened and tight. Fast or phasic fibres give dynamic, voluntary movement; they fatigue more rapidly and tend to weakness. Postural and phasic muscles are often antagonistic ... Hypertrophy and atrophy occur at the same time in antagonistic muscles, which may

lead to changes in resting length, with contracture of the postural muscles and stretching of the phasic muscles.

Postural muscles

Those postural muscles which have been noted as responding to stress by shortening are listed in Box 2.5. The scalenes are a borderline set of muscles – they start life as phasic muscles but can become, through overuse/abuse, more postural in their function (Fig. 2.9A and B).

Can postural muscles and phasic muscles change from one form into the other?

While Lewit and Janda (Lewit 1999) have suggested that postural muscles under stress will shorten, and phasic muscles similarly stressed will weaken, it is now becoming clear that the function of a muscle can modify its structure. This helps to explain some mysteries – for example why the scalenes are sometimes short, and sometimes weak, and sometimes both, and yet are classified generally as phasic muscles, and sometimes as 'equivocal' (maybe postural and maybe phasic).

Lin et al (1994), writing in *The Lancet*, examined motor muscle physiology in growing children, reviewing current understanding of the postural/phasic muscle interaction: muscles, Lin observed, are considered to be developmentally

Box 2.5 Postural muscles that shorten under stress

Gastrocnemius, soleus, medial hamstrings, short adductors of the thigh, hamstrings, psoas, piriformis, tensor fascia lata, quadratus lumborum, erector spinae muscles, latissimus dorsi, upper trapezius, sternomastoid, levator scapulae, pectoralis major and the flexors of the arms

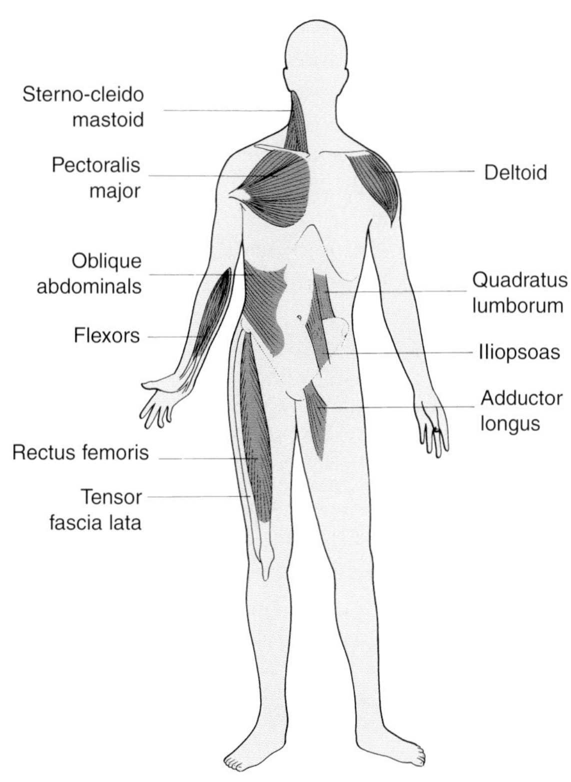

Figure 2.9A The major postural muscles of the anterior aspect of the body.

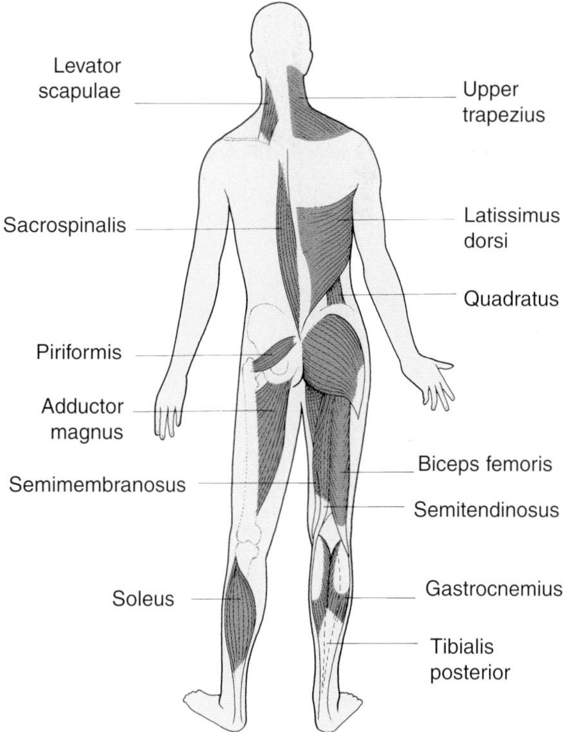

Figure 2.9B The major postural muscles of the posterior aspect of the body.

static, which is surprising considering in vitro information relating to the development and adaptability of muscles derived from mammals. For example Buller (1960) showed that a committed muscle fibre type could be transformed from slow twitch to fast twitch, and vice versa, in cross innervation experiments, confirming that impulse traffic down the nerve conditions the fibre type.

The implication of this research is that if a group of muscles such as the scalenes are dedicated to movement (which they should be) and not to stabilisation (which they may have to be if 'postural' stresses are imposed), they can become postural in type, and so will develop a tendency to shorten if stressed. This is precisely what seems to happen in people with chronic upper-chest breathing patterns or asthma.

Characteristics of postural and phasic muscles

The characteristics which identify a muscle as belonging to one or other of these two groups, in this particular model, are given in Table 2.1.

Embedded in the descriptions of these muscle groupings in some of the writing about them is the assumption that postural muscles have a predominance of type I fibres, and phasic muscles type II. All muscles comprise both red (type I) and white (type II), slow and fast, fibres which produce both postural and phasic functions; however, the classification of a muscle into either a 'postural' or 'phasic' group is made on the basis of their *predominant* activity, their major functional tendency.

Norris (personal communication, 1999) states:

> Gastrocnemius is a mobiliser or 'task muscle' [see discussion of stabiliser/mobiliser categorisations later in this chapter], and has a predominance of type II fibres in most people. However, training may affect the appearance of muscle as a type I or type II. For example hard fast calf training will selectively recruit the type II fibres and cause them to hypertrophy. The muscle now acts as if it had more type II fibres (because they are bigger and more 'practised' at recruitment). Although the actual fibre number is unchanged it appears functionally to the clinician (not using EMG) that it has. The change can therefore be one of hypokinetics or hyperkinetics.

Table 2.1 Postural/phasic muscle characteristics

	Postural muscles	Phasic muscles
Type	Slow twitch – red	Fast twitch – white
Respiration	Anaerobic	Aerobic
Function	Static/supportive	Phasic/active
Dysfunction	Shorten	Weaken
Treatment	Stretch/relax	Facilitate/strengthen

Put more simply, function modifies structure, and this may be the result of use patterns, as in the gastrocnemius example, or of positional (postural) adaptation, as in the effect on suboccipital musculature resulting from chronic 'chin-poke' posture related to strernocleidomastoid shortness.

Rehabilitation implications

Janda suggests that before any attempt is made to strengthen weak muscles, any hypertonicity in their antagonists should be addressed by appropriate treatment which relaxes (and if appropriate lengthens) them – for example, by stretching using MET. Relaxation of hypertonic muscles leads to an automatic restoration of strength to their antagonists, once inhibitory hypertonic effects have been removed. Should a hypertonic muscle also be weak, it commonly regains strength following stretch/relaxation (Janda 1978). Commenting on this phenomenon, chiropractic rehabilitation expert Craig Liebenson (1990b) states:

> Once joint movement is free, hypertonic muscles relaxed, and connective tissue lengthened, a muscle-strengthening and movement coordination program can begin. It is important not to commence strengthening too soon because tight, overactive muscles reflexively inhibit their antagonists, thereby altering basic movement patterns. It is inappropriate to initiate muscle strengthening programs while movement performance is disturbed, since the patient will achieve strength gains by use of 'trick' movements.

(Dr Liebenson discusses these and other treatment and rehabilitation topics more fully in Chapter 5.)

Skiers' muscles as an example

Just how common such imbalances are was illustrated by Schmid (1984), who studied the main postural and phasic muscles in eight members of the male Olympic ski teams from Switzerland and Liechtenstein. He found that among this group of apparently superbly fit individuals, fully six of the eight members had demonstrably short right iliopsoas muscles, five also had left iliopsoas shortness, and the majority also displayed weakness of the rectus abdominis muscles.

A number of other muscle imbalances were noted, and the conclusion was that athletic fitness offers no more protection from muscular dysfunction than does a sedentary lifestyle (possibly quite the contrary!).

Liebenson (1990b) has discussed the work of Sommer (1985), who found that competitive basketball and volleyball players frequently produce patellar tendinitis and other forms of knee dysfunction due to the particular stresses they endure because of muscular imbalances. Their ability to jump is often seriously impaired by virtue of shortened psoas and quadriceps muscles with associated weakness of gluteus maximus. This imbalance leads to decreased hip extension and hyperextension of the knee joint. Once muscular balance is restored, a more controlled jump is possible, as is a reduction in reported fatigue. The element of fatigue should not be forgotten in this equation, since hypertonic muscles are working excessively both to perform their functions and often to compensate for weakness in associated muscles.

Evjenth & Hamberg (1984) succinctly summarise: 'Every patient with symptoms involving the locomotor system, particularly symptoms of pain and/or constrained movement, should be examined to assess joint and muscle function. If examination shows joint play to be normal, but reveals shortened muscles or muscle spasm, then treatment by stretching [and by implication MET] is indicated.'

Stabilisers and mobilisers (Box 2.6)

British physiotherapist researcher Chris Norris (2000) comments on the postural/phasic model:

> The terms postural and phasic, used by Jull and Janda (1987), can be misleading. In their categorisation, the hamstring muscles are placed in the postural grouping while the gluteals are placed in the phasic grouping. The reaction described for these muscles is that the postural group (represented by the hamstrings in this case) tend to tighten, are biarticular, have a lower irritability threshold, and a tendency to develop trigger points. This type of action would suggest a phasic (as opposed to tonic) response, and is typical of a muscle used to develop power and speed in sport for example, a task carried out by the hamstrings. The so called 'phasic group' is said to lengthen, weaken and be uniarticular, a description perhaps better suited to the characteristics of a muscle used for postural holding. The description of the muscle responses described by Jull and Janda (1987) is accurate, but the terms postural and phasic do not seem to adequately describe the groupings.

The issue of 'naming' what is observed, in terms of muscle behaviour, seems to be a key feature of the debate. Norris (2000) suggests that mobiliser muscles are more or less the same, in most of their characteristics, as Janda's postural muscles. Similarly, stabilisers are equated with phasic muscles. Apart from the apparent semantic contradiction (i.e. it is hard to liken a 'stabiliser' to 'phasic' activity), this suggests that the intrinsic model is accurate, whatever the names ascribed to the muscle categories. Some muscles do tend to shorten, and some do tend to weaken (and in some cases lengthen) whatever names we call them.

The language discrepancy between the *mobiliser/stabiliser* and the *postural/phasic* designations of muscles does not, however, exhaust the complications facing practitioners trying to make sense of modern research. They also have to contend with elements such as *deep/superficial*, *monoarticular/polyarticular*, *global/local*.

Global and local muscles

Bergmark (1989) and Richardson et al (1999) have categorised muscles in yet another way. They describe some muscles as *local* ('central') and others as being *global* ('guy rope'). Global muscles are likened to the ropes supporting a ship's mast. In this model central muscles are seen as lying deep or as possessing deep components which attach to the spine. Global muscles are seen as having the capacity to control the

Box 2.6 Mobiliser and stabiliser characteristics (Richardson et al 1992, 1999)

Mobiliser features	**Stabiliser features**
Fusiform	Aponeurotic
Fast twitch	Slow twitch
Produce angular rotation	Maintain joint balance
Relatively small proprioceptive role	Major proprioceptive role
Produce torque and power activities	Antigravity endurance tasks
Phasic activity	Tonic activity
Concentric muscle functions	Eccentric and isometric functions
Fatigue easily	Resistant to fatigue
Often superficial	Often more deeply placed
Activated at 30-40% MVC (maximum voluntary contraction)	Activated above 40% MVC
Tighten and shorten	**Selectively weaken and lengthen**

Examples of these muscle designations

Mobilisers (which selectively shorten and tighten):

- Rectus abdominis
- Lateral fibres external oblique
- Erector spinae
- Gastrocnemius/soleus
- Iliocostalis
- Hamstrings
- Upper trapezius
- Adductors of the thigh
- Levator scapulae
- Iliopsoas
- Suboccipitals
- Rectus femoris
- Pectoralis major and minor

Stabilisers (which selectively weaken and lengthen):

- Gluteus medius and maximus
- Vastus medius oblique
- Transversus abdominis
- Internal obliques
- Multifidus
- Serratus anterior
- Deep neck flexors
- Lower trapezius
- Quadratus lumborum (see notes on this controversial muscle in this chapter, p. 47, and in Box 4.8)

spine's resistance to bending, as well as being able to influence spinal alignment, balancing and accommodating to the forces imposed on the spine:

- *Global muscles*: anterior portion of the internal obliques, external obliques, rectus abdominis, the lateral fibres of the quadratus lumborum and the more lateral portions of the erector spinae (Bogduk & Twomey 1991).
- *Local muscles*: multifidi, intertrasversarii, interspinales, transversus abdominis, the posterior portion of the internal oblique, the medial fibres of quadratus lumborum and the more central portion of the erector spinae.

Richardson et al (1999) describe (discussing low back pain) the essentially practical nature of their focus on the 'local' and 'global' characterisation model:

> Basically, there are two broad approaches for improving the spinal protection role of the muscles which can be gleaned from anatomical and biomechanical studies on lumbopelvic stabilization. The first utilizes the principle of minimizing forces applied to the lumbar spine during functional activities. The second is to ensure that the deep local muscle system is operating to stabilize the individual spinal segments.

This model is therefore essentially pragmatic: 'Lighten the stress load and improve stabilising function' would summarise its objectives, and few clinicians would argue with these.

Identification of those muscles under-performing in their stabilisation roles (usually deep rather than superficial), followed by re-education of the appropriate use of these, plays a major part in the protocols which emerge from this approach. Little attention is described as being paid to overactive antagonists which might be inhibiting underactive deep muscles. However, as well as a brief encouragement to deal with ergonomic factors, these authors do state that:

> Global [i.e. superficial] muscle function can cause potentially harmful effects if there is overactivity in certain muscles of this system. Methods of treatment aimed at decreasing any unnecessary activity in these muscles will assist in minimizing harmful forces. Logically this could only be safely pursued if the protective function of the deep-local muscles was being reestablished at the same time.

The argument therefore seems to boil down to whether short, tight structures, whatever name they are given, are treated first, or whether the weak structures (whatever they are named) receive primary attention, or whether some form of synchronised approach is adopted. Readers will make their own choices.

Dual role of certain muscles

In the mobiliser/stabiliser model some muscles seem to act as both. Norris (2000) states:

> The quadratus lumborum has been shown to be significant as a stabiliser in lumbar spine movements (McGill et al 1996) while tightening has also been described (Janda 1983). It seems likely that the muscle may act functionally [differently] in its medial and lateral portions, with the medial portion being more active as a stabiliser of the lumbar spine and the lateral more active as a mobiliser. Such sub-division is seen in a number of other muscles, for example the gluteus medius where the posterior fibres are more posturally involved (Jull 1994); the internal oblique where the posterior fibres attaching to the lateral raphe are considered stabilisers (Bergmark 1989); the external oblique where the lateral fibres work during flexion in parallel with the rectus abdominis (Kendall et al 1993).

How strong should an MET contraction be?

Of particular interest in application of MET, as described in this text, is the observation (see Box 2.6), that postural/mobiliser muscles activate with contractions below 30% of maximum voluntary contraction (MVC). Hoffer & Andreasson (1981) demonstrated that efforts below 25% MVC provide maximal joint stiffness. More importantly, McArdle et al (1991) have shown that a prolonged tonic holding contraction and a low MVC (under 30–40% MVC) selectively recruits tonic (postural) fibres. This vital information will be noted again in the technique segments of the book.

Easing the confusion

This text remains faithful to the model described by Janda and others in describing muscles as being either *postural* or *phasic*. This does not mean rejection of alternative concepts (stabiliser/mobiliser, global/local, etc.) as described by Norris, Richardson and others. It is simply that although renaming something may serve a purpose in research terms, it does not seem to offer any particular advantage clinically in relation to the identification of shortness or weakness, or of the appropriate application of MET to such structures.

Chiropractic rehabilitation expert Craig Liebenson (personal communication, 1999) suggests a way in which the clinician can avoid the possibility of confusion. Simply define particular muscles as 'having a tendency to shortening or weakening'. Whether they are classified as postural or phasic, or as mobilisers or stabilisers, then becomes irrelevant to what needs doing.

Norris (2000) supports the possibility of confusion arising out of attempts at muscle categorisation:

> Any relatively simplistic categorisation of muscle is fraught with problems. The danger with muscle imbalance categorisation is that practitioners will expect set changes to occur and fail to adequately assess a patient. When this occurs, important deviations from the 'imbalance norm' can be missed and treatment outcomes will be impaired. Although muscle imbalance categorisation can usefully assist the astute practitioner, they are not cast in stone. Assessment will still be required but can be refined to reveal the subtleties of muscle reaction to altered use and pathology.

He points out that if the practitioner can identify that a muscle is weak (i.e. has poor inner range holding), rehabilitation methods are needed to remedy this. Further, if a muscle is inappropriately tight or short, safe methods (such as MET) exist to release and/or lengthen it. And of course once muscle balance has been restored, habitual posture and use patterns need to be addressed.

Box 2.7 offers summaries of some of the patterns which can be associated with imbalances between stabilisers and mobilisers, and possible observational evidence which can be confirmed by tests (Norris 1995a–e, 1998; see also Ch. 5 for functional assessments, Boxes 2.8 and 2.9 and Fig. 2.10).

Where do joints fit into the picture?

Janda has an answer to this emotive question when he says that it is not known whether dysfunction of muscles causes joint dysfunction or vice versa (Janda 1988). He points out, however, that since clinical evidence abounds that joint mobilisation (thrust or gentle mobilisation) influences the muscles which are in anatomic or functional relationships with the joint, it may well be that normalisation of the excessive tone of the muscles in this way is what is providing the benefit, and that, by implication, normalisation of the muscle tone by other means (such as MET) would provide an equally useful basis for a beneficial outcome and joint normalisation. Since reduction in muscle spasm/contraction commonly results in a reduction in joint pain, the answer to many such problems would seem to lie in appropriate soft tissue attention.

Box 2.7 Patterns of imbalance

Patterns of imbalance as some muscles weaken and lengthen, and synergists become overworked, while antagonists shorten (see this chapter for cross syndromes, and Ch. 5 for Janda's functional tests for muscle imbalance):

Lengthened or underactive stabiliser	Overactive synergist	Shortened antagonist
1. Gluteus medius	TFL, quadratus lumborum, piriformis	Thigh adductors
2. Gluteus maximus	Iliocostalis lumborum and hamstrings	Iliopsoas, rectus femoris
3. Transverse abdominis	Rectus abdominis	Iliocostalis lumborum
4. Lower trapezius	Levator scapulae/upper trapezius	Pectoralis major
5. Deep neck flexors	SCM	Suboccipitals
6. Serratus anterior	Pectoralis major/minor	Rhomboids
7. Diaphragm		Scalenes, pectoralis major

Box 2.8 Observation

Observation can often provide evidence of an imbalance involving cross-patterns of weakness/lengthening and shortness (see this chapter for cross syndromes, and Ch. 5 for Janda's functional tests for muscle imbalance).

For example:

Muscle inhibition/weakness/lengthening	*Observable sign*
Transverse abdominis	Protruding umbilicus
Serratus anterior	Winged scapula
Lower trapezius	Elevated shoulder girdle('Gothic' shoulders)
Deep neck flexors	Chin 'poking'
Gluteus medius	Unlevel pelvis on one-legged standing
Gluteus maximus	Sagging buttock(s)

Tests can be used to assess muscle imbalance.
Postural inspection provides a quick screen, muscle length tests, movement patterns, and inner holding endurance times (see Box 2.9)

Box 2.9 Inner range holding (endurance) tests (Fig. 2.10)

'Inner holding isometric endurance' tests can be performed for muscles which have a tendency to lengthen, in order to assess their ability to maintain joint alignment in a neutral zone. Usually a lengthened muscle will demonstrate a loss of endurance when tested in a shortened position. This can be tested by the practitioner passively pre-positioning the muscle in a shortened position and assessing the duration of time that the patient can hold the muscle in the shortened position. There are various methods used, including:

- Ten repetitions of the holding position for 10 seconds at a time
- Alternatively, a single 30-second hold can be requested
- If the patient cannot hold the position actively from the moment of passive pre-positioning, this is a sign of inappropriate antagonist muscle shortening
- Norris (1999) states that 'Optimal endurance is indicated when the full inner range position can be held for 10 to 20 seconds. Muscle lengthening is present if the limb falls away from the inner range position immediately.'

Norris (1999) describes examples of inner range holding tests (see also Fig. 2.10) for:

Iliopsoas
Patient is seated
Practitioner lifts one leg into greater hip flexion so that foot is well clear of floor
Patient is asked to hold this position.

Gluteus maximus
Patient is prone
Practitioner lifts one leg into extension at the hip (knee flexed to 90°)
Patient is asked to hold the leg in this position.

Posterior fibres of gluteus medius
Patient is side-lying with uppermost leg flexed at hip and knee so that both the knee and foot are resting on the floor/surface
Practitioner places the flexed leg into a position of maximal unforced external rotation at the hip, foot still resting on the floor
Patient is asked to maintain this position.

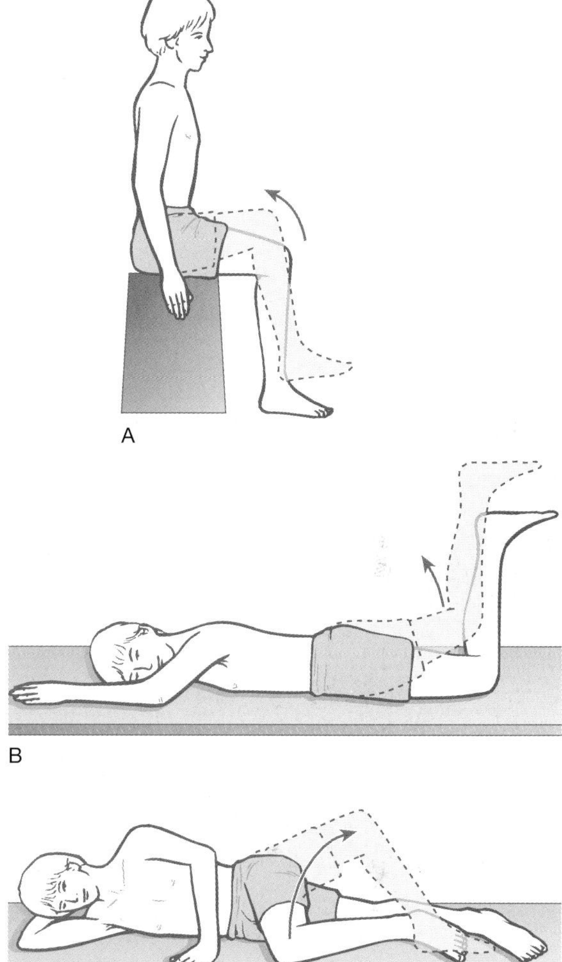

Figure 2.10 **A** Iliopsoas holding test. **B** Gluteus maximus holding test. **C** Posterior fibres gluteus medius holding test.

Liebenson (1990b) takes a view with a chiropractic bias: 'The chief abnormalities of [musculoskeletal] function include muscular hypertonicity and joint blockage. Since these abnormalities are functional rather than structural they are reversible in nature … once a particular joint has lost its normal range of motion, the muscles around that joint will attempt to minimise stress at the involved segment.'

After describing the processes of progressive compensation as some muscles become hypertonic while inhibiting their antagonists, he continues, 'What may begin as a simple restriction of movement in a joint can lead to the development of muscular imbalances and postural change. This chain of events is an example of what we try to prevent through adjustments of subluxations.'

We are left then with one view which has it that muscle release will frequently normalise joint restrictions, as well as a view which holds the opposite – that joint normalisation sorts out soft tissue problems, leaving direct work on muscles for rehabilitation settings and for attention if joint mobilisation fails to deal with long-term changes (fibrosis, etc.).

It is possible that both views are to some extent correct. However, what emphasis therapists/practitioners give to their prime focus – be it joint or be it soft tissues – the certainty is that what is required is anything but a purely local view, as Janda helps us to understand.

PATTERNS OF DYSFUNCTION

When a chain reaction evolves in which some muscles shorten and others weaken, predictable patterns involving imbalances develop, and Czech researcher Vladimir Janda describes the so-called upper and lower 'crossed' syndromes (see below and Tables 2.2 and 2.3).

Upper crossed syndrome (Fig. 2.11)

This involves the basic imbalance shown in Table 2.2. As the changes listed in Table 2.2 take place, they alter the relative positions of the head, neck and shoulders as follows:

1. The occiput and C1/2 will hyperextend, with the head being pushed forward.
2. The lower cervical to 4th thoracic vertebrae will be posturally stressed as a result.
3. Rotation and abduction of the scapulae occurs.
4. An altered direction of the axis of the glenoid fossa will develop, resulting in the humerus needing to be stabilised by additional levator scapula and upper trapezius activity, with additional activity from supraspinatus as well.

Table 2.2 Upper crossed syndrome

Pectoralis major and minor Upper trapezius Levator scapulae Sternomastoid	All tighten and shorten
while Lower and middle trapezius Serratus anterior and rhomboids	All weaken

Table 2.3 Lower crossed syndrome

Hip flexors Iliopsoas, rectus femoris TFL, short adductors Erector spinae group of the trunk	All tighten and shorten
while Abdominal and gluteal muscles	All weaken

The result of these changes is greater cervical segment strain plus referred pain to the chest, shoulders and arms. Pain mimicking angina may be noted plus a decline in respiratory efficiency.

The solution, according to Janda, is to be able to identify the shortened structures and to release (stretch and relax) them, followed by re-education towards more appropriate function.

Lower crossed syndrome (Fig. 2.12)

This involves the basic imbalance shown in Table 2.3. The result of the chain reaction in Table 2.3 is that the pelvis tips forward on the frontal plane, flexing the hip joints and producing lumbar lordosis and stress at L5–S1 with pain and irritation. A further stress commonly appears in the sagittal plane in which quadratus lumborum tightens and gluteus maximus and medius weaken.

When this 'lateral corset' becomes unstable, the pelvis is held in increased elevation, accentuated when walking, resulting in L5–S1 stress in the sagittal plane. One result is low back pain. The combined stresses described produce instability at the lumbodorsal junction, an unstable transition point at best.

Also commonly involved are the piriformis muscles which in 20% of individuals are penetrated by the sciatic nerve so that piriformis syndrome can produce direct sciatic pressure and pain. Arterial involvement of piriformis shortness produces ischaemia of the lower extremity, and through a relative fixation of the sacrum, sacroiliac dysfunction and pain in the hip.

The solution for an all too common pattern such as this is to identify the shortened structures and to release them, ideally using variations on the theme of MET, followed by re-education of posture and use.

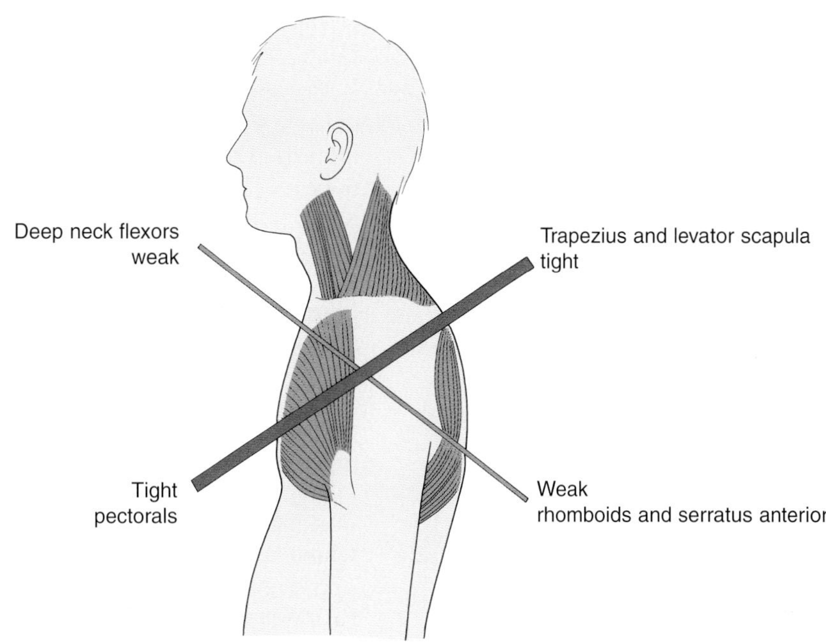

Figure 2.11 The upper crossed syndrome, as described by Janda.

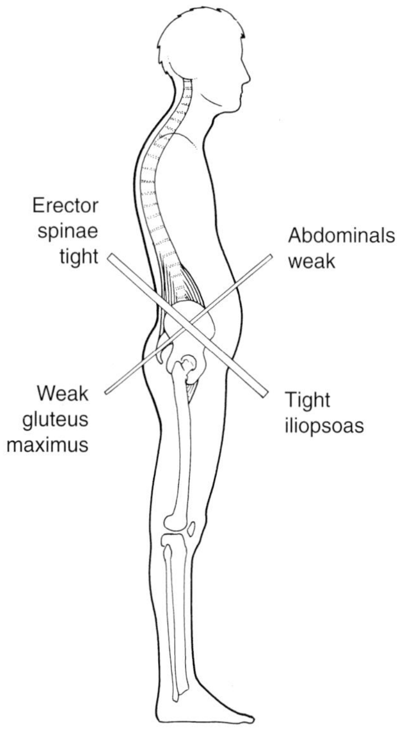

Figure 2.12 The lower crossed syndrome, as described by Janda.

Chain reaction leads to facial and jaw pain

In case it is thought that such imbalances are of merely academic interest, a practical example of the negative effects of the chain reactions described above is given by Janda (1986b) in an article entitled 'Some aspects of extracranial causes of facial pain'.

Janda's premise is that temporomandibular joint (TMJ) problems and facial pain can be analysed in relation to the patient's whole posture. He has hypothesised that the muscular pattern associated with TMJ problems may be considered as locally involving hyperactivity and tension in the temporal and masseter muscles while, because of this hypertonicity, reciprocal inhibition occurs in the suprahyoid, digastric and mylohyoid muscles. The external pterygoid in particular often develops spasm. This imbalance between jaw adductors and jaw openers alters the ideal position of the condyle and leads to a consequent redistribution of stress on the joint, leading to degenerative changes.

Janda describes the typical pattern of muscular dysfunction of an individual with TMJ problems as involving upper trapezius, levator scapula, scaleni, sternomastoid, suprahyoid, lateral and medial pterygoid, masseter and temporal muscles, all of which show a tendency to tighten and to develop spasm.

He notes that while the scalenes are unpredictable, and while commonly, under overload conditions, they become atrophied and weak, they may also develop spasm, tenderness and trigger points.

The postural pattern in a TMJ patient might involve (Fig. 2.13; see also Fig. 2.12):

1. Hyperextension of knee joints
2. Increased anterior tilt of pelvis
3. Pronounced flexion of hip joints
4. Hyperlordosis of lumbar spine
5. Rounded shoulders and winged (rotated and abducted) scapulae
6. Cervical hyperlordosis
7. Forward thrust of head
8. Compensatory over-activity of upper trapezius and levator scapulae
9. Forward thrust of head resulting in opening of mouth and retraction of mandible.

This series of changes provokes increased activity of the jaw adductor and protractor muscles, creating a vicious cycle of dysfunctional activity.

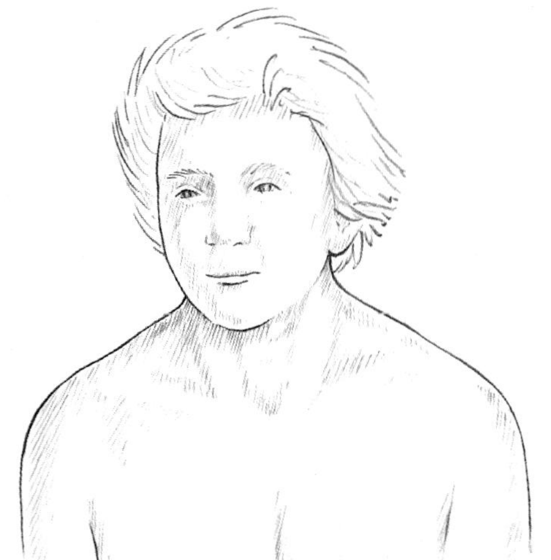

Figure 2.13 A typical pattern of upper thoracic and cervical stress as described by Janda would involve a degree of TMJ stress. Note the 'Gothic shoulders' which result from upper trapezius hypertonicity and shortening.

Intervertebral joint stress in the cervical spine follows.

The message which can be derived from this evidence is that patterns first need to be identified before they can be assessed for the role they might be playing in the patient's pain and restriction conditions, and certainly before these can be successfully and appropriately treated. (Dr Liebenson discusses a number of Vladimir Janda's observation assessment methods in Chapter 5.)

Patterns of change with inappropriate breathing (Fig. 2.14A and B)

Garland (1994) describes the somatic changes which follow from a pattern of hyperventilation, upper chest breathing.

When faced with persistent upper chest breathing patterns we should be able to identify reduced diaphragmatic efficiency and commensurate restriction of the lower rib cage as these evolve into a series of changes with accessory breathing muscles being inappropriately and excessively used:

- A degree of visceral stasis and pelvic floor weakness will develop, as will an imbalance between increasingly weak abdominal muscles and increasingly tight erector spinae muscles.
- Fascial restriction from the central tendon via the pericardial fascia, all the way up to the basiocciput, will be noted.
- The upper ribs will be elevated and there will be sensitive costal cartilage tension.
- The thoracic spine will be disturbed by virtue of the lack of normal motion of the articulation with the ribs, and sympathetic outflow from this area may be affected.
- Accessory muscle hypertonia, notably affecting the scalenes, upper trapezius and levator scapulae, will be palpable and observable.
- Fibrosis will develop in these muscles, as will myofascial trigger points.
- The cervical spine will become progressively rigid with a fixed lordosis being a common feature in the lower cervical spine.

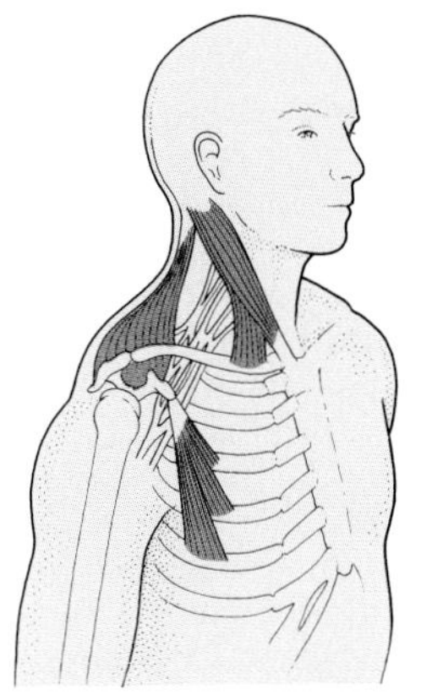
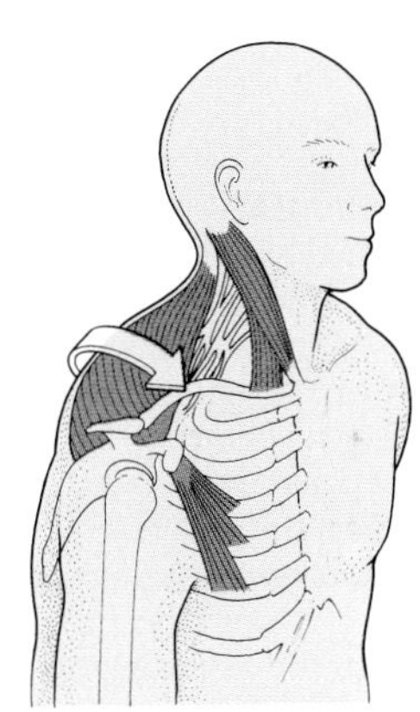

Figure 2.14A A progressive pattern of postural and biomechanical dysfunction develops, resulting in, and aggravated by, inappropriate breathing function.

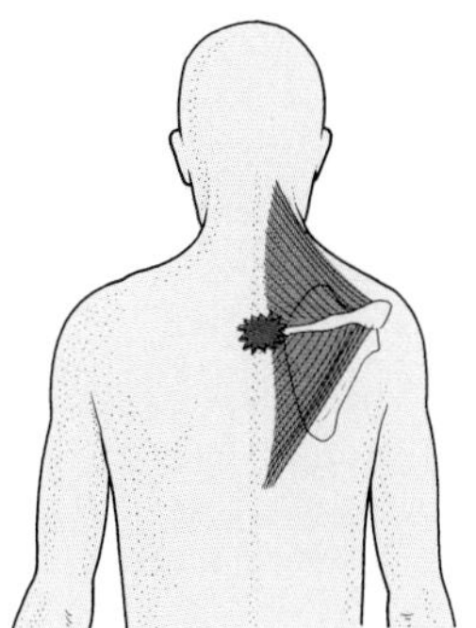
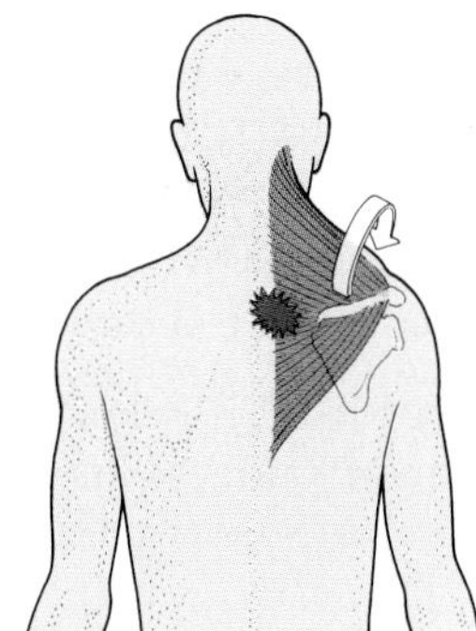

Figure 2.14B The local changes in the muscles of an area being stressed in this way will include the evolution of fibrotic changes and myofascial trigger points.

- A reduction in the mobility of the 2nd cervical segment and disturbance of vagal outflow from this region is likely.
- Although not noted in Garland's list of dysfunction (in which he states 'psychology overwhelms physiology'), we should bear in mind that the other changes which Janda has listed in his upper crossed syndrome (see above) are also likely consequences, including the potentially devastating effects on shoulder function of the altered position of the scapulae and glenoid fossae as this pattern evolves.
- Also worth noting in relation to breathing function and dysfunction are two important muscles not included in Garland's list: quadratus lumborum and iliopsoas, both of which merge fibres with the diaphragm. Since these are both postural muscles, with a propensity to shortening when stressed, the impact of such shortening, either uni- or bilaterally, can be seen to have major implications for respiratory function, whether the primary feature of such a dysfunction lies in diaphragmatic or in muscular distress.

Recall that among possible stress factors which will result in shortening of postural muscles is disuse, and that a situation in which upper chest breathing has replaced diaphragmatic breathing as the norm would lead to reduced diaphragmatic excursion and consequent reduction in activity for those aspects of quadratus lumborum and psoas which are integral with it, and shortening would be a likely result of this.

Recall also Schmid's skiers (see p. 44), whose most obvious shortening feature was psoas – it is hard to imagine that their overall performance efficiency would not be impaired by the impact of bilaterally short psoas structures (as found in 75% of those examined) dragging on their diaphragms as they hurtle down the mountainsides.

Garland concludes his listing of somatic changes associated with hyperventilation by saying, 'Physically and physiologically [all of] this runs against a biologically sustainable pattern, and in a vicious cycle, abnormal function (use) alters normal structure, which disallows return to normal function.' He also points to the likelihood of counselling (for associated anxiety or depression, perhaps) and breathing retraining being far more likely to be successfully initiated if the structural component(s) – as listed – are dealt with in such a way as to minimise the effects of the somatic changes described.

The words of the pioneer osteopathic physician Carl McConnell (1902) remind us of wider implications:

> Remember that the functional status of the diaphragm is probably the most powerful mechanism of the whole body. It not only mechanically engages the tissues of the pharynx to the perineum, several times per minute, but is physiologically indispensable to the activity of every cell in the body. A working knowledge of the crura, tendon, and the extensive

ramification of the diaphragmatic tissues, graphically depicts the significance of structural continuity and functional unity. The wealth of soft tissue work centering in the powerful mechanism is beyond compute, and clinically it is very practical.

Fascia and the thorax

In both Garland's and McConnell's discussion of respiratory function mention has been made of fascia, the importance of which was indicated earlier in this chapter in relation to some of the thoughts of Rolf and Cathie. An additional reference to the ubiquitous nature and vital importance of this structure comes from Leon Page (1952), who discusses the involvement of fascia in the thoracic region:

> The cervical fascia extends from the base of the skull to the mediastinum and forms compartments enclosing oesophagus, trachea, carotid vessels and provides support for the pharynx, larynx and thyroid gland. There is direct continuity of fascia from the apex of the diaphragm to the base of the skull, extending through the fibrous pericardium upward through the deep cervical fascia and the continuity extends not only to the outer surface of the sphenoid, occipital and temporal bones but proceeds further through the foramina in the base of the skull around the vessels and nerves to join the dura.

Goldthwaite's overview

Goldthwaite, in his classic 1930s discussion of posture, links a wide array of problems to the absence of balanced posture (Goldthwaite 1945). Clearly some of what he hypothesises remains conjecture, but we can see just how much impact postural stress can have on associated tissues, starting with diaphragmatic weakness:

> The main factors which determine the maintenance of the abdominal viscera in position are the diaphragm and the abdominal muscles, both of which are relaxed and cease to support in faulty posture. The disturbances of circulation resulting from a low diaphragm and ptosis may give rise to chronic passive congestion in one or all of the organs of the abdomen and pelvis, since the local as well as general venous drainage may be impeded by the failure of the diaphragmatic pump to do its full work in the drooped body. Furthermore, the drag of these congested organs on their nerve supply, as well as the pressure on the sympathetic ganglia and plexuses, probably causes many irregularities in their function, varying from partial paralysis to overstimulation. All these organs receive fibres from both the vagus and sympathetic systems, either one of which may be disturbed. It is probable that one or all of these factors are active at various times in both the stocky and the slender anatomic types, and are responsible for many functional digestive disturbances. These disturbances, if continued long enough, may lead to diseases later in life. Faulty body mechanics in early life, then, becomes a vital factor in the production of the vicious cycle of chronic diseases and presents a chief point of attack in its prevention ... In this upright position, as one becomes older, the tendency is for the abdomen to relax and sag more and more, allowing a ptosic condition of the abdominal and pelvic organs unless the supporting lower abdominal muscles are taught to contract properly. As the abdomen relaxes, there is a great tendency towards a drooped chest, with narrow rib angle, forward shoulders, prominent shoulder blades, a forward position of the head, and probably pronated feet. When the human machine is out of balance, physiological function cannot be perfect; muscles and ligaments are in an abnormal state of tension and strain. A well-poised body means a machine working perfectly, with the least amount of muscular effort, and therefore better health and strength for daily life.

Note how closely Goldthwaite mirrors the picture Janda paints in his upper and lower crossed syndromes (see above, pp. 50–51), and 'posture and facial pain' description (p. 51).

Patterns of function and patterns of dysfunction are seen in the various examples given to provide us with fertile soil in which to seek a crop of dysfunctional tissues, ripe for therapeutic harvesting.

Korr's trophic influence research

Irwin Korr has spent half a century investigating the scientific background to osteopathic methodology and theory, and among his most important research has been that which demonstrated the role of neural structures in delivery of trophic substances (Korr 1986, Korr et al 1967). The various patterns of stress which we have covered in this chapter are capable of drastically affecting this. He states:

> Also involved in somatic dysfunction are neural influences that are based on the transfer of specific proteins synthesised by the neuron to the innervated tissue. This delivery is accomplished by axonal

transport and junctional traversal. These 'trophic' proteins are thought to exert long-term influences on the developmental, morphologic, metabolic and functional qualities of the tissues – even on their viability. Biomechanical abnormalities in the musculoskeletal system can cause trophic disturbances in at least two ways (1) by mechanical deformation (compression, stretching, angulation, torsion) of the nerves, which impedes axonal transport; and (2) by sustained hyperactivity of neurons in facilitated segments of the spinal cord [see below, p. 56] which slows axonal transport and which because of metabolic changes, may affect protein synthesis by the neurons. It appears that manipulative treatment would alleviate such impairments of neurotrophic function.

IDENTIFICATION AND NORMALISATION OF PATTERNS OF DYSFUNCTION

Observation, palpation, specific tests – these are the ways in which such patterns may be identified and assessed so that treatment can take account of more than the local dysfunction and can place the patient's symptoms within the context of whole-body dysfunctional patterns which represent the sum of their present adaptation and compensation efforts.

Patterns of imbalance can be observed in predictable areas, relating to specific forms of dysfunction (headache, thoracic inlet, low back, etc.) and the reader is directed to Dr Liebenson's analysis of this approach to assessment in Chapter 5.

If an imbalance pattern is recognisable, and, within that, emphasis is given to what is hypertonic and what (within both hypertonic and hypotonic muscles) is reflexively active, as in the case of myofascial trigger points, a therapeutic starting point is possible which leads physiologically towards the normalisation and resolution – if only partially – of the somatic dysfunction patterns currently on display.

As whatever is tense and tight to an undesirable degree is released and stretched, so will antagonists regain tone, and a degree of balance be restored. As local myofascial trigger areas are resolved, so will reflexively initiated pain and sympathetic overactivity be minimised. The stress burden will be lightened, energy will be saved, function will improve, joint stress will be reduced, exacerbation of patterns of dysfunction will be modified.

This is not the end of the story, however, since re-education as to more appropriate use is clearly the ideal long-term objective if the causes of dysfunction related to misuse, abuse or overuse of the musculoskeletal system are to be addressed. However, it is suggested that such re-education – whether postural or functional (as in breathing retraining), or sensory-motor rehabilitation where faulty motor patterns are well established – will be more successfully achieved if chronic mechanical restrictions have been minimised.

Liebenson (1990b) comments: 'In rehabilitation it is important to identify and correct overactive or shortened musculature prior to attempting a muscle strengthening regimen .... The effectiveness of any rehabilitation program is enhanced if hypertonic muscles are relaxed, and if necessary stretched, prior to initiating a strengthening program' (see Ch. 5 for an introduction to Dr Liebenson's rehabilitation methods).

There are certainly other ways of normalising hypertonicity than use of MET, even if only temporarily, such as use of inhibitory ischaemic compression (Chaitow 1991b), positional release methods (Jones 1982) or joint manipulation (Lewit 1999). Indeed, many experts in manual medicine hold that manipulation of associated joints will automatically and spontaneously resolve soft tissue hypertonicity (Janda 1978, Mennell 1952); however, neither manipulation of joints nor use of methods which do not in some way stretch the tissues will reduce and encourage towards normal those structures which have become fibrotically altered, whereas MET will do so if used appropriately.

The major researchers into myofascial trigger points, Travell & Simons, influenced by the work of Karel Lewit, also suggest that use of MET is an ideal means of normalising these centres of neurological mayhem (Travell & Simons 1992).

Trigger points

It is necessary to include a brief overview of myofascial trigger points in any consideration of patterns of dysfunction.

The reflex patterns – and facilitation

In the body, when an area is stressed repetitively and chronically, the local nerve structures in that area tend to become overexcitable, more easily activated, hyperirritable – a process known as facilitation.

There are two forms of facilitation and if we are to make sense of muscle dysfunction, we have to understand these.

Segmental facilitation (Korr 1976, Patterson 1976)

Organ dysfunction will result in facilitation of the paraspinal structures at the level of the nerve supply to that organ. If there is any form of cardiac disease, for example, there will be a 'feed-back' of impulses along these same nerves towards the spine, and the muscles alongside the spine at that upper thoracic level will become hypertonic. If the cardiac problem continues, the area will become facilitated, with the nerves of the area, including those passing to the heart, becoming hyperirritable (Fig. 2.15).

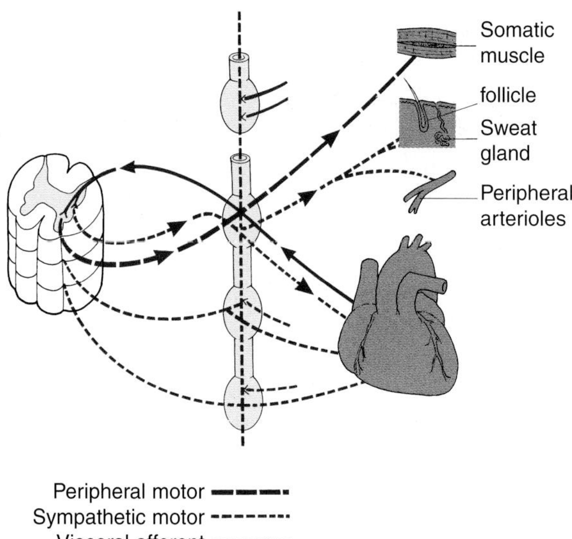

Figure 2.15 Schematic representation of the neurological influences involved in the process of facilitation resulting from visceral dysfunction (cardiac disease in this example). Hyperirritable neural feedback to the CNS will result, which influences muscle, skin (both palpable) and venous structures in associated areas, as well as the neural supply to the organ itself.

Electromyographic readings of the muscles alongside the spine at the upper thoracic level would show this region to be very active compared with that above and below it, and the muscles alongside the spine at that level would be hypertonic and probably painful to pressure.

Once facilitated, if there were any additional stress impacting the individual, of any sort, whether emotional physical, chemical, climatic, mechanical or whatever, or absolutely anything which imposed stress on the person as a whole – not just this particular part of their body – there would be a marked increase in neural activity in the facilitated area and not in the rest of the spinal structures.

Korr has called such an area a 'neurological lens' – it concentrates the nerve activity to the facilitated area, so creating more activity and also a local increase in muscle tone at that level of the spine. Similar segmental (spinal) facilitation occurs in response to any organ problem, obviously affecting only the part of the spine from which the nerves to that organ emerge. Other causes of segmental (spinal) facilitation can include stress imposed on a part of the spine through injury, overactivity, repetitive stress, poor posture or structural imbalance (short leg for example).

Korr (1978) tells us that when subjects who have had facilitated segments identified 'were exposed to physical, environmental and psychological stimuli similar to those encountered in daily life, the sympathetic responses in those segments was exaggerated and prolonged. The disturbed segments behaved as though they were continually in or bordering on a state of "physiologic alarm".'

In assessing and treating somatic dysfunction, the phenomenon of segmental facilitation needs to be borne in mind since the causes and treatment of these frequently lie outside the scope of practice of manual practitioners and therapists. In many instances, however, appropriate manipulative treatment, including use of MET, can help to 'de-stress' facilitated areas.

How to recognise a facilitated area

A number of observable and palpable signs indicate an area of segmental (spinal) facilitation.

Beal (1983) tells us that such an area will usually involve two or more segments (unless traumatically induced, in which case single segments are possible). The paraspinal tissues will palpate as rigid or 'board-like'. With the patient supine and the palpating hands under the patient's paraspinal area to be tested (standing at the head of the table, for example, and reaching under the shoulders for the upper thoracic area), any ceilingward 'springing' attempt on these tissues will result in a distinct lack of elasticity, unlike more normal tissues above or below the facilitated area (Beal 1983).

Grieve (1986), Gunn & Milbrandt (1978), and Korr (1948) have all helped to define the palpable and visual signs which accompany facilitated dysfunction:

- A gooseflesh appearance is observable in facilitated areas when the skin is exposed to cool air – the result of a facilitated pilomotor response.
- A palpable sense of 'drag' is noticeable as a light touch contact is made across such areas, due to increased sweat production resulting from facilitation of the sudomotor reflexes.
- There is likely to be cutaneous hyperaesthesia in the related dermatome, as the sensitivity is increased – for example, to a pin prick – due to facilitation.
- An 'orange peel' appearance is noticeable in the subcutaneous tissues when the skin is rolled over the affected segment, due to subcutaneous trophoedema.
- There is commonly localised spasm of the muscles in a facilitated area, which is palpable segmentally as well as peripherally in the related myotome. This is likely to be accompanied by an enhanced myotatic reflex due to the process of facilitation.

Local (trigger point) facilitation in muscles (Fig. 2.16)

A similar process of facilitation occurs when particularly easily stressed parts of muscle (origins and insertions for example) are overused, abused, misused, disused in any of the many ways discussed earlier in this chapter.

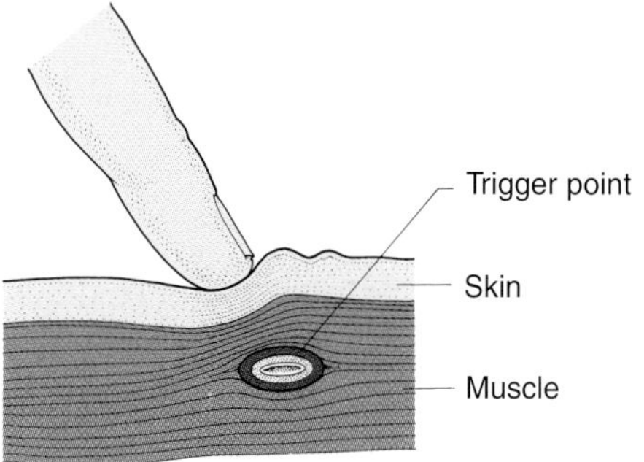

Figure 2.16 Trigger points are areas of local facilitation which can be housed in any soft tissue structure, most usually muscle and/or fascia. Palpation from the skin or at depth may be required to localise these.

Localised areas of hypertonicity will develop, sometimes accompanied by some oedema, sometimes with a stringy feel – but always with a sensitivity to pressure.

Many of these palpably painful, tender, sensitive, localised, facilitated points are myofascial trigger points which are not only painful themselves when pressed, but will also when active transmit or activate pain (and other) sensations some distance away from themselves, in 'target' tissues.

In the same manner as the facilitated areas alongside the spine, these trigger points will be made more active by any stress, of whatever type, impacting on the body as a whole – not just on the area in which they lie. When not actively sending pain to a distant area, trigger points (local tender or pain areas) are said to be 'latent'. The same signs as described for spinal/segmental facilitation can be observed and palpated in these areas, with 'drag' palpation being among the most rapid means of identifying such local dysfunction.

The leading researchers into pain, Melzack & Wall (1988), have stated that there are few, if any, chronic pain problems which do not have trigger point activity as a major part of the picture, perhaps not always as a prime cause but almost always as a maintaining feature.

What causes the trigger point to develop?

Janet Travell and David Simons are the two physicians who, above all others, have helped our understanding of trigger points. Simons has described the evolution of trigger points as follows (Lewit & Simons 1984):

> In the core of the trigger lies a muscle spindle which is in trouble for some reason. Visualise a spindle like a strand of yarn in a knitted sweater ... a metabolic crisis takes place which increases the temperature locally in the trigger point, shortens a minute part of the muscle (sarcomere) – like a snag in a sweater, and reduces the supply of oxygen and nutrients into the trigger point. During this disturbed episode an influx of calcium occurs and the muscle spindle does not have enough energy to pump the calcium outside the cell where it belongs. Thus a vicious cycle is maintained and the muscle spindle can't seem to loosen up and the affected muscle can't relax.

Simons has tested his concept and found that, at the core of trigger points, there is an oxygen deficit compared with the muscle tissue which surrounds it.

Travell has confirmed that the following factors can all help to maintain and enhance trigger point activity: nutritional deficiency (especially vitamin C, B-complex vitamins and iron); hormonal imbalances (low thyroid, menopausal or premenstrual situations for example); infections (bacteria, viruses or yeast); allergies (wheat and dairy in particular); low oxygenation of tissues (aggravated by tension, stress, inactivity, poor respiration) (Simons & Travell 1983).

Facilitation and the central nervous system

Facilitation, both segmental and local, is a feature of the shortening of muscles, as a whole, or in part.

Korr has shown that muscle spindles in areas of dysfunction are hypersensitive to change in muscle length, possibly due to incorrect spinal cord setting of the gamma-neuron control of the intrafusal muscle fibres. If influences from higher centres further exaggerate this high 'gamma-gain', exacerbation of local restriction is likely. It is only when gamma-gain is restored to normal, possibly via manipulation, that normality is achieved. This scenario may be accompanied by another feature of internal discord in which, because of multiple stresses being imposed on them, musculoskeletal reporting stations (proprioceptors in soft tissues, including skin) are presenting 'garbled' and conflicting information, so making appropriate adaptive responses impossible (Korr 1975).

An example is a situation in which high-gain spindles would be reporting greater than real muscle lengths, and this information was simultaneously being contradicted by reports from joint receptors. The CNS responses to mixed signals would be inappropriate and could lead to increased dysfunction, spasm, etc. This set of events forms the basis of functional and 'strain/counterstrain' methods of soft tissue normalisation (Jones 1981).

Fibromyalgia and trigger points

Is the result of trigger point activity known as myofascial pain syndrome (MPS) the same as fibromyalgia syndrome (FMS)?

According to a leading researcher into this realm, P. Baldry (1993), the two conditions are similar or identical in that both fibromyalgia and myofascial pain syndrome:

- Are affected by cold weather
- May involve increased sympathetic nerve activity and may involve conditions such as Raynaud's phenomenon
- Have tension headaches and paraesthesia as major associated symptoms
- Are unaffected by anti-inflammatory pain-killing medication whether of the cortisone type or standard formulations.

However, fibromyalgia and myofascial pain syndrome are different in that:

- MPS affects males and females equally, fibromyalgia mainly females
- MPS is usually local to an area such as the neck and shoulders, or low back and legs, although it can affect a number of parts of the body at the same time; fibromyalgia is a generalised problem, often involving all four 'corners' of the body at the same time
- Muscles which contain areas which feel 'like a tight rubber band' are found in around 30%

of people with MPS but more than 60% of people with FMS
- People with FMS have poorer muscle endurance (they get tired faster) than do people with MPS
- MPS can sometimes be bad enough to cause disturbed sleep; in fibromyalgia the sleep disturbance has a more causative role, and is a pronounced feature of the condition
- MPS produces no morning stiffness whereas fibromyalgia does
- There is not usually fatigue associated with MPS while it is common in fibromyalgia
- MPS can sometimes lead to depression (reactive) and anxiety whereas in a small percentage of fibromyalgia cases (some leading researchers believe) these conditions can be the trigger for the start of the condition
- Conditions such as irritable bowel syndrome, dysmenorrhoea and a feeling of swollen joints are noted in fibromyalgia but seldom in MPS
- Low dosage tricyclic antidepressant drugs are helpful in dealing with the sleep problems, and many of the symptoms, of fibromyalgia, but not of MPS
- Exercise programmes (cardiovascular fitness) can help some fibromyalgia patients, according to experts, but this is not a useful approach in MPS
- The outlook for people with MPS is excellent, since the trigger points usually respond quickly to manipulative (stretching in particular) techniques or acupuncture, whereas the outlook for fibromyalgia is less positive, with a lengthy treatment and recovery phase being the norm.

Summary (Block 1993, Goldenberg 1993, Rothschild 1991)

Trigger points are certainly part – in some cases the major part – of the pain suffered by people with muscle pain in general, as well as fibromyalgia, and when they are, MET offers a useful means of treatment, since a trigger point will reactivate if the muscle in which it lies cannot easily reach its normal resting length (Fig. 2.17).

Summary of trigger point characteristics

- Janet Travell defines trigger points as 'hyperirritable foci lying within taut bands of muscle which are painful on compression and which refer pain or other symptoms at a distant site'.
- Embryonic trigger points will develop as satellites of existing triggers in the target area, and in time these will produce their own satellites.
- According to Professor Melzack, nearly 80% of trigger points are in exactly the same positions as known acupuncture points, as used in traditional Chinese medicine.
- Painful points which do not refer symptoms to a distant site are simply latent triggers requiring additional stress to create greater facilitation and turn them into active triggers.
- The taut band in which triggers lie will twitch if a finger is run across it, and is tight but not fibrosed, since it will soften and relax if the appropriate treatment is applied – something fibrotic tissue cannot do.
- Muscles which contain trigger points will often hurt when they are contracted (i.e. when they are working).
- Trigger points are areas of increased energy consumption and lowered oxygen supply due to inadequate local circulation. They will therefore add to the drain on energy and any fatigue being experienced.
- The muscles in which trigger points lie cannot reach their normal resting length (i.e. they are held in a shortened position).
- Until muscles can reach this normal resting length without pain or effort, any treatment of the trigger points will only achieve temporary relief, since they will reactivate when re-stressed sufficiently.
- Stretching of the muscles, using either active or passive methods, is useful in treating both the shortness and the trigger point since this can reduce the contraction (taut band) as well as increasing circulation to the area.
- There are many ways of treating trigger points including acupuncture, procaine injections, direct manual ischaemic pressure, stretching, ice therapy, some of which (pressure, acupuncture)

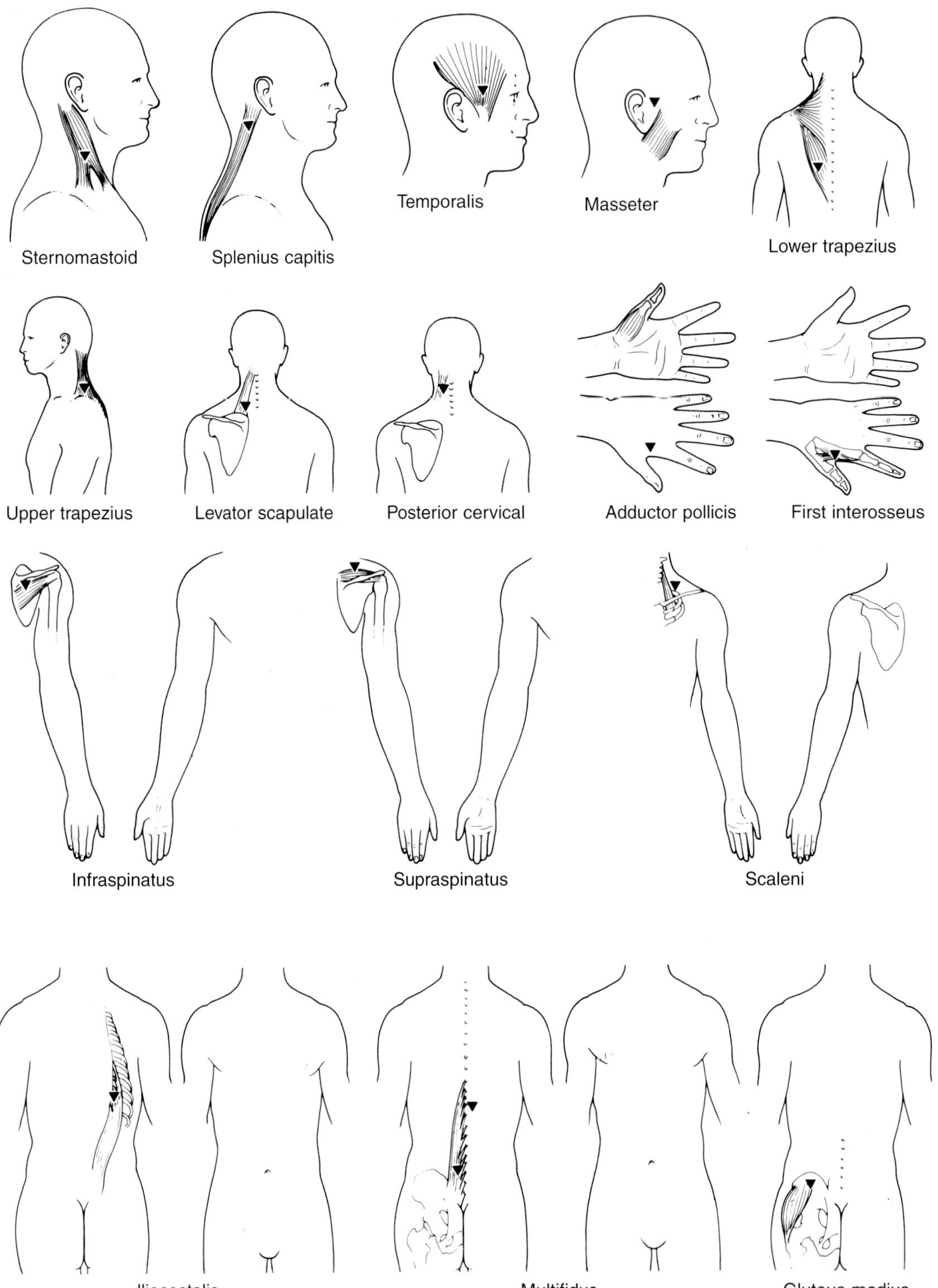

Figure 2.17 A selection of the most commonly found examples of representations of trigger point sites and their reference (or target) areas. Trigger points found in the same sites in different people will usually refer to the same target areas.

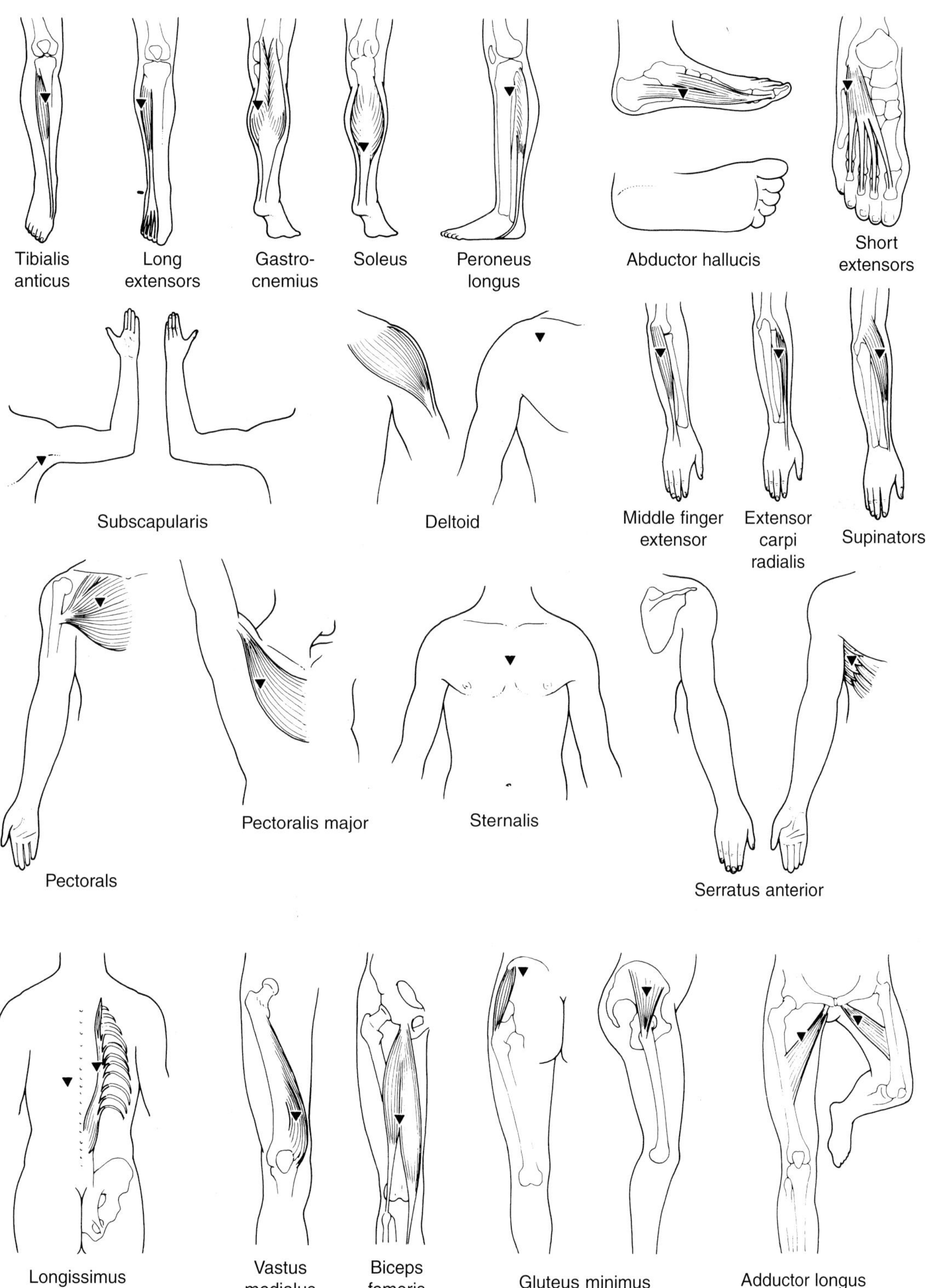
Tibialis anticus
Long extensors
Gastro-cnemius
Soleus
Peroneus longus
Abductor hallucis
Short extensors
Subscapularis
Deltoid
Middle finger extensor
Extensor carpi radialis
Supinators
Pectorals
Pectoralis major
Sternalis
Serratus anterior
Longissimus
Vastus medialus
Biceps femoris
Gluteus minimus
Adductor longus

cause the release of endorphins, which explains one of the ways in which pain is reduced – another involves the substitution of one sensation (pressure, needle) for another in which pain messages are partially or totally blocked from reaching or being registered by the brain.

- Other treatment methods (stretching for example) alter the dynamics of the circulatory imbalance affecting trigger points and appear to deactivate them.
- The target area to which a trigger refers pain will be the same in everyone if the trigger point is in the same position – but this distribution of pain does not relate directly to neural pathways or to acupuncture meridian pathways.
- The way in which a trigger point relays pain to a distant site is thought to involve one of a variety of neurological mechanisms, and probably involves the brain 'mislocating' pain messages which it receives via several different pathways.
- The sites of trigger points lie in parts of muscles (postural or phasic) most prone to mechanical stress, producing circulatory inadequacy and lack of oxygen – among other changes.
- Trigger points become self-perpetuating (a cycle of pain–increased tone–pain) and will never go away unless adequately treated.

Integrated neuromuscular inhibition technique (INIT)

The author (Chaitow 1994) has described an integrated sequence in which, after location of an active (referring symptoms) trigger point, this receives ischaemic compression, followed by positional release (osteopathic functional or strain/counterstrain methods), followed (in the same position of ease) by the imposition by the patient of an isometric contraction which is either stretched subsequently (postfacilitation stretch) or simultaneously (isolytic stretch). This combination of methods effectively deactivates trigger points (see Ch. 7).

Efficient stretching and releasing of whatever soft tissues are short and tight requires an approach which incorporates choices from the variety of different uses of MET as described above. In the following chapters presentation will be made of sequences of assessment and MET treatment methods for the major postural muscles as identified by the work of Lewit, Janda and others, as well as other applications of variations on the theme of MET.

REFERENCES

Bailey M, Dick L 1992 Nociceptive considerations in treating with counterstrain. Journal of the American Osteopathic Association 92: 334–341

Baldry P E 1993 Acupuncture trigger points and musculoskeletal pain. Churchill Livingstone, London

Barlow W 1959 Anxiety and muscle tension pain. British Journal of Clinical Practice 13(5): 339–350

Basmajian J 1978 Muscles alive. Williams and Wilkins, Baltimore

Beal M 1983 Palpatory testing of somatic dysfunction in patients with cardiovascular disease. Journal of the American Osteopathic Association 82: 822–831

Beighton P et al 1983 Hypermobility of joints. Springer-Verlag, Berlin

Bennet C 1952 Physics. Barnes and Noble, New York

Bergmark A 1989 Stability of the lumbar spine: a study in mechanical engineering. Acta Orthopaedica Scandinavica 230(suppl): 20–24

Block S 1993 Fibromyalgia and the rheumatisms. Controversies in Clinical Rheumatology 19(1): 61–78

Bogduk N, Twomey L 1991 Clinical anatomy of the lumbar spine, 2nd edn. Churchill Livingstone, Edinburgh

Brookes D 1984 Cranial osteopathy. Thorsons, London

Buller A 1960 Interactions between motor neurons and muscles. Journal of Physiology (London) 150: 417–439

Cantu R, Grodin A 1992 Myofascial manipulation. Aspen Publications, Maryland

Cathie A 1974 Selected writings. Academy of Applied Osteopathy Yearbook 1974, pp 15–126

Chaitow L 1991a Palpatory literacy. Thorsons/Harper Collins, London

Chaitow L 1991b Soft tissue manipulation. Healing Arts Press, Rochester

Chaitow L 1994 INIT in treatment of pain and trigger points – an introduction. British Journal of Osteopathy 13: 17–21

Cisler T 1994 Whiplash as a total body injury. Journal of the American Osteopathic Association 94(2): 145–148

Cyriax J 1962 Textbook of orthopaedic medicine. Cassell, London

Dahl J B, Erichsen C J, Fuglsang-Frederiksen A, Kehlet H 1992 Pain sensation and nociceptive reflex excitability in surgical patients and human volunteers. British Journal of Anaesthesia 69: 117–121

DiGiovanna E 1991 An osteopathic approach to diagnosis and treatment. Lippincott, Philadelphia
Evjenth O, Hamberg J 1984 Muscle stretching in manual therapy. Alfta Rehab, Sweden
Fahrni H 1966 Backache relieved. Thomas, Springfield
Garland W 1994 Presentation to Respiratory Function Congress, Paris, 1994
Goldenberg D 1993 Fibromyalgia, chronic fatigue syndrome and myofascial pain syndrome. Current Opinions in Rheumatology 5: 199–208
Goldthwaite J 1945 Essentials of body mechanics. Lippincott, Philadelphia
Greenman P 1989 Principles of manual medicine. Williams and Wilkins, Baltimore
Grieve G 1986 Modern manual therapy. Churchill Livingstone, London
Gunn C, Milbrandt W 1978 Early and subtle signs in low back sprain. Spine 3: 267–281
Gutstein R 1955 A review of myodysneuria (fibrositis). American Practitioner and Digest of Treatments 6(4): 570–577
Guyton A 1987 Basic neuroscience, anatomy and physiology. W B Saunders, Philadelphia
Hoffer J, Andreasson C 1981 Inefficient muscular stabilization of the lumbar spine associated with low back pain. Spine 21: 2640–2650
Hubbard D R, Berkoff G M 1993 Myofascial trigger points show spontaneous needle EMG activity. Spine 18: 1803–1807
Isaacson J 1980 Living anatomy – an anatomic basis for osteopathic theory. Journal of the American Osteopathic Association 79(12): 752–759
Janda V 1960 Postural and phasic muscles in the pathogenesis of low back pain. In: Proceedings XI Congress Rehabilitation International, Dublin
Janda V 1978 Muscles – central nervous motor regulation and back problems. In: Korr I (ed) Neurobiological mechanisms in manipulative therapy. Plenum Press, New York
Janda V 1983 Muscle function testing. Butterworths, London
Janda V 1984 Low back pain – trends, controversies. Presentation, Turku, Finland, 3–4 September 1984
Janda V 1985 Pain in the locomotor system. In: Glasgow E (ed) Aspects of manipulative therapy. Churchill Livingstone, London
Janda V 1986a Muscle weakness and inhibition in back pain syndromes. In: Grieve G (ed) Modern manual therapy of the vertebral column. Churchill Livingstone, Edinburgh
Janda V 1986b Some aspects of extracranial causes of facial pain. Journal of Prosthetic Dentistry 56(4): 484–487
Janda V 1988 In: Grant R (ed) Physical therapy of the cervical and thoracic spine. Churchill Livingstone, New York
Janda V 1989 Differential diagnosis of muscle tone in respect of inhibitory techniques. Presentation, Physical Medicine Research Foundation, 21 September 1989
Janda V 1991 Muscle spasm – a proposed procedure for differential diagnosis. Manual Medicine 1001: 6136–6139
Johansson H 1991 Pathophysiological mechanisms involved in genesis and spread of muscular tension. A hypothesis. Medical Hypotheses 35: 196
Jones L 1964 Spontaneous release by positioning. The DO 4: 109–116
Jones L 1981 Strain and counterstrain. American Academy of Osteopathy, Newark
Jones L 1982 Strain and counterstrain. Academy of Applied Osteopathy, Boulder
Jull G 1994 Active stabilisation of the trunk. Course notes, Edinburgh
Jull G, Janda V 1987 Muscles and motor control in low back pain: assessment and management. In: Twomey L (ed) Physical therapy of the low back. Churchill Livingstone, New York
Kendall F P, McCreary E K, Provance P G 1993 Muscles: testing and function, 4th edn. Williams and Wilkins, Baltimore
Knott M, Voss D 1968 Proprioceptive neuromuscular facilitation. Hoeber, New York
Komendatov G 1945 Proprioceptivnije reflexi glaza i golovy u krolikov. Fiziologiceskij Zurnal 31: 62
Korr I 1947 The neural basis of the osteopathic lesion. Journal of the American Osteopathic Association 48: 191–198
Korr I 1948 The emerging concept of the osteopathic lesion. Journal of the American Osteopathic Association 48: 127–138
Korr I 1975 Proprioceptors and somatic dysfunction. Journal of the American Osteopathic Association 74: 638–650
Korr I 1976 Spinal cord as organiser of the disease process. Academy of Applied Osteopathy Yearbook 1976, Newark, Ohio
Korr I 1978 Sustained sympatheticotonia as a factor in disease. In: Korr I (ed) The neurobiological mechanisms in manipulative therapy. Plenum Press, New York
Korr I 1980 Neurobiological mechanisms in manipulation. Plenum Press, New York
Korr I 1986 Somatic dysfunction, osteopathic manipulative treatment, and the nervous system. Journal of the American Osteopathic Association 86(2): 109–114
Korr I, Wilkinson P, Chornock F 1967 Axonal delivery of neuroplasmic components to muscle cells. Science 155: 342–354
Kraus H 1970 Clinical treatment of back and neck pain. McGraw Hill, New York
Kuchera M et al 1990 Athletic functional demand and posture. Journal of the American Osteopathic Association 90(9): 843–844
Latey P 1996 Feelings, muscles and movement. Journal of Bodywork and Movement Therapies 1(1): 44–52
Lewit K 1974 Functional pathology of the motor system. Proceedings of the Fourth Congress of the International Federation of Manual Medicine, Prague
Lewit K 1980 Relation of faulty respiration to posture with clinical implications. Journal of the American Osteopathic Association 79(8): 525–529
Lewit K 1996 Role of manipulation in spinal rehabilitation. In: Liebenson C (ed) Rehabilitation of the spine. Williams and Wilkins, Baltimore
Lewit K 1999 Manipulation in rehabilitation of the motor system. Butterworth, London
Lewit K, Simons D 1984 Myofascial pain – relief by post-isometric relaxation. Archives of Physical Medicine and Rehabilitation 65: 462–466
Liebenson C 1990a Muscular relaxation techniques. Journal of Manipulative and Physiological Therapeutics 12(6): 446–454
Liebenson C 1990b Active muscular relaxation techniques (part 2). Journal of Manipulative and Physiological Therapeutics 13(1): 2–6

Liebenson C 1996 Rehabilitation of the spine. Williams and Wilkins, Baltimore

Lin J P et al 1994 Physiological maturation of muscles in childhood. Lancet (June): 1386–1389

McArdle W, Katch F, Katch V 1991 Exercise physiology, energy, nutrition and human performance, 3rd edn. Lea Febiger, Philadelphia

McConnell C 1902 Yearbook of the Osteopathic Institute of Applied Technique 1902, pp 75–78

McGill S M, Juker, D, Kropf P 1996 Quantitative intramuscular myoelectric activity of quadratus lumborum during a wide variety of tasks. Clinical Biomechanics 11: 170–172

Mathews P 1981 Muscle spindles. In: Brooks V (ed) Handbook of physiology. American Physiological Society, Bethseda

Melzack R, Wall P 1988 The challenge of pain. Penguin, New York

Mennell J 1952 The science and art of manipulation. Churchill Livingstone, London

Mense S 1993 Nociception from skeletal muscle in relation to clinical muscle pain. Pain 54: 241–290

Myers T 1997 The anatomy trains. Journal of Bodywork and Movement Therapies 1(2): 91–191

Myers T 1998 A structural approach. Journal of Bodywork and Movement Therapies 2(1): 14–20

Myers T 2001 Anatomy trains: myofascial meridians for manual and movement therapists. Churchill Livingstone, Edinburgh

Neuberger A et al 1953 Metabolism of collagen. Biochemistry Journal 53: 47–52

Norris C M 1995a Spinal stabilisation. 1. Active lumbar stabilisation – concepts. Physiotherapy 81(2): 61–64

Norris C M 1995b, Spinal stabilisation. 2. Limiting factors to end-range motion in the lumbar spine. Physiotherapy 81(2): 64–72

Norris C M 1995c Spinal stabilisation. 3. Stabilisation mechanisms of the lumbar spine. Physiotherapy 81(2): 72–79

Norris C M 1995d Spinal stabilisation. 4. Muscle imbalance and the low back. Physiotherapy 81(3): 127–138

Norris C M 1995e Spinal stabilisation. 5. An exercise program to enhance lumbar stabilisation. Physiotherapy 81(3): 138–146

Norris C M 1998 Sports injuries, diagnosis and management, 2nd edn. Butterworths, London

Norris C M 1999 Functional load abdominal training. Journal of Bodywork and Movement Therapies 3(3): 150–158

Norris C 2000 The muscle designation debate. Journal of Bodywork and Movement Therapies 4 (4):225–241

Page L 1952 Academy of Applied Osteopathy Yearbook

Patterson M 1976 Model mechanism for spinal segmental facilitation. Academy of Applied Osteopathy Yearbook 1976, Newark, Ohio

Pauling L 1976 The common cold and 'flu. Freeman, London

Prior T 1999 Biomechanical foot function: a podiatric perspective (part 2). Journal of Bodywork and Movement Therapies 3(3): 169–184

Richardson C, Jull G, Toppenburg R, Comerford C 1992 Techniques for active lumbar stabilisation for spinal protection. Australian Journal of Physiotherapy 38(2): 106–112

Richardson C, Jull G, Hodges P, Hides J 1999 Therapeutic exercise for spinal segmental stabilisation in low back pain. Churchill Livingstone, Edinburgh

Rolf I 1962 Structural dynamics. British Academy of Osteopathy Yearbook 1962, Maidstone

Rolf I 1977 Rolfing – the integration of human structures. Harper and Row, New York

Rothschild B 1991 Fibromyalgia – an explanation. Comprehensive Therapy 17(6): 9–14

Sandman K 1984 Psychophysiological factors in myofascial pain. Journal of Manipulative and Physiological Therapeutics 7(4): 237–242

Scariati P 1991 Myofascial release concepts. In: DiGiovanna E (ed) An osteopathic approach to diagnosis and treatment. Lippincott, London

Schiable H G, Grubb B D 1993 Afferent and spinal mechanisms of joint pain. Pain 155: 5–54

Schmid H 1984 Muscular imbalances in skiers. Manual Medicine (2): 23–26

Selye H 1976 The stress of life. McGraw-Hill, New York

Simons D 1994 Ch 28 In: Vecchiet L, Albe-Fessard D, Lindblom U, Giamberardino M (eds) New trends in referred pain and hyperalgesia, pain research and clinical management, vol 7. Elsevier Science Publishers, Amsterdam

Simons D, Travell J 1983 The trigger point manual. Williams and Wilkins, Baltimore

Sommer H 1985 Patellar chodropathy and apicitis – muscle imbalances of the lower extremity. Butterworths, London

Stedman 1998 Stedman's electronic medical dictionary. Version 4. Williams and Wilkins, Baltimore

Travell J, Simons D 1983 Myofascial pain and dysfunction – the trigger point manual (vol 1). Williams and Wilkins, Baltimore

Travell J, Simons D 1992 The trigger point manual (vol 2). Williams and Wilkins, Baltimore

Triano J, Schultz A B 1987 Correlation of objective measure of trunk motion and muscle function with low-back disability ratings. Spine 12: 561

Van Buskirk R 1990 Nociceptive reflexes and the somatic dysfunction. Journal of the American Osteopathic Association 90(9): 792–809

van Wingerden J-P 1997 The role of the hamstrings in pelvic and spinal function. In: Vleeming A, Mooney V, Dorman T, Snijders C, Stoekart R (eds) Movement, stability and low back pain. Churchill Livingstone, New York

Vleeming A, Mooney A, Dorman T, Snijders C, Stoekart R 1989 Load application to the sacrotuberous ligament: influences on sacroiliac joint mechanics. Clinical Biomechanics 4: 204–209

Waddell G 1998 The back pain revolution. Churchill Livingstone, Edinburgh

Walsh E G 1992 Muscles, masses and motion: the physiology of normality, hypotonicity, spasticity, and rigidity. MacKeith Press, Blackwell Scientific Publications, Oxford

Walther D 1988 Applied kinesiology. SDC Systems, Pueblo

Ward R 1997 Foundations of osteopathic medicine. Williams and Wilkins, Baltimore

World Health Organization 1981 Third Report on Rehabilitation. WHO, Geneva

Zink G, Lawson W 1979 Osteopathic structural examination and functional interpretation of the soma. Osteopathic Annals 7(12): 433–440

CHAPTER CONTENTS

3

How to use MET

Chapter 1 described a number of variations on the theme of MET (and stretching) as used by clinicians such as Karel Lewit, Vladimir Janda, Craig Liebenson, Aaron Mattes, Edward Stiles, Robert McAtee and others. Chapter 4 will describe a sequence for the evaluation/assessment of the major postural (or *mobiliser*) muscles of the body – for relative shortness – along with details of suggested MET approaches for normalising, stretching and relaxing those muscles. Additionally there will be examples of the use of pulsed MET (repetitive mini-contractions based on the work of T. J. Ruddy (1962)) in facilitating proprioceptive re-education of weak and shortened structures.

In this chapter, suggestions are given as to how to begin to learn the application of MET methods, both for muscles and for joints (specific muscle by muscle and particular joint descriptions of MET treatment can be found in later chapters).

A primary requirement for the practitioner is the identification by means of assessment of a need for the use of MET. Is there an identifiable restriction which requires releasing, modifying? This brings us to the need for sound palpation skills.[1]

[1] In this text the practitioner is presented in descriptions of technique and exercises as being male (because the author is), whereas the patient/client is described variously as male or female. It is hoped that this gender bias regarding the practitioner does not offend the reader, since no offence is intended.

PALPATION SKILLS

Ease and bind

The concept and reality of tissues providing the palpating hands or fingers with a sense of their relative tension or 'bind', as opposed to their state of relaxation or 'ease', is one which the beginner needs to grasp and the advanced practitioner probably takes for granted. There can never be enough focus on these two characteristics, which allow the tissues to speak as to their current degree of comfort or distress. In the previous chapter (p. 36) the 'loose–tight' concept was presented. Ward (1997) states that 'Tightness suggests tethering, while looseness suggests joint and/or soft tissue laxity, with or without neural inhibition.'

Osteopathic pioneer H. V. Hoover (1969) describes ease as a state of equilibrium, or 'neutral', which the practitioner senses by having at least one completely passive 'listening' contact (either the whole hand or a single of several fingers or thumb) in touch with the tissues being assessed. Bind is, of course, the opposite of ease and can most easily be noted by lightly palpating the tissues surrounding, or associated with, a joint as this is taken towards the end of its range of movement – its resistance barrier (Box 3.1).

Greenman (1996) states:

> The examiner must be able to identify and characterize normal and abnormal range of movement and normal and abnormal barrier to movement to make a diagnosis. Most joints have motion in multiple planes, but for descriptive purposes we describe barriers to movement within one plane of motion for one joint. The total range of motion from one extreme to the other is limited by the anatomical integrity of the joint and its supporting ligaments, muscles and fascia … somewhere within the total range of movement is found a midline neutral point.

This is the point of maximum ease which the exercise described below attempts to identify.

In order to 'read' hypertonicity (bind) and the opposite, a relaxed (ease) state, palpation skills need to be refined. As a first step, Goodridge suggests the following test, which examines medial hamstring and short adductor status. This exercise offers the opportunity for becoming comfortable with the reality of ease and bind in a practical manner (Goodridge 1981).[2]

Box 3.1 Barriers

A variety of different terms can be used to describe what is perceived when a restriction barrier is reached or engaged. These terms relate to a large degree to the type of tissue providing the restriction, and to the nature of the restriction. For example:

- Normal end of range for soft tissues is felt as a progressive build-up of tension, leading to a gradually reached barrier, as all slack is removed.
- If a fluid restriction (oedema, congestion, swelling) causes reduction in range of motion, the end-feel will have a 'boggy', yielding yet spongy feel.
- If muscle physiology has changed (hypertonicity, spasm, contracture), the end-feel will produce a tight, tugging sensation.
- If fibrotic tissue is responsible for a reduction in range, end-feel will be rapid and harsh but with a slight elasticity remaining.
- In hypermobile individuals, or structures, the end-feel will be loose and the range greater than normal.
- If bony tissue is responsible for reduction in range (arthritis for example), end-feel will be sudden and hard without any elasticity remaining.
- Pain may also produce a restriction in range, and the end-feel resulting from sudden pain will be rapid and widespread, as surrounding tissues protect against further movement.

The barrier used in MET treatment is a 'first sign of resistance' barrier, in which the very first indication of the onset of 'bind' is noted. This is the place at which further movement would produce stretching of *some* fibres of the muscle(s) involved. This is where MET isometric contractions, whether these involve the agonists or antagonists, commence in acute (and joint) problems, and short of which contractions commence in chronic problems.

Test for palpation of ease and bind during assessment of adductors of the thigh

(Fig. 3.1A and 3.1B; see also Fig. 1.3)

Goodridge (1981) presents a basic method for beginning to become familiar with MET. Before

[2] This test and its interpretation and suggested treatment, using MET (should shortness be noted), will be fully explained in Chapter 4, but in this setting it is being used as an exercise for the purposes of the practitioner becoming familiar with the sense of 'ease and bind', and not for actually testing the muscles involved for dysfunction.

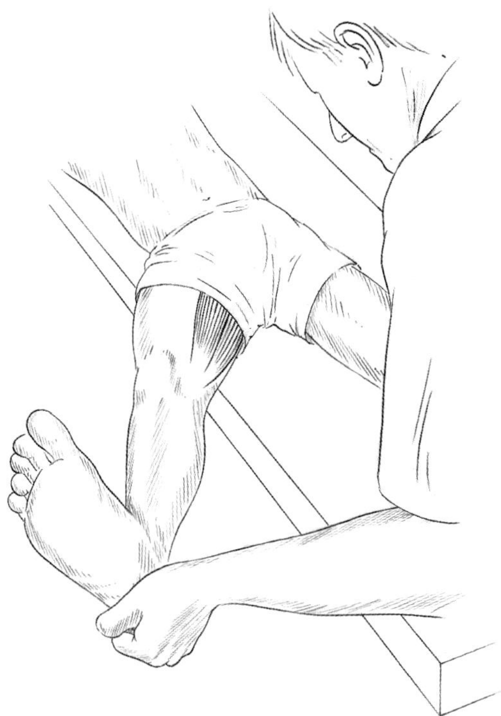

Figure 3.1A Assessment of 'bind'/restriction barrier with the first sign of resistance in the adductors (medial hamstrings) of the right leg. In this example, the practitioner's perception of the transition point, where easy movement alters to demand some degree of effort, is regarded as the barrier.

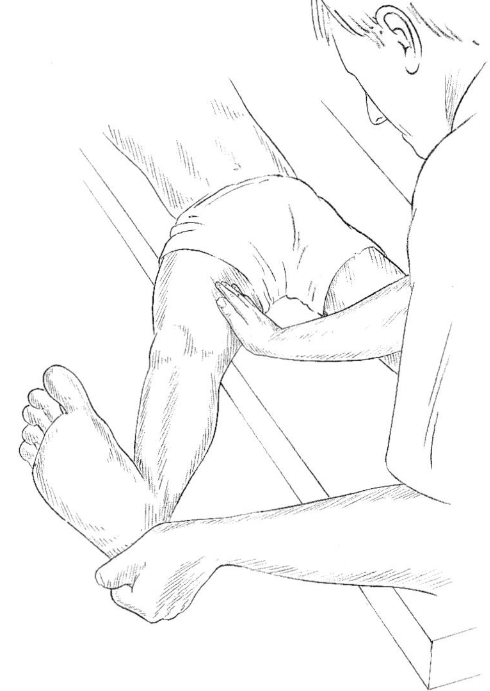

Figure 3.1B Assessment of 'bind'/restriction barrier with the first sign of resistance in the adductors (medial hamstrings) of the right leg. In this example, the barrier is identified when the palpating hand notes a sense of bind in tissues which were relaxed (at ease) up to that point.

starting this exercise, ensure that the patient/model lies supine, so that the non-tested leg is abducted slightly, heel over end of table. The leg to be tested should be close to the edge of the table. (Ensure that the tested leg is in the anatomically correct position, knee in full extension and with no external rotation of the leg, which would negate the test.)

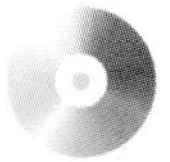

Goodridge's ease/bind palpation exercise, part 1 (Goodridge 1981)

1. The practitioner slowly eases the straight leg into abduction, 'After grasping the supine patient's foot and ankle, in order to abduct the lower limb, the practitioner closes his eyes during the abduction, and feels, in his own body, from his hand through his forearm, into his upper arm, the beginning of a sense of resistance.'

2. 'He stops when he feels it, opens his eyes, and notes how many degrees in an arc the patient's limb has travelled.'

What Goodridge (1981) is trying to establish is that the practitioner senses the *very beginning, the first sign* of the end of the range of free movement, where easy, 'free-floating' motion ceases, and effort on the part of the practitioner moving the part begins. This barrier is not a pathological one, but represents the first sign of resistance, the place at which tissues require some degree of passive effort to move them. This is also the place at which the first signs of bind should be palpated.

It is suggested that the process described by Goodridge be attempted several (indeed many) times, so that the practitioner gets a sense of where resistance begins.

The exercise is then performed again as described below.

Goodridge's ease/bind palpation exercise, part 2

The patient lies close to the edge of the table on the side of the leg being tested. The practitioner stands between the patient's partially abducted leg and the table, facing the head of the table, so that all control of the tested leg is achieved by using the lateral (non table-side) hand which holds and supports the leg at the ankle. The other (table-side) hand rests passively on the inner thigh, palpating the muscles which are being tested (adductors and medial hamstrings).

This palpating hand (often called a 'listening' hand in osteopathy) must be in touch with the skin, moulded to the contours of the tissues being assessed, but should exert no pressure, and should be completely relaxed.

As in part 1 of this exercise, abduction of the tested leg is introduced by the non table-side hand/arm, until the first sign of resistance is noted by the hand which is providing the motive force (i.e. the one holding the leg). As this point of resistance is approached, a tightening of the tissues ('a sense of bind') in the mid-inner thigh should be noted under the palpating hand.

If this sensation is not clear, then the leg should be taken back towards the table, and slowly abducted again, but this time it should be taken past the point where easy movement is lost, and effort begins, and towards its end of range. Here 'bind' will certainly be sensed.

As the leg is once more taken back towards the table, a softening, a relaxation, an 'ease', will be noted in these same tissues.

The same sequence should then be performed with the other leg, so that the practitioner becomes increasingly familiar with the sense of these two extremes (ease and bind).

It is important to try to note the very moment at which the transition from ease to bind (and bind to ease) occurs, not to an extreme degree, but where it begins, whether movement is from ease to bind or vice versa.

Normal excursion of the straight leg into abduction is around 45°, and by testing both legs in the manner described it is possible to evaluate whether they are both tight and short, or whether one is and the other is not. Even if both are tight and short, one may be more restricted than the other. This is the one to treat first using MET.

MET exercise

It is suggested that before using MET clinically you should perform palpation exercises relating to ease and bind (as described above) on many other muscles as they are being both actively and passively moved, until skill in reading this change in tone has been acquired. Once you feel that the beginnings of bind in the adductors can be ascertained by palpation, and having decided which leg to treat, you can attempt simple use of MET.

The point at which the very first sign of bind was noted (or where the hand carrying the leg felt the first sign that effort was required during abduction) is the resistance barrier (see also Box 3.1, above). In subsequent chapters this barrier will be referred to over and over again. It is the place where an MET isometric contraction can begin in some applications of the methods (notably PIR – see below). It is also the place which is mentally/visually marked if the practitioner wishes to start a contraction from an easier mid-range position, but which it is necessary to note as the place at which resistance was a feature before the isometric contraction.

Identification and appropriate use of the first sign of the barrier of resistance (i.e. where bind is first noted) is a fundamental and absolutely critical part of the successful use of MET, along with other key features which include the degree of effort used by the patient, and whether subsequently (after the contraction) the tissues are taken to a new barrier, or through the old one to introduce passive stretching.

The following exercises in MET variations include the key features emphasised by some of the leading clinicians who have contributed to MET modern methodology:

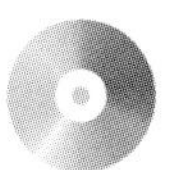

Basic exercise in MET using postisometric relaxation (PIR) in acute context

- The patient's limb is positioned where resistance is first perceived during abduction, and at this point the practitioner employs MET to lessen the sense of resistance and increase the range of movement.
- The patient/model is asked to use no more than 20% of available strength to try to take the leg gently back towards the table (i.e. to adduct the leg) against firm, unyielding resistance offered by the practitioner.
- In this example the patient is trying to take the limb away from the barrier, while the practitioner holds the limb firmly at the barrier.
- The patient/model should be contracting the agonists, the muscles which require release (and which, once released, would allow greater and less restricted abduction).
- As the patient/model induces and holds the contraction she is commonly asked to hold an inhaled breath.
- The isometric contraction should be introduced slowly, and resisted without any jerking, wobbling, or bouncing.
- Maintaining the resistance to the contraction should produce no strain in the practitioner.
- The contraction should be held for between 7 and 10 seconds – the time it is thought necessary for the 'load' on the Golgi tendon organs to become active and to neurologically influence the intrafusal fibres of the muscle spindles, which inhibits muscle tone, so providing the opportunity for the area (muscle, joint) to be taken to a new resting length/resistance barrier with far less effort, or to stretch it through the barrier of resistance, if this is appropriate (see below) (Scariati 1991).
- An instruction is given to the patient, 'Now let your breath go, and release your effort, slowly and completely', while the practitioner maintains the limb at the same resistance barrier.
- The patient/model is asked to breathe in and out once more, and to completely relax, and as she exhales the limb is gently guided to the new resistance barrier, where bind is once more sensed (the range should almost always be able to be increased by a significant degree).
- After use of the isometric contraction (which induces postisometric relaxation (PIR) in the previously contracted tissues) there exists a latency period of anything from 15 to 30 seconds during which the muscle can be taken to its new resting length, or stretched more easily than would have been the case before the contraction (Guissard et al 1988).

The exercise can be repeated, precisely as described above, to see whether even more release is possible, working from the new resistance barrier to whatever new range is gained following the each successive contraction. This approach represents an example of Lewit's PIR method, as described in Chapter 1 (Lewit 1999), and is ideal for releasing tone, for relaxing spasm, particularly in acute conditions.

Basic exercise in MET using postisometric relaxation (PIR) in chronic context

Where fibrosis is a feature, or for chronic conditions, a more vigorous approach can be used in order to actually stretch the muscle(s) rather than simply taking them to a new barrier. This would be closer to Janda's (1993) approach ('postfacilitation stretch' as described in Ch. 1, p. 10), which calls for the starting of the contraction from a more 'slack', mid-range position, rather than at the actual barrier.

- Janda suggests stretching the tissues immediately following cessation of the contraction, and holding the stretch for at least 10 seconds, before allowing a rest period of up to half a minute. He also suggests the procedure be repeated if necessary.

Modification of Janda's approach

- The recommendation for use of MET for chronic fibrotic tissues, based on the author's experience, is that following a contraction of between 10 and 12 seconds, commencing from a mid-range position rather than at a barrier, using more than 20% but not more than 50% of the patient's available strength (Janda asks for full strength), a short (2–3 seconds) rest period is allowed for complete postisometric relaxation (PIR), before stretch is introduced which takes the tissues to a point *just beyond* the previous barrier of resistance.

• It is useful to have the patient gently assist in taking the (now) relaxed area towards and through the barrier. Patient participation in movement towards stretch activates the antagonists, and therefore reduces the danger of a stretch reflex (Mattes 1990).

• The procedure of contraction, relaxation, followed by patient assisted stretch is repeated (with or without a rest period between contractions) until no more gain in length of restricted tissues is being achieved.

The differences between Janda's and Lewit's use of PIR

- Lewit starts at, and Janda short of, the restriction barrier
- Janda utilises a longer and stronger contraction
- Janda takes the tissues beyond, rather than just to, the new barrier of resistance (with or without patient assistance).

Janda's approach is undoubtedly successful but carries with it a possibility of very mildly traumatising the tissues (albeit that this is an approach only recommended for chronic and not acute situations). The stronger contraction which he asks for, and the rapid introduction of stretching following the contraction, are the areas which it is suggested should be modified (as described above) with little loss of successful outcome, and with a greater degree of safety.

Reciprocal inhibition (RI)

An alternative physiological mechanism, reciprocal inhibition (RI), produces a very similar latency ('refractory') period to that produced by PIR.

RI is advocated for acute problems, especially where the muscle(s) requiring release are traumatised or painful, and cannot easily or safely be used in sustained contractions such as those described in the notes on PIR above.

To use RI, the tissues requiring treatment should be placed just short of their resistance barrier (as identified by palpation) (Liebenson 1989). This requirement relates to two factors:

1. The greater ease of initiating a contraction from a mid-range position as opposed to the relative difficulty of doing so when at an end of range position
2. Reduced risk of inducing cramp from a mid-range position, particularly in lower extremity structures such as the hamstrings, and especially if longer or stronger contractions than the norm (20% strength, 10–12 seconds) are being used.

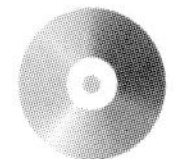

Basic exercise in MET using reciprocal inhibition (RI) in acute and chronic contexts

The example involves abduction of the limb, as outlined above:

• The first sense of restriction/bind is evaluated as the limb is abducted, at which point the limb is returned a fraction towards a mid-range position (by a few degrees only).

• From this position the patient/model is asked to attempt to *abduct* the leg themselves, using no more than 20% of strength, taking it towards the restriction barrier, while the practitioner resists this effort.

• Following the end of the contraction (which may be accompanied by breath holding as described earlier), the patient/model is asked to 'release and relax', followed by a further exhaled breath and further relaxation, at which time the limb is guided by the practitioner *to* (acute problem) or *through* (chronic problem) the new barrier *with* (chronic) or *without* (acute) the patient's/model's assistance.

MET – SOME COMMON ERRORS AND CONTRAINDICATIONS

Greenman (1989) summarises several of the important component elements of MET as follows:

- There is a patient-active muscle contraction
  - from a controlled position
  - in a specific direction
  - met by practitioner applied distinct counterforce
  - involving a controlled intensity of contraction.

The common errors which he notes, and which are as important to memorise as are the directions for use of MET, include those listed below:

Patient errors during MET

(Usually based on inadequate instruction from the practitioner!)

1. Contraction is too hard (remedy: give specific guidelines, e.g. 'use only 20% of strength', or whatever is most appropriate).
2. Contraction is in the wrong direction (remedy: give simple but accurate instructions).
3. Contraction is not sustained for long enough (remedy: instruct the patient/model to hold the contraction until told to ease off, and give an idea ahead of time as to how long this will be).
4. The individual does not relax completely after the contraction (remedy: have them release and relax and then inhale and exhale once or twice, with the suggestion 'now relax completely').

To this list the author would add:

5. Starting and/or finishing the contraction too hastily. There should be a slow build-up of force and a slow letting go; this is easily achieved if a rehearsal is carried out first to educate the patient into the methodology.

Practitioner errors in application of MET

These include:

1. Inaccurate control of position of joint or muscle in relation to the resistance barrier (remedy: have a clear image of what is required and apply it).
2. Inadequate counterforce to the contraction (remedy: meet and match the force in an isometric contraction; allow movement in an isotonic concentric contraction; and overcome the contraction in an isolytic manoeuvre).
3. Counterforce is applied in an inappropriate direction (remedy: ensure precise direction needed for best effect).
4. Moving to a new position too hastily after the contraction (there is usually more than 20 seconds of refractory muscle tone release during which time a new position can easily be adopted – haste is unnecessary and counterproductive).
5. Inadequate patient instruction is given (remedy: get the words right so that the patient can cooperate). Whenever force is applied by the patient in a particular direction, and when it is time to release that effort, the instruction must be to do so gradually. Any quick effort is self-defeating.
6. The coinciding of the forces at the outset (patient and practitioner) as well as at release is important. The practitioner must be careful to use enough, but not too much, effort, and to ease off at the same time as the patient.
7. The practitioner fails to maintain the stretch position for a period of time which allows connective tissue to begin to lengthen (ideally 20–30 seconds, but certainly not just a few seconds).

Contraindications and side-effects of MET

If pathology is suspected, no MET should be used until an accurate diagnosis has been established. Pathology (osteoporosis, arthritis, etc.) does not rule out the use of MET, but its presence needs to be established so that dosage of application can be modified accordingly (amount of effort used, number of repetitions, stretching introduced or not, etc.).

As to side-effects, Greenman (1989) explains:

> All muscle contractions influence surrounding fascia, connective tissue ground substance and interstitial fluids, and alter muscle physiology by reflex mechanisms. Fascial length and tone is altered by muscle contraction. Alteration in fascia influences not only its biomechanical function, but also its

biochemical and immunological functions. The patient's muscle effort requires energy and the metabolic process of muscle contraction results in carbon dioxide, lactic acid and other metabolic waste products which must be transported and metabolised. It is for this reason that the patient will frequently experience some increase in muscle soreness within the first 12 to 36 hours following MET treatment. Muscle energy procedures provide safety for the patient since the activating force is intrinsic and the dosage can be easily controlled by the patient, but it must be remembered that this comes at a price. It is easy for the inexperienced practitioner to overdo these procedures and in essence to overdose the patient.

DiGiovanna (1991) states that side-effects are minimal with MET:

MET is quite safe. Occasionally some muscle stiffness and soreness after treatment. If the area being treated is not localised well or if too much contractive force is used pain may be increased. Sometimes the patient is in too much pain to contract a muscle or may be unable to cooperate with instructions or positioning. In such instances MET may be difficult to apply.

If beginners to MET:

- Stay within the very simple guideline which states categorically *cause no pain when using MET*
- Stick to light (20% of strength) contractions
- Do not stretch over-enthusiastically, but only take muscles a short way past their restriction barrier when stretching
- Have the patient assist in this stretch.

No side-effects are likely apart from the soreness mentioned above, and this is a normal part of all manual methods of treatment.

While the author advocates that the above recommendations be kept as a guideline for all therapists and practitioners exploring the MET approach, not all texts advocate a completely painless use of stretching and the contrary view needs to be recorded.

Sucher (1990), for example, suggests that discomfort is inevitable with stretching techniques, especially when self-applied at home: 'There should be some discomfort, often somewhat intense locally ... however, symptoms should subside within seconds or minutes following the stretch.' Kottke (1982) says, 'Stretching should be past the point of pain, but there should be no residual pain when stretching is discontinued.'

Clearly what is noted as pain for one individual will be described as discomfort by another, making this a subjective exercise. Hopefully, sufficient emphasis has been given to the need to keep stretching associated with MET light, just past the restriction barrier, and any discomfort tolerable to the patient.

Breathing and MET

Many of the guidelines for application of isometric contraction call for patient participation over and above their 'muscle energy' activity, most notably involving the holding of a breath during the contraction/effort and the release of the breath as the new position or stretch is passively or actively adopted. Is there any valid evidence to support this apparently clinically useful element of MET methodology?

There is certainly 'common practice' evidence, for example in weight training, where the held breath is a feature of the harnessing and focusing of effort, and in yoga practice, where the released breath is the time for adoption of new positions. Fascinating as such anecdotal material might be, it is necessary to explore the literature for evidence which carries more weight, and fortunately this is available in abundance.

Cummings & Howell (1990) have looked at the influence of respiration on myofascial tension and have clearly demonstrated that there is a mechanical effect of respiration on resting myofascial tissue (using the elbow flexors as the tissue being evaluated). They also quote the work of Kisselkova & Georgiev, who reported that resting EMG activity of the biceps brachii, quadriceps femoris and gastrocnemius muscles 'cycled with respiration following bicycle ergonometer exercise, thus demonstrating that non respiratory muscles receive input from the respiratory centres' (Kisselkova & Georgiev 1976). The conclusion was that 'these studies document both a mechanically and a neurologically mediated influence on the tension produced by myofascial tissues, which gives objective verification of the clinically observed influence of respiration on the musculoskeletal system, and validation of its potential role in manipulative therapy.'

So there is an influence, but what variables does it display? Lewit helps to create subdivisions in the simplistic picture of 'breathing in enhances effort' and 'breathing out enhances movement', and a detailed reading of his book *Manipulative Therapy in Rehabilitation of the Motor System* (Lewit 1999) is highly recommended for those who wish to understand the complexities of the mechanisms involved.

Among the simpler connections which he discusses, and for which evidence is provided, are the following facts:

- The abdominal muscles are assisted in their action during exhalation, especially against resistance
- Movement into flexion of the lumbar and cervical spine is assisted by exhalation
- Movement into extension (i.e. straightening up from forward bending; bending backwards) of the lumbar and cervical spine is assisted by inhalation
- Movement into extension of the thoracic spine is assisted by exhalation (try it and see how much more easily the thoracic spine extends as you exhale than when you inhale)
- Thoracic flexion is enhanced by inhalation
- Rotation of the trunk in the seated position is enhanced by inhalation and inhibited by exhalation
- Neck traction (stretching) is easier during exhalation but lumbar traction (stretching) is eased by inhalation and retarded by exhalation.

The author suggests that breathing assistance to isometric contractions only be employed if they prove helpful to the patient, and in specific situations, for example involving the scalenes where they are directly involved in producing a contraction of the muscles.

Degree of effort with isometric contraction

Most MET contractions are light and only rarely, when large muscle groups are involved, might contractions involving up to 50% of a patient's strength be called for.

There is evidence that recruitment of phasic muscle fibres occurs when an effort much in excess of 30% of strength is used (Liebenson 1996). Since in most instances it is the postural fibres which require stretching, little advantage would be gained by inducing reduced tone in phasic fibres. To increase the recruitment of postural fibres there is more benefit in sustaining a mild contraction for a longer period rather than increasing the force of a contraction. (For more on this topic see the discussion of MVC in Ch. 1).

In the case of the scalene muscles, a held inhalation automatically produces an isometric contraction. Therefore in treating these muscles with MET a held breath would seem to be essential.

MET VARIATIONS

Strength testing – Mitchell's view

Before applying MET to an apparently short muscle, Mitchell suggests (Mitchell et al 1979) that it and its pair should be assessed for relative strength. If the muscle which requires lengthening tests as weaker than its pair, he calls for the reasons for this relative weakness to be evaluated and treated. For example an antagonist might be inhibiting it, and this factor should be dealt with so that the muscle which is due to receive MET attention is strengthened. At this time, according to Mitchell and colleagues (1979), MET as described can most suitably be used.

Goodridge (1981) concurs with this view, and states that:

> When a left–right asymmetry in range of motion exists, in the extremities that asymmetry may be due to either a hypertonic or hypotonic condition. Differentiation is made by testing for strength, comparing left and right muscle groups. If findings suggest weakness is the cause of asymmetry in range of motion, the appropriate muscle group is treated to bring it to equal strength with its opposite number before range of motion is retested to determine whether shortness in a muscle group may also contribute to the restriction.

One common reason for a muscle testing as 'weak' (compared with norms or with its pair) involves increased tone in its antagonist, which would automatically inhibit the weaker muscle. One approach at restoring relative balance might therefore involve the antagonists to any muscle which tests as weak first receiving attention – possibly using MET – to reduce excessive tone and/or to initiate stretching. Following MET treatment of those muscles found to be short and/or hypertonic, subsequent assessment may show that previously weak or hypotonic antagonists have strengthened but still require toning. This can be achieved using isotonic contractions, or Ruddy's methods (see below), or some other form of rehabilitation. Reference to strength testing will be made periodically in descriptions of MET application to particular muscles in Chapter 4 whenever this factor seems important clinically, especially in regard to its mention by Mitchell (Mitchell et al 1979).

Janda's view

Janda (1993) provides evidence of the relative lack of accuracy involved in strength testing, preferring instead an assessment of balanced or unbalanced function and relative shortness in particular structures, considered in the context of overall musculoskeletal function, as a means of deciding what needs attention. This seems to be close to the 'loose–tight' concept discussed in Chapter 2 (Ward 1997). Janda effectively dismisses the idea of using strength tests to any degree in evaluating functional imbalances (Janda 1993, Kraus 1970), when he states:

> Individual muscle strength testing is unsuitable because it is insufficiently sensitive and does not take into account evaluation of coordinated activity between different muscle groups. In addition in patients with musculoskeletal syndromes, weakness in individual muscles may be indistinct, thus rendering classical muscle testing systems unsatisfactory. This is probably one of the reasons why conflicting results have been reported in studies of patients with back pain.

Janda is also clear in his opinion that weak, short muscles will regain tone if stretched appropriately.

Mitchell and Janda and 'the weakness factor'

Mitchell's (1979) recommendation regarding strength testing prior to use of MET complicates the approach advocated by the author, which is to use indications of overactivity or stress, or, even more importantly, signs of malcoordination and imbalance, as clues to a postural (mobiliser) muscle being short. 'Functional' tests, such as those devised by Janda and described by Liebenson in Chapter 5, or objective evidence of dysfunction (using one of the many such tests described in Ch. 4) can be used to provide such evidence. Put simply:

- If a postural (mobiliser, see Ch. 2) muscle is overused, misused, abused or disused, it will modify by shortening. Evidence of overactivity, inappropriate firing sequences and/or excessive tone all suggest that a muscle is dysfunctional.
- If such a muscle falls within one of the groups described in Chapter 2 as postural or mobiliser, then it may be considered to have shortened.
- The degree of such shortening may then be assessed using palpation and basic tests as described in Chapter 4.

Additional evidence of a need to use MET induced stretching can be derived from basic palpation which indicates the presence of fibrosis and/or myofascial trigger point activity, or of inappropriate electromyographic (EMG) activity (should such technology be available).

Ideally therefore some observable and/or palpable evidence of functional imbalance will be available which can guide the therapist/practitioner as to the need for MET or other interventions in particular muscles.[3] For example, in testing for overactivity, and by implication shortness, in quadratus lumborum (QL), an attempt may be made to assess the muscle firing sequence involved in raising the leg laterally in a side-lying posture. There is a 'correct' and an 'incorrect' (or balanced and unbalanced) sequence; if the latter is noted, stress is proved and, since this is a postural muscle (or at least the lateral aspect of it is, see discussion of QL in Ch. 2), shortness can be assumed.

[3] This topic is discussed further in Chapter 5 which is devoted to Dr Liebenson's views on rehabilitation and which further discusses aspects of Vladimir Janda's functional tests. Some of Janda's, as well as Lewit's, functional assessments are also included in the specific muscle evaluations given in Chapter 4.

The reader must decide whether to introduce Mitchell's (Mitchell et al 1979) element of strength testing into any assessment protocol which they adopt. The recommendation by Mitchell and colleagues (1979) that muscle strength be taken into account before MET is used will not be detailed in each paired muscle discussed in the text, and is highlighted here (and in a few specific muscles where these noted authors and clinicians place great emphasis on its importance) in order to remind the reader of the possibility of its incorporation into the methodology of MET use.

The author has not found that application of weakness testing (as part of the work-up before deciding on the suitability or otherwise of MET use for particular muscles) significantly improves results. He does, however, recognise that in individual cases it might be a useful approach, but considers that systematic weakness testing may be left until later in a treatment programme, after dealing with muscles which show evidence of shortness.

Strength testing methodology

In order to test a muscle for strength a standard procedure is carried out as follows:

- The area should be relaxed and not influenced by gravity
- The area/muscle/joint should be positioned so that whatever movement is to be used can be easily performed
- The patient should be asked to perform a concentric contraction which is evaluated against a scale, as outlined in Box 3.2.

The degree of resistance required to prevent movement is a subjective judgement unless mechanical resistance and/or electronic measurement is available. For more detailed knowledge of muscle strength testing, texts such as Janda's *Muscle Function Testing* (Janda 1983) are recommended.

Box 3.2 Scale for evaluation of concentric contractions

Grade 0 = no contraction/paralysis

Grade 1 = no motion noted but contraction felt by palpating hand

Grade 2 = some movement possible on contraction, if gravity influence eliminated ('poor')

Grade 3 = Motion possible against gravity's influence ('fair')

Grade 4 = Movement possible during contraction against resistance ('good')

Ruddy's methods – 'pulsed MET'

In the 1940s and 50s, osteopathic physician T. J. Ruddy developed a method which utilised a series of rapid pulsating contractions against resistance, which he termed 'rapid resistive duction'. As described in Chapter 1, it was in part this work which Fred Mitchell Snr used as his base for the development of MET, along with PNF methodology. Ruddy's method (Ruddy 1962) called for a series of muscle contractions against resistance, at a rhythm a little faster than the pulse rate. This approach can be applied in all areas where isometric contractions are suitable, and is particularly useful for self-treatment following instruction from a skilled practitioner.

According to Greenman (1996), who studied with him, ' He [Ruddy] used these techniques in the cervical spine and around the orbit in his practice as an ophthalmologist–otorhinolaryngologist.'

Ruddy's work is now known as 'pulsed MET'. Its simplest use involves the dysfunctional tissue/joint being held at its resistance barrier, at which time the patient, ideally (or the practitioner if the patient cannot adequately cooperate with the instructions), against the resistance of the practitioner, introduces a series of rapid (2 per second), minute efforts towards (or sometimes away from) the barrier. The barest initiation of effort is called for with, to use Ruddy's words, 'no wobble and no bounce'. The use of this 'conditioning' approach involves contractions which are 'short, rapid and rhythmic, gradually increasing the amplitude and degree of resistance, thus conditioning the proprioceptive system by rapid movements'.

In describing application of this method to the neck (in a case of vertigo) Ruddy gives instruction as to the directions in which the series of resisted efforts should be made. These must include 'movements ... in a line of each major direction, forwards, backwards, right forward and right backwards or along an antero-posterior line in four directions along the multiplication "X" sign, also a half circle, or rotation right and left.'

If reducing joint restriction or elongation of a soft tissue is the objective then, following each series of 20 mini-contractions, the slack should be taken out of the tissues and another series of contractions should be commenced from the new barrier, possibly in a different direction – which can and should be varied according to Ruddy's guidelines, to take account of all the different elements in any restriction. Despite Ruddy's suggestion that the amplitude of the contractions be increased over time, the effort itself must never exceed the barest beginning of an isometric contraction.

The effects are likely, Ruddy suggests, to include improved oxygenation and improved venous and lymphatic circulation through the area being treated. Furthermore, he believes that the method influences both static and kinetic posture because of the effects on proprioceptive and interoceptive afferent pathways, and that this helps maintain 'dynamic equilibrium', which involves 'a balance in chemical, physical, thermal, electrical and tissue fluid homeostasis'.

In a setting in which tense, hypertonic, possibly shortened musculature has been treated by stretching, it may prove useful to begin facilitating and strengthening the inhibited, weakened antagonists by means of Ruddy's methods. This is true whether the hypertonic muscles have been treated for reasons of shortness/hypertonicity alone, or because they accommodate active trigger points within their fibres. The introduction of a pulsating muscle energy procedure such as Ruddy's, involving these weak antagonists, therefore offers the opportunity for:

- Proprioceptive re-education
- Strengthening facilitation of the weak antagonists
- Further inhibition of tense agonists
- Enhanced local circulation and drainage
- In Liebenson's words, 'reeducation of movement patterns on a reflex, subcortical basis' (Liebenson 1996).

Ruddy's work was a part of the base on which Mitchell Snr and others constructed MET and his work is worthy of study and application since it offers, at the very least, a useful means of modifying the employment of sustained isometric contraction and has particular relevance to acute problems and safe self-treatment settings. Examples of Ruddy's method will be described in later chapters.

Isotonic concentric strengthening MET methods

Contractions which occur against, and overcome, resistance allow tensions to develop within a muscle which vary as the joint angle alters. The effect is to tone and strengthen the muscle(s) involved in the contraction. For example:

- The practitioner positions the limb, or area, so that the muscle group will be at resting length, and thus will develop a strong contraction.
- The practitioner explains the direction of movement required, as well as the intensity and duration of that effort. The patient strongly contracts the muscle with the objective of moving the muscle through a complete range, quickly (about 2 seconds).
- The practitioner offers counterforce which is less than that of the patient's contraction, and maintains this throughout the contraction. This is repeated several times, with a progressive increase in practitioner's counterforce (the patient's effort in the strengthening mode is always maximal).
- Where weak muscles are being toned via such isotonic methods, the practitioner allows the concentric contraction of the muscles (i.e. offers only partial resistance to the contractile effort).
- Such exercises always involve practitioner effort which is less than that applied by the patient. The subsequent isotonic concentric contraction of the weakened muscles should allow approximation of the origins and insertions to be achieved under some degree of control by the practitioner.
- Isotonic efforts are usually suggested as being of short duration, ultimately employing maximal effort on the part of the patient. The use of concen-

tric isotonic contractions to tone a muscle or muscle group can be expanded to become an isokinetic, whole joint movement (see below).

Isotonic eccentric alternatives

Norris (1999) suggests that there is evidence that when rapid movement is used in isotonic concentric activities it is largely phasic, type II, fibres which are being recruited. In order to tone postural (type 1) muscles which may have lost their endurance potential, *eccentric isotonic exercises, performed slowly,* are more effective. Norris states: 'Low resistance, slow movements should be used ... eccentric actions have been shown to be better suited for reversal of serial sarcomere adaptation.' Rapidly applied isometric eccentric manoeuvres ('isolytic') are described later in this chapter.

Strengthening a joint complex with isokinetic MET

A variation on the use of simple isotonic concentric contractions, as described above, is to use isokinetic contraction (also known as progressive resisted exercise). In this the patient, starting with a weak effort but rapidly progressing to a maximal contraction of the affected muscle(s), introduces a degree of resistance to the *practitioner's* effort to put a joint, or area, through a full range of motion. An alternative or subsequent exercise involves the practitioner partially resisting the patient's active movement of a joint through a rapid series of as full a range of movements as possible.

Mitchell (Mitchell et al 1979) describes an isokinetic exercise as follows: 'The counterforce is increased during the contraction to meet changing contractile force as the muscle shortens and its force increases.' These are, he says, especially valuable in improving efficient and coordinated use of muscles, and in enhancing the tonus of the resting muscle. 'In dealing with paretic muscles, isotonics (in the form of progressive resistance exercise) and isokinetics, are the quickest and most efficient road to rehabilitation.'

The use of isokinetic contraction is reported to be a most effective method of building strength, and to be superior to high repetition, lower resistance exercises (Blood 1980). It is also felt that a limited range of motion, with good muscle tone, is preferable (to the patient) to normal range with limited power. Thus the strengthening of weak musculature in areas of limitation of mobility is seen as an important contribution in which isokinetic contractions may assist.

Isokinetic contractions not only strengthen the (largely phasic, type II) fibres which are involved, but have a training effect which enables them to operate in a more coordinated manner. There is often a very rapid increase in strength. Because of neuromuscular recruitment, there is a progressively stronger muscular effort as this method is repeated. Contractions and accompanying mobilisation of the region should take no more than 4 seconds at each contraction in order to achieve maximum benefit with as little fatiguing as possible of either the patient or the practitioner. Prolonged contractions should be avoided.

The simple and safest applications of isokinetic methods involve small joints such as those in the extremities, largely because they are more easily controlled by the practitioner's hands. Spinal joints are more difficult to mobilise and to control when muscular resistance is being utilised at full strength. The options in achieving increased tone and strength via these methods therefore involves a choice between a partially resisted isotonic contraction, or the overcoming of such a contraction, at the same time as the full range of movement is being introduced. Both of these options can involve maximum contraction of the muscles by the patient. Home treatment of such conditions is possible via self-treatment, as in other MET methods.[4]

DiGiovanna (1991) suggests that isokinetic exercise increases the work which a muscle can subsequently perform more efficiently and rapidly than either isometric or isotonic exercises.

To summarise:

- To tone weak phasic (stabiliser, see Ch. 2) muscles, perform concentric isotonic exercises using full strength, rapidly (4 seconds maximum).

[4] Both isotonic concentric and eccentric contractions will take place during the isokinetic movement of a joint.

- To tone weak postural (mobiliser, see Ch. 2) muscles, slowly perform eccentric isotonic (i.e. isolytic, see below) exercises using increasing degrees of effort. In order to tone postural fibres, slow speed, eccentric resistance is most effective (Norris 1999).

Reduction of fibrotic changes with isolytic (isotonic eccentric) MET

As discussed above, when a patient initiates a contraction and it is overcome by the practitioner, this is termed an 'isotonic *eccentric* contraction' (e.g. when a patient tries to flex the arm and the practitioner overrides this effort and straightens it during the contraction of the flexor muscles). In such a contraction the origins and insertions of the muscles (and therefore the joint angles) are separated, despite the patient's effort to approximate them. This is termed an isolytic contraction, in that it involves the stretching and to an extent the breaking down (sometimes called 'controlled microtrauma') of fibrotic tissue present in the affected muscles.

Microtrauma is inevitable, and this form of 'controlled' injury is seen to be useful especially in relation to altering the interface between elastic and non-elastic tissues – between fibrous and non-fibrous tissues. Mitchell (Mitchell et al 1979) states that 'Advanced myofascial fibrosis sometimes requires this "drastic" measure, for it is a powerful stretching technique.'

'Adhesions' of this type are broken down by the application of force by the practitioner which is just a little greater than that of the patient. This procedure can be uncomfortable, and patients should be advised of this, as well as of the fact that they need only apply sufficient effort to ensure that they remain comfortable. Limited degrees of effort are therefore called for at the outset of isolytic contractions.

However, in order to achieve the greatest degree of stretch (in the condition of myofascial fibrosis for example), it is necessary for the largest number of fibres possible to be involved in the isotonic contraction. Thus there is a contradiction in that in order to achieve this large involvement, the degree of contraction should be a maximal one, which could produce pain which, while undesirable in most manual treatment, may be deemed necessary in this instance.

Additionally, in many instances the procedure might be impossible to achieve if a large muscle group (e.g. hamstrings) is involved were a maximal contraction to be used, especially if the patient is strong and the practitioner slight or at least inadequate to the task of overcoming the force of the contracting muscle(s). Less than optimal contraction is therefore called for, repeated several times perhaps, but confined to specific muscles where fibrotic change is greatest (e.g. tensor fascia lata (TFL)) and to patients who are not frail, pain-sensitive or in other ways unsuitable for what is the most vigorous MET method.

Unlike isotonic eccentric contractions, which have the aim of strengthening weak postural (mobiliser) muscles and which are performed slowly (as discussed earlier in this chapter), isolytic contractions aimed at stretching fibrotic tissues are performed rapidly.

Summary of choices for MET in treating muscle problems

To return to Goodridge's introduction to MET (see earlier in this chapter) – using the adductors as our target tissues we can now see that a number of choices are open to the practitioner once the objective has been established, for example to lengthen shortened adductor muscles.

If the objective is to lengthen shortened adductors, on the right, several methods could be used:

- The patient could contract the right abductors, against equal practitioner counterforce, in order to relax the adductors by reciprocal inhibition.
- The patient could contract the right adductors, against equal practitioner counterforce, in order to achieve post isometric relaxation.
- The patient could contract the right adductors while the practitioner offered greater counterforce, thus *rapidly* overcoming the isotonic contraction (producing an eccentric isotonic, or isolytic, contraction), introducing microtrauma to fibrotic tissues.
- The limb could be abducted to the restriction barrier where Ruddy's 'pulsed MET' could be

introduced. The practitioner offers counterforce as the patient 'pulses' towards the barrier 20 times in 10 seconds.

In all of these methods the shortened muscles would have been taken to their appropriate barrier before commencing the contraction – either at the first sign of resistance if PIR and movement to a new barrier was the objective, or in a mid-range (just short of the first sense of 'bind') position if RI or a degree of postfacilitation stretching was considered more appropriate.

For an isolytic stretch the contraction commences from the resistance barrier, as do all isokinetic and 'Ruddy' activities.

If the objective were to strengthen weakened adductors, on the right:

- Since these are defined as postural (mobiliser) muscles, the patient could be asked to *slowly* adduct the limb from its barrier, as the operator allowed the patient's effort to overcome resistance, so toning the muscle while it was contracting.

The essence of muscle energy methods then is the harnessing of the patient's own muscle power. The next prerequisite is the application of counterforce, in an appropriate and predetermined manner.

In isometric methods this counterforce must be unyielding. No test of strength must ever be attempted. Thus the patient should never be asked to 'try as hard as he can' to move in this or that direction. It is important before commencing that this instruction, and the rest of the procedure, be carefully explained, so that the patient has a clear idea of his role. The direction, limited degree of effort and duration must all be clear, as must the associated instructions regarding breathing patterns and eye movements (if these are being used).

Joints and MET

MET uses muscles and soft tissues for its effects; nevertheless, the impact of these methods on joints is clearly profound since it is impossible to consider joints independently of the muscles which support and move them. For practical purposes, however, an artificial division is made in the text of this book, and in Chapter 6 there will be specific focus given to topics such as MET in treatment of joint restriction and dysfunction; preparing joints for manipulation with MET; as well as the vexed question of the primacy of muscles or joints in dysfunctional settings. The opinions of experts such as Hartman, Stiles, Evjenth, Lewit, Janda, Goodridge and Harakal will be outlined in relation to these and other joint-related topics.

A chiropractic view is provided in Chapter 5, which looks at rehabilitation implications of MET as its prime interest, but which also touches on the treatment protocol which chiropractic expert Craig Liebenson suggests in relation to dysfunctional imbalances which involve joint restriction/blockage.

Self-treatment

Lewit (1991) is keen to involve patients in home treatment, using MET. He describes this aspect thus:

> Receptive patients are taught how to apply this treatment to themselves, as autotherapy, in a home programme. They passively stretched the tight muscle with their own hand. This hand next provided counter pressure to voluntary contraction of the tight muscle (during inhalation) and then held the muscle from shortening, during the relaxation phase. Finally, it supplied the increment in range of motion (during exhalation) by taking up any slack that had developed.

How often should self-treatment be prescribed?

Gunnari & Evjenth (1983) recommend frequent applications of mild stretching or, if this is not possible, more intense but less frequent self-stretching at home. They state that 'Therapy is more effective if it is supplemented by more frequent self-stretching. In general, the more frequent the stretching, the more moderate the intensity; less frequent stretching, such as that done every other day, may be of greater intensity.'

Self-treatment methods are not suitable to all regions (or for all patients) but there are a large number of areas which lend themselves to such methods. Use of gravity as a counter pressure source is often possible in self-treatment. For example, in order to stretch quadratus lumborum (see Fig. 3.2A–C), the patient stands, legs apart and sidebending, in order to impose a degree of stretch to the shortened muscle. By inhaling and slightly easing the trunk towards an upright position, against the weight of the body, which gravity is pulling towards the floor, and then releasing the breath at the same time as trying to sidebend further towards the floor, a lengthening of quadratus will have been achieved.

Lewit (1999) suggests, in such a movement, that the movement against gravity be accompanied by movement of the eyes in the direction away from which bending is taking place, while the attempt to bend further – after the contraction – should be enhanced by looking in the direction towards which bending is occurring. Use of eye movements in this way facilitates the effects. Several attempts by the patient to induce greater freedom of movement in any restricted direction by means of such simple measures should achieve good results.

The use of eye movements relates to the increase in tone which occurs in muscles as they prepare for movement when the eyes move in a given direction. Thus, if the eyes look down there will be a general increase in tone (slight, but measurable) in the flexors of the neck and trunk. In order to appreciate the influence of eye movement on muscle tone the reader might experiment by fixing their gaze to the left as they attempt to turn their head to the right. This should be followed by gazing right and simultaneously turning the head to the right.

The principles of MET are now hopefully clearer and the methods seen to be applicable to a large range of problems.

Rehabilitation, as well as first-aid and some degree of normalisation of both acute and chronic soft tissue and joint problems are all possible, given correct application. Combined with NMT, this offers the practitioner the chance of achieving safe and effective therapeutic intervention.

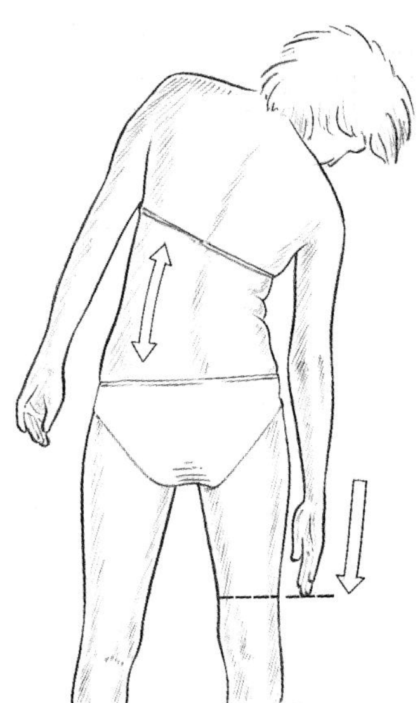

Figure 3.2A MET self-treatment for quadratus lumborum. Patient assesses range of sidebending to the right.

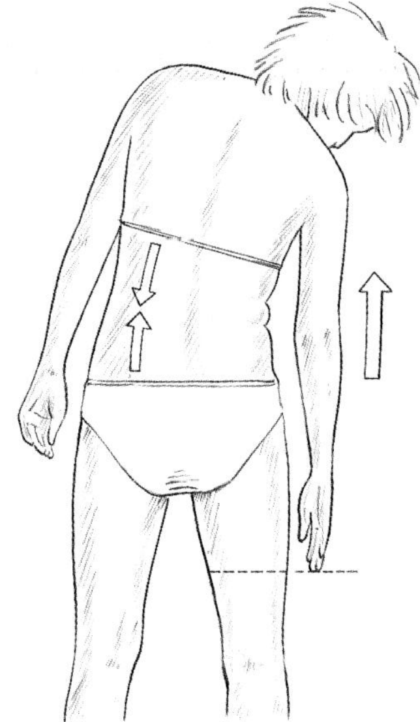

Figure 3.2B Patient contracts quadratus lumborum by straightening slightly, thereby introducing an isometric contraction against gravity.

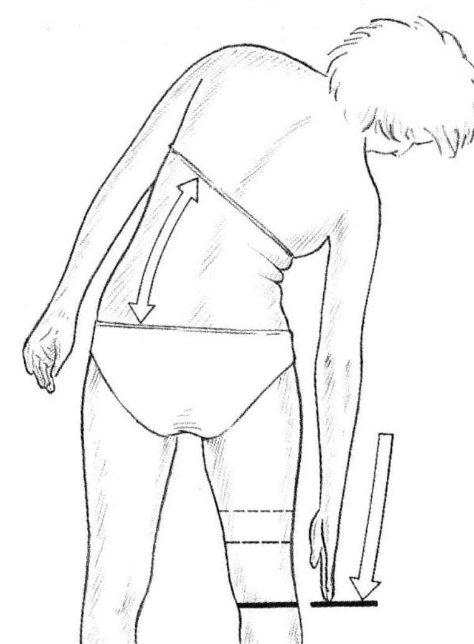

Figure 3.2C After 7–10 seconds, the contraction is released and the patient will be able to sidebend further, stretching quadratus lumborum towards its normal resting length.

When should MET be applied to a muscle?

When should MET (PIR, RI or postfacilitation stretch) be applied to a muscle to relax and/or stretch it?

1. When it is demonstrably shortened – unless the shortening is attributable to associated joint restriction, in which case this should receive primary attention, possibly also involving MET (see Ch. 6).
2. When it contains areas of shortening, such as are associated with myofascial trigger points or palpable fibrosis. It is important to note that trigger points evolve within stressed (hypertonic) areas of phasic, as well as postural muscles, and that these tissues will require stretching, based on evidence which shows that trigger points reactivate unless shortened fibres in which they are housed are stretched to a normal resting length as part of a therapeutic intervention (Simons et al 1998).
3. When periosteal pain points are palpable, indicating stress at the associated muscle's origin and/or insertion (Lewit 1999).
4. In cases of muscular imbalance, in order to reduce hypertonicity when weakness in a muscle is attributable, in part or totally, to inhibition deriving from a hypertonic antagonist muscle (group).

Evaluation

It is seldom possible to totally isolate one muscle in an assessment, and reasons other than muscle shortness can account for apparent restriction (intrinsic joint dysfunction for example). Other methods of evaluation as to relative muscle shortness are also called for, including direct palpation.

The 'normal' range of movements of particular muscles should be taken as guidelines only, since individual factors will often determine that what is 'normal' for one is not so for another.

Wherever possible, an understanding is called for of functional patterns which are observable, for example in the case of the upper fixators of the shoulder/accessory breathing muscles. If a pattern of breathing is observed which indicates a predominance of upper chest involvement, as opposed to diaphragmatic, this in itself would indicate that this muscle group was being 'stressed' by overuse. Since stressed postural (mobiliser) muscles will shorten, an automatic assumption of shortness can be made in such a case regarding the scalenes, levator scapulae, etc. (see Ch. 2 for a fuller discussion of Janda's evidence for this and for Garland's description of structural changes relating to this pattern of breathing).

Once again let it be clear that the various tests and assessment methods suggested in Chapter 4, even when utilising evidence of an abnormally short range of motion, are meant as indicators of, and not certainties, as to shortness (Gunnari & Evjenth 1983). As Evjenth observes: 'If the preliminary analysis identifies shortened muscles, then a provisional trial treatment is performed. If the provisional treatment reduces pain and improves the affected movement pattern, the preliminary analysis is confirmed, and treatment may proceed.'

MUSCLE ENERGY TECHNIQUE – SUMMARY OF VARIATIONS

1. Isometric contraction – using reciprocal inhibition (acute setting, without stretching)

Indications

- Relaxing acute muscular spasm or contraction
- Mobilising restricted joints
- Preparing joint for manipulation.

Contraction starting point For acute muscle or any joint problem, commence at 'easy' restriction barrier (first sign of resistance).

Modus operandi Antagonist(s) to affected muscle(s) is used in isometric contraction, so obliging shortened muscles to relax via reciprocal inhibition. Patient is attempting to push towards the barrier of restriction against practitioner/therapist's precisely matched counterforce.

Forces Practitioner/therapist's and patient's forces are matched. Initial effort involves approximately 20% of patient's strength (or less); an increase to no more than 50% on subsequent contractions if appropriate. Increasing the duration of the contraction (up to 20 seconds) may be more effective than any increase in force.

Duration of contraction Initially 7–10 seconds, increasing to up to 20 seconds in subsequent contractions if greater effect required, and if no pain is induced by the effort.

Action following contraction Area (muscle/joint) is taken to its new restriction barrier without stretch after ensuring complete relaxation. Perform movement to new barrier on an exhalation.

Repetitions Repeat three to five times or until no further gain in range of motion is possible.

2. Isometric contraction – using postisometric relaxation (acute setting, without stretching)

Indications

- Relaxing acute muscular spasm or contraction
- Mobilising restricted joints
- Preparing joint for manipulation.

Contraction starting point At resistance barrier.

Modus operandi The affected muscles (agonists) are used in the isometric contraction, therefore the shortened muscles subsequently relax via postisometric relaxation. If there is pain on contraction this method is contraindicated and the previous method (use of antagonist) is employed. Practitioner/therapist is attempting to push towards the barrier of restriction against the patient's precisely matched counter-effort.

Forces Practitioner/therapist's and patient's forces are matched. Initial effort involves approximately 20% of patient's strength; an increase to no more than 50% on subsequent contractions is appropriate. Increase of the duration of the contraction (up to 20 seconds) may be more effective than any increase in force.

Duration of contraction Initially 7–10 seconds, increasing to up to 20 seconds in subsequent contractions if greater effect required.

Action following contraction Area (muscle/joint) is taken to its new restriction barrier without stretch after ensuring patient has completely relaxed. Perform movement to new barrier on an exhalation.

Repetitions Repeat three to five times or until no further gain in range of motion is possible.

3. Isometric contraction – using postisometric relaxation (chronic setting, with stretching, also known as postfacilitation stretching)

Indications

- Stretching chronic or subacute restricted, fibrotic, contracted soft tissues (fascia, muscle) or tissues housing active myofascial trigger points.

Contraction starting point Short of resistance barrier.

Modus operandi Affected muscles (agonists) are used in the isometric contraction, therefore the shortened muscles subsequently relax via postisometric relaxation, allowing an easier stretch to be performed. Practitioner/therapist is attempting to push through barrier of restriction against the patient's precisely matched counter-effort.

Forces Practitioner/therapist's and patient's forces are matched. Initial effort involves approximately 30% of patient's strength; an increase to no more than 50% on subsequent contractions is appropriate. Increase of the duration of the contraction (up to 20 seconds) may be more effective than any increase in force.

Duration of contraction Initially 7–10 seconds, increasing to up to 20 seconds in subsequent contractions if greater effect required.

Action following contraction Rest period of 5 seconds or so, to ensure complete relaxation before commencing the stretch, is useful. On an exhalation the area (muscle) is taken to its new restriction barrier and a small degree beyond, painlessly, and held in this position for at least 10 and up to 60 seconds. The patient should, if possible, participate in helping move the area to and through the barrier, effectively further inhibiting the structure being stretched and retarding the likelihood of a myotatic stretch reflex.

Repetitions Repeat three to five times or until no further gain in range of motion is possible, with each isometric contraction commencing from a position short of the barrier.

4. Isometric contraction – using reciprocal inhibition (chronic setting, with stretching)

Indications

- Stretching chronic or subacute restricted, fibrotic, contracted soft tissues (fascia, muscle) or tissues housing active myofascial trigger points
- This approach is chosen if contraction of the agonist is contraindicated because of pain.

Contraction starting point A little short of resistance barrier.

Modus operandi Antagonist(s) to affected muscles are used in the isometric contraction, therefore the shortened muscles subsequently relax via reciprocal inhibition, allowing an easier stretch to be performed. Patient is attempting to push through barrier of restriction against the practitioner/therapist's precisely matched counter-effort.

Forces Practitioner/therapist's and patient's forces are matched. Initial effort involves approximately 30% of patient's strength; an increase to no more than 50% on subsequent contractions is appropriate. Increase of the duration of the contraction (up to 20 seconds) may be more effective than any increase in force.

Duration of contraction Initially 7–10 seconds, increasing to up to 20 seconds in subsequent contractions if greater effect required.

Action following contraction Rest period of 5 seconds or so, to ensure complete relaxation before commencing the stretch, is useful. On an exhalation the area (muscle) is taken to its new restriction barrier and a small degree beyond, painlessly, and held in this position for at least 10 and up to 60 seconds. The patient should, if possible, participate in helping move the area to and through the barrier, effectively further inhibiting the structure being stretched and retarding the likelihood of a myotatic stretch reflex.

Repetitions Repeat three to five times or until no further gain in range of motion is possible, with each isometric contraction commencing from a position short of the barrier.

5. Isotonic concentric contraction (for toning or rehabilitation)

Indications

- Toning weakened musculature.

Contraction starting point In a mid-range easy position.

Modus operandi The contracting muscle is allowed to do so, with some (constant) resistance from the practitioner/therapist.

Forces The patient's effort overcomes that of the practitioner/therapist since patient's force is greater than practitioner/therapist resistance. Patient uses maximal effort available, but force is built slowly not via sudden effort. Practitioner/therapist maintains a constant degree of resistance.

Duration 3–4 seconds.

Repetitions Repeat five to seven times, or more if appropriate.

6. Isotonic eccentric contraction (isolytic, for reduction of fibrotic change, to introduce controlled microtrauma)

Indications

- Stretching tight fibrotic musculature.

Contraction starting point At restriction barrier.

Modus operandi The muscle to be stretched is contracted and is rapidly prevented from doing so by the practitioner/therapist, via superior practitioner/therapist effort, and the contraction is overcome and reversed so that a contracting muscle is stretched. The process should take no more than 4 seconds. Origin and insertion do not approximate. Muscle is stretched to, or as close as possible to, full physiological resting length.

Forces Practitioner/therapist's force is greater than patient's. Less than maximal patient's force is employed at first. Subsequent contractions build towards this, if discomfort is not excessive.

Duration of contraction 2–4 seconds.

Repetitions Repeat three to five times if discomfort is not excessive.

⚠ **CAUTION:** Avoid using isolytic contractions on head/neck muscles or at all if patient is frail, very pain-sensitive, or osteoporotic.

7. Isotonic eccentric contraction (isolytic, for strengthening weak postural muscles)

Indications

- Strengthening weakened postural muscle.

Contraction starting point At restriction barrier.

Modus operandi The muscle is contracted and is prevented from doing so by the practitioner/therapist, via superior practitioner/therapist effort, and the contraction is slowly overcome and reversed, so that a contracting muscle is stretched. Origin and insertion do not approximate. Muscle is stretched to, or as close as possible to, full physiological resting length.

Forces Practitioner/therapist's force is greater than patient's. Less than maximal patient's force is employed at first. Subsequent contractions build towards this, if discomfort is not excessive.

Duration of contraction 5–7 seconds.

Repetitions Repeat three to five times if discomfort is not excessive.

⚠ **CAUTION:** Avoid using isotonic eccentric contractions on head/neck muscles or at all if patient is frail, very pain-sensitive, or osteoporotic.

8. Isokinetic (combined isotonic and isometric contractions)

Indications

- Toning weakened musculature
- Building strength in all muscles involved in particular joint function
- Training and balancing effect on muscle fibres.

Starting point of contraction Easy mid-range position.

Modus operandi Patient resists with moderate and variable effort at first, progressing to maximal effort subsequently, as practitioner/ therapist puts joint rapidly through as full a range of movements as possible. This approach differs from a simple isotonic exercise by virtue of whole ranges of motion, rather than single motions being involved, and because resistance varies, progressively increasing as the procedure progresses.

Forces Practitioner/therapist's force overcomes patient's effort to prevent movement. First movements (taking an ankle, say, into all its directions of motion) involve moderate force, progressing to full force subsequently. An alternative is to have the practitioner/therapist (or machine) resist the patient's effort to make all the movements.

Duration of contraction Up to 4 seconds.

Repetitions Repeat two to four times.

REFERENCES

Blood S 1980 Treatment of the sprained ankle. Journal of the American Osteopathic Association 79(11): 689

Cummings J, Howell J 1990 The role of respiration in the tension production of myofascial tissues. Journal of the American Osteopathic Association 90(9): 842

DiGiovanna E 1991 Treatment of the spine. In: DiGiovanna E (ed) An osteopathic approach to diagnosis and treatment. Lippincott, Philadelphia

Goodridge J 1981 MET – definition, explanation, methods of procedure. Journal of the American Osteopathic Association 81(4): 249

Greenman P 1989 Principles of manual medicine. Williams and Wilkins, Baltimore

Greenman P 1996 Principles of manual medicine, 2nd edn. Williams and Wilkins, Baltimore

Guissard N et al 1988 Muscle stretching and motorneurone excitability. European Journal of Applied Physiology 58: 47–52

Gunnari H, Evjenth O 1983 Sequence exercise. [Norwegian] Dreyers Verlag, Oslo

Hoover H 1969 A method for teaching functional technique. Yearbook of Academy of Applied Osteopathy 1969, Newark, Ohio

Janda V 1993 Assessment and treatment of impaired movement patterns and motor recruitment. Presentation to Physical Medicine Research Foundation, Montreal, October 9–11, 1993

Kisselkova, Georgiev J 1976 Journal of Applied Physiology 46: 1093–1095

Kottke F 1982 Therapeutic exercise to maintain mobility. In: Krusen's handbook of physical medicine and rehabilitation, 3rd edn. W B Saunders, Philadelphia

Kraus H 1970 Clinical treatment of back and neck pain. McGraw Hill, New York

Lewit K 1991 Manipulative therapy in rehabilitation of the motor system. Butterworths, London

Lewit K 1999 Manipulative therapy in rehabilitation of the motor system, 3rd edn. Butterworths, London

Liebenson C 1989 Active muscular relaxation methods. Journal of Manipulative and Physiological Therapeutics 12(6): 446–451

Liebenson C 1996 Rehabilitation of the spine. Williams and Wilkins, Baltimore
Mattes A 1990 Active and assisted stretching. Mattes, Sarasota
Mitchell F, Moran P, Pruzzo N 1979 An evaluation and treatment manual of osteopathic muscle energy technique. Valley Park, Missouri
Norris C 1999 Functional load abdominal training (part 1). Journal of Bodywork and Movement Therapies 3(3): 150–158
Ruddy T J 1962 Osteopathic rhythmic resistive technic. Academy of Applied Osteopathy Yearbook 1962, pp 23–31
Scariati P 1991 Neurophysiology relevant to osteopathic manipulation. In: DiGiovanna E (ed) An osteopathic approach to diagnosis and treatment. Lippincott, Philadelphia
Simons D, Travell J, Simmons L 1998 Myofascial pain and dysfunction: the trigger point manual (vol 1), 2nd edn. Williams and Wilkins, Baltimore
Sucher B 1990 Thoracic outlet syndrome – a myofascial variant (part 2). Journal of the American Osteopathic Association 90(9): 810–823
Ward R 1997 Foundations of osteopathic medicine. Williams and Wilkins, Baltimore

CHAPTER CONTENTS

4

Sequential assessment and MET treatment of main postural muscles

OBJECTIVES OF MANUAL TREATMENT

What are the focuses and objectives of manual treatment in general, and manipulation in particular?

- Lewit (1985a) summarises what he believes manipulation is concerned with in the phrase 'restricted mobility', with or without pain.
- Evjenth (1984) is equally succinct, and states that what is needed to become proficient in treating patients with symptoms of pain or 'constrained movement' is 'experience gained by thoroughly examining every patient'. The only real measure of successful treatment is, he states, 'restoration of muscle's normal pattern of movement with freedom from pain'.
- Janda (1988) seems mainly to be concerned with 'imbalances' and the implications of dysfunctional patterns in which some muscles become weaker and others progressively tighter.
- Greenman (1996) reports on the conclusion of a 1983 workshop in which manual experts from around the world considered the question. The conclusion was that 'The goal of manipulation is to restore maximal pain-free movement of the musculoskeletal system in postural balance'.

Previous chapters have discussed concepts relating to 'tight–loose', 'ease–bind' and particular muscle groups – however categorised – being subject, as part of their adaptation to the stresses of life, to shortening, while others are subject to weakening and/or lengthening. It is in the context of such adaptation, compensation and decompensation that soft tissue and articular changes can be identified by means of diligent palpation and assessment. Hopefully attention will also be paid to any habits of use which have contributed to the dysfunctional pattern being treated.

Restoration of a more normal function demands the availability of therapeutic tools by means of which change can be engineered. Accompanying biomechanical (manipulation, etc.) solutions and strategies which retard the chances of recurrence should be introduced, possibly involving particular focus on key muscles requiring strengthening, or enhanced posture, or breathing function. Such 're-education' depends for success at least partly on the structural and functional imbalances which are present at the outset being modified to allow change (towards improved posture, fuller breathing, etc.). No one with restricted and shortened accessory breathing/upper fixator muscles can learn to breathe correctly until these have been to an extent normalised. No one with short lumbar erector spinae and weak abdominal muscles can learn to use their spine in a posturally correct manner until these muscular imbalances have been to an extent normalised.

The structure–function continuum demands that therapeutic attention be paid to both aspects. Function cannot change until structure allows it to do so, and structure will continue to modify and adapt at the expense of optimal function until dysfunctional patterns of use change.

Part of a solution is offered by the methods used in muscle energy technique (MET), in which the short and tight structures are identified and lengthened while the weak and 'sagging' muscles are encouraged to enhanced tone and strength. Rehabilitation and re-education methods can then work in a relatively unhindered environment as new habits of use are learned.

Greenman (1996) offers a summary of this clinical approach: 'After short tight muscles are stretched, muscles that are inhibited can undergo retraining ... as in all manual medicine procedures, after assessment, stretching, and strengthening, reevaluation of faulty movement patterns ... is done.'

EVALUATING MUSCLE SHORTNESS

Many of the problems of the musculoskeletal system seem to involve pain related to aspects of muscle shortening (Lewit 1999). Where weakness (or lack of tone) is found to be a major element, it will often be noted that antagonists to these muscles are hypertonic and/or shortened, reciprocally inhibiting their tone. It is the author's experience and opinion that prior to any effort to strengthen weak muscles, shortened ones should be dealt with by appropriate means, after which spontaneous toning usually occurs in the previously 'weak' muscles. If muscle tone remains inadequate, then, and only then, should exercise and/or isotonic procedures be initiated. This is not a universally accepted model, with many clinicians preferring to work on weak structures first, so reducing tone in their (usually) hypertonic antagonists. Attention to weak structures as a primary therapeutic effort may usefully reduce hypertonicity in antagonists; however, such treatment methods cannot reverse the fibrotic state of many chronically shortened structures, and until this is achieved the author contends that enhanced strength of previously weak phasic (stabiliser, see Ch. 2) muscles offers little overall benefit towards the objective of restoring functional balance.

Janda (1983) tells us that tight muscles usually maintain their strength; however, in extreme cases of tightness some decrease in strength occurs. In such cases stretching (MET) of the tight muscle usually leads to a rapid recovery of strength (as well as toning of their antagonists via removal of reciprocal inhibition). As noted in Chapter 3, weak postural muscles benefit from slowly applied isotonic eccentric methods (Norris 1999).

It is therefore important that we learn to assess short, tight muscles in a systematic, standardised manner.

Janda (1983) suggests that, in order to obtain a reliable evaluation of muscle shortness:

- The starting position, method of fixation and direction of movement must be observed carefully
- The prime mover must not be exposed to external pressure

- If possible, the force exerted on the tested muscle must not work over two joints
- The examiner should perform, at an even speed, a slow movement that brakes slowly at the end of the range
- To keep the stretch and the muscle irritability about equal, the movement must not be jerky
- Pressure or pull must always act in the required direction of movement
- Muscle shortening can only be correctly evaluated if the joint range is not decreased, as might be the case should an osseous limitation or joint blockage exist (Janda 1983).

It is also in shortened muscles, as a rule, that reflex activity is noted. This takes the form of local dysfunction – variously called trigger points, tender points, zones of irritability, hyperalgesic zones, neurovascular and neurolymphatic reflexes, etc. (Chaitow 1991). Localising these is possible via normal palpatory methods. Identification and treatment of tight muscles may also be systematically carried out using the methods described later in this chapter.[1]

Box 4.1 'Acute' and 'chronic'

The words 'acute' and 'chronic' should alert the reader to the differences in methodology which these variants call for in applying MET, especially in terms of the starting position for contractions and whether or not stretching should take place after the contraction.

In acute conditions the isometric contraction starts at the barrier, whereas in chronic conditions the contraction starts short of the barrier. After the contraction the practitioner takes the area to the new barrier in acute conditions, or through the previous resistance barrier into slight sustained stretch in chronic conditions.

The term 'acute' may be applied to strain or injury which has occurred within the past 3 weeks, or where the symptoms such as pain are acute, or where active inflammation is present.

Use of the antagonists to the affected muscle(s) offers an alternative to activation of an isometric contraction in such muscles if this proves painful or difficult for the patient to perform.

A further alternative is to use Ruddy's repetitive pulsing contractions, rather than a sustained contraction, if the latter is painful or difficult for the patient to perform (see Ch. 3).

IMPORTANT NOTES ON ASSESSMENTS AND USE OF MET

1. When the term 'restriction barrier' is used in relation to soft tissue structures, it is meant to indicate the place where you note the first signs of resistance (as palpated by sense of 'bind', or sense of effort required to move the area, or by visual or other palpable evidence) and not the greatest possible range of movement obtainable. (Refer to the ease/bind palpation exercise involving the adductors in Ch. 3 and Fig. 3.1A, B.)

2. In all treatment descriptions involving MET (apart from the first set of assessment tests involving gastrocnemius and soleus) it will be assumed that the 'shorthand' reference to 'acute' and 'chronic' will be adequate to alert the reader to the variations in methodology which these variants call for (see Box 4.1). The appropriate barriers for use in acute and chronic situations were summarised in the descriptions of MET variations in Chapter 3.

3. Assistance from the patient is valuable as movement is made to or through a barrier, provided that the patient can be educated to gentle cooperation and can learn not to use excessive effort.

4. In most MET treatment guidelines in this chapter the method described will involve isometric contraction of the agonist(s) – i.e. the muscle(s) which require stretching. It is assumed that the reader is now familiar with the possibility of using the antagonists to achieve reciprocal inhibition (RI) before initiating stretch or movement to a new barrier, and will use this alternative when appropriate (if there is pain on use of agonist; if there has been prior trauma to the agonist; in an attempt to see if more release can be made available after the initial use of the agonist isometrically).

5. Isolytic (eccentric isotonic) contractions will be suggested in a few instances, most notably in treating tensor fascia lata (TFL), but these are not

[1] Note that the assessment methods presented are not themselves diagnostic but provide strong indications of probable shortness of the muscles being tested.

generally recommended for application in sensitive patients or in potentially 'fragile' areas such as the muscles associated with the cervical spine.

6. Careful reading of Chapters 1 and 3 in particular is urged before commencing practice of the methods listed below.

7. There should be no pain experienced during application of MET, although mild discomfort (stretching) is acceptable.

8. The methods of assessment and treatment of postural muscles given here are far from comprehensive or definitive. There are many other assessment approaches, and numerous treatment/stretch approaches, using variations on the theme of MET, as evidenced by the excellent texts by Janda, Basmajian, Lewit, Liebenson, Greenman, Grieve, Mattes, Hartman, Evjenth and Dvorak, among others. The methods recommended below provide a sound basis for the application of MET to specific muscles and areas, as do the methods suggested for spinal, pelvic, neck and shoulder regions in following chapters (Chs 5 and 6). By developing the skills with which to apply the methods, as described, a repertoire of techniques can be acquired offering a wide base of choices that will be appropriate in numerous clinical settings.

9. Some of the discussion of particular muscles will include notes containing information unrelated to the main objective, which is to outline assessment and MET treatment possibilities. These notes are included where the particular information they carry is likely to be useful clinically.

10. Breathing cooperation can, and should, be used as part of the methodology of MET. This, however, will not be repeated as an instruction in each example of MET use below. Basically, if appropriate (that is, if the patient is cooperative and capable of following instructions), the patient should be given the instructions outlined in Box 4.2. A note which gives the instruction to 'use appropriate breathing', or some variation on it, will be found in the following text describing various MET applications, and this refers to the guidelines outlined in Box 4.2.

11. Various eye movements are sometimes advocated during contractions and stretches, particularly by Lewit who uses these methods to great effect. The only specific recommendations for this in this chapter will be found in regard to muscles such as the scalenes and sternomastoid, where the use of eye movements is particularly valuable in terms of the gentleness of the contractions they induce.

12. 'Pulsed muscle energy technique' is based on Ruddy's work (see Ch. 3). It can be substituted for any of the methods described in the text below for treating shortened soft tissue structures, or for increasing the range of motion in joints (Ruddy 1962).

13. There are times when 'co-contraction' is useful, involving contraction of both the agonist and the antagonist. Studies have shown that this approach is particularly useful in treatment of the hamstrings, when both these and the quadriceps are isometrically contracted prior to stretch (Moore at al 1980).

14. It is seldom necessary to treat all the shortened muscles which are identified via the methods described below. For example, Lewit and Simons mention that isometric relaxation of the suboccipital muscles will also relax the sternocleidomastoid muscles; treatment of the thoracolumbar muscles induces relaxation of iliopsoas, and vice versa; treatment (MET) of the sternocleidomastoid and scalene muscles relaxes the pectorals. These interactions are worthy of greater study.

Box 4.2 Notes on breathing during MET

Patients who are cooperative and capable of following instructions should be asked to:

- Inhale as they slowly build up an isometric contraction
- Hold the breath during the 7–10 second contraction, and
- Release the breath as they slowly cease the contraction
- Inhale and exhale fully once more, following cessation of all effort, as they are asked to 'let go completely'

During this second exhalation the tissues are taken to their new barrier in an acute condition, or the barrier is passed as the muscle is stretched in a chronic condition (with patient assistance if possible).

Stretching – what is happening?

The notes in Chapter 2 which relate to fascia and the characteristics of connective tissue are particularly relevant to MET application in general, and the stretching element of MET in particular.

In a chronic condition, when stretching beyond the initial resistance barrier is introduced following an isometric contraction, the objective is clearly to lengthen the shortened structure being treated. Application of MET comprises *neurological* as well as *biomechanical* elements.

The isometric contraction involves two neurological components:

- Postisometric relaxation (PIR) will follow contraction of the agonist, as a result of Golgi tendon organ mediation
- Reciprocal inhibition (RI) will occur affecting the antagonist, as a result of spindle mediation.

Reciprocal inhibition is again a feature when the patient actively assists an area into stretch, so reducing the likelihood of the myotatic stretch reflex being activated, while at the same time reciprocally inhibiting the tissues which are being taken past their restriction barrier.

Once stretching has actually commenced, biomechanical effects are initiated as sustained, low intensity force is applied to lengthen the tissues and 'creep' (see Ch. 2) begins. The longer the stretched status is maintained, the greater the viscoelastic effect on connective tissue and the more 'permanent' the increased length is likely to be (Taylor et al 1990).

The author suggests that practitioners using MET methods, following an isometric contraction, should hold tissues in a slightly stretched state (where appropriate, i.e. in chronic soft tissue problems) for not less than 10 seconds, and ideally for 30 seconds or more, to allow this slow lengthening process to begin.

It is also suggested that a second stretch be introduced (and sometimes a third, although experience suggests that very little additional gain is likely if the first two stretches have been adequately performed), always following an isometric contraction.

MET for joints, and post-treatment discomfort

When treating restricted joints using MET (see Ch. 6) *no stretching* should be introduced following isometric contractions. The MET approach suggested is precisely that indicated (see Chs 2 and 3) for acute soft tissue problems. The barrier is engaged and, following isometric contraction, a new barrier is moved to, without force or stretching.

Unlike the time required to hold soft tissues at stretch in order to achieve a lengthening, no such feature is part of the protocol for treatment of joints using MET. Once the new barrier is reached, having taken out available slack without force after the isometric contraction, the subsequent contraction is called for and the process is repeated.

The author has found that a variety of directions of resisted effort are useful in attempting to achieve release and mobilisation of a restricted joint. Patient-directed efforts towards the restriction barrier, as well as away from it, and using a combination of forces, often of a 'spiral' nature, should be experimented with, if a joint does not release using the most obvious directions of contraction. Additionally the author suggests the use of Ruddy's pulsed MET approaches as variations on the theme of MET to release blocked joints.

Greenman (1996) advocates three to five repetitions of contractions when treating joints with MET, and warns that discomfort should be anticipated for 12–36 hours after the treatment. He explains why this occurs:

> [MET] muscle contractions influence the surrounding fascia, connective tissue ground substance, and interstitial fluids, and alter muscle physiology by reflex mechanisms. Fascial length and tone is altered by muscle contraction. Alteration in fascia influences not only its biomechanical function but also the biochemical and immunological functions. The patient's muscle effort requires energy and the metabolic process of muscle contraction results in carbon dioxide, lactic acid, and other metabolic waste products that must be transported and metabolized.

The author recommends that effleurage be applied to the tissues following MET, in order to reduce the degree of discomfort which Greenman suggests is likely.

Postural muscle assessment sequence checklist

The checklist in Box 4.3 can be used to follow (and record results of) the simple sequence of postural muscle assessment as described in detail later in this chapter.

SEQUENTIAL ASSESSMENT AND MET TREATMENT OF POSTURAL MUSCLES

These assessment and treatment recommendations represent a synthesis of information derived from personal clinical experience and from the numerous sources which are cited, or are based on the work of researchers, clinicians and therapists who are named (Basmajian 1974, Cailliet 1962, Dvorak & Dvorak 1984, Fryette 1954, Greenman 1989, 1996, Janda 1983, Lewit 1992, 1999, Mennell 1964, Rolf 1977, Williams 1965).[2]

Box 4.3 Postural muscle assessment sequence

NAME ______________________________

E = Equal (circle both if both are short)

L or R are circled if left or right are short

Spinal abbreviations indicate low lumbar, lumbodorsal junction, low-thoracic, mid-thoracic and upper thoracic areas (of flatness and therefore reduced ability to flex – short erector spinae)

01. Gastrocnemius E L R
02. Soleus E L R
03. Medial hamstrings E L R
04. Short adductors E L R
05. Rectus femoris E L R
06. Psoas E L R
07. Hamstrings
    a) upper fibres E L R
    b) lower fibres E L R
08. Tensor fascia lata E L R
09. Piriformis E L R
10. Quadratus lumborum E L R
11. Pectoralis major E L R
12. Latissimus dorsi E L R
13. Upper trapezius E L R
14. Scalenes E L R
15. Sternocleidomastoid E L R
16. Levator scapulae E L R
17. Infraspinatus E L R
18. Subscapularis E L R
19. Supraspinatus E L R
20. Flexors of the arm E L R
21. Spinal flattening:
    a) seated legs straight LL LDJ LT MT UT
    b) seated legs flexed LL LDJ LT MT UT
22. Cervical spine extensors short? Yes No

1. Assessment and treatment of gastrocnemius and soleus

Assessment of tight gastrocnemius (01) and soleus (02) (Fig. 4.1A, B)

The patient is supine with feet extending over the edge of the table. For right leg examination the practitioner's left hand grasps the Achilles tendon just above the heel, avoiding pressure on the tendons. The heel lies in the palm of the hand, fingers curving round it. The practitioner's right hand is placed so that the fingers rest on the dorsum of the foot (these are not active and do not apply any pulling stretch), with the thumb on the sole, lying along the medial margin. (This position is important – it is a mistake to place the thumb too near the centre of the sole of the foot.)

Stretch is introduced by means of a pull on the heel with the left hand, taking out the slack of the muscle, while at the same time the right hand maintains the cephalad pressure via the thumb (along its entire length).

A range of movement should be achieved which takes the sole of the foot to a 90° angle to the leg without any force being applied. If this is not possible (i.e. force is required to achieve the 90° angle between the sole of the foot and the leg), there is shortness in gastrocnemius and/or soleus. Further screening is required to identify precisely which (see soleus test below).

It is possible to use the (left) hand, which has removed slack from the muscles via traction, to palpate for a sense of bind, as the foot is dorsiflexed. The leg must remain resting on the table all the while and the right hand holding/palpating the muscle insertion and the heel should be

[2] The 'code' number assigned to each muscle links it to the postural muscle assessment sequence checklist in Box 4.3.

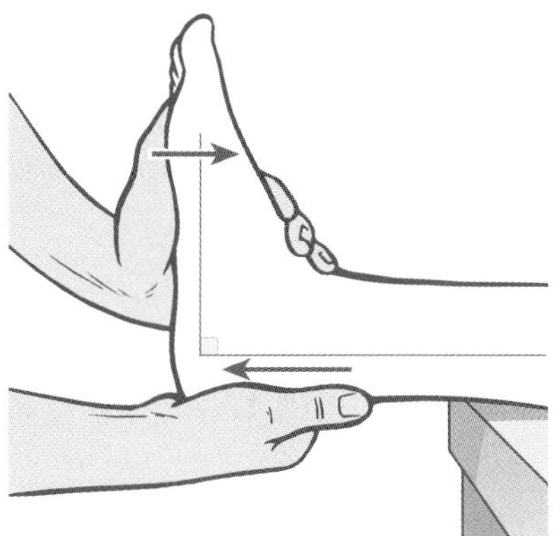

Figure 4.1A Assessment or treatment of gastrocnemius and soleus. During assessment the sole of the foot should achieve a vertical position without effort once slack is taken out via traction on the heel. Treatment would involve taking the tissues to or through (acute/chronic) the identified barrier following an isometric contraction.

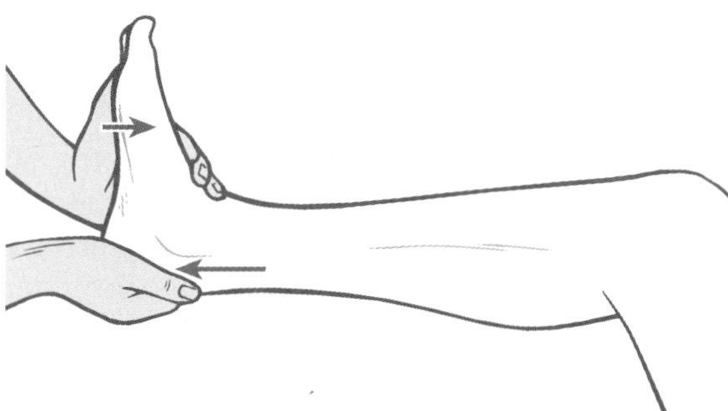

Figure 4.1B With the knee flexed, the same assessment is evaluating the status of soleus alone. Treatment would involve taking the tissues to or through (acute/chronic) the identified barrier following an isometric contraction.

placed so that it is an extension of the leg, not allowing an upward (towards the ceiling) pull when stretch is introduced.

An alternative method is to have the patient seated on the table, legs outstretched, and to have her bend towards the toes with arms extended. If toe touching is possible, but toes are *plantarflexed*, then there is probably shortness of the gastrocnemius–soleus muscles.

Assessment of tight soleus (02)

The method described above assesses both gastrocnemius and soleus. To assess only the soleus, precisely the same procedure is adopted, with the knee passively flexed (over a cushion, for example).

If the sole of the foot fails to easily come to a 90° angle with the leg, without force, once slack has been taken out of the tissues via traction through the long axis of the calf from the heel, soleus is considered short. If the test in which the leg was straight indicated shortness of gastrocnemius or soleus, and the test in which the knee was flexed was normal, then gastrocnemius alone is short.

A screening test for soleus involves the patient being asked to squat, trunk in slight flexion, feet placed shoulder width apart, so that the buttocks rest between the legs (which face forwards rather than outwards). If the soleus muscles are normal then it should be possible to go fully into this position with the heels remaining flat on the floor. If not, and the heels rise from the floor as the squat is performed, the soleus muscles are probably shortened.

MET treatment of shortened gastrocnemius and soleus (Fig. 4.1A, B)

The exact same position is adopted for treatment as for testing, with the knee flexed over a rolled towel or cushion if soleus is being treated, and the knee straight if gastrocnemius is being treated.

If the condition is acute (defined as a dysfunction/injury of less than 3 weeks' duration) the area is treated with the foot dorsiflexed to the restriction barrier.

If it is a chronic problem (longer duration than 3 weeks) the barrier is assessed and the muscle treated in a position of ease, in the mid-range, away from the restriction barrier.

Starting from the appropriate position, at the restriction barrier or just short of it, based on the degree of acuteness or chronicity, the patient is asked to exert a small effort (no more than 20% of available strength) towards plantarflexion, against unyielding resistance, with appropriate breathing (see Box 4.2).

This effort isometrically contracts either gastrocnemius or soleus (depending on whether the knee is unflexed or flexed). This contraction is held for 7–10 seconds (or longer – up to 20 seconds – if the condition is chronic) together with a held breath (if appropriate).

On slow release, on an exhalation, the foot/ankle is dorsiflexed (be sure to flex the whole foot and not just the toes) to its new restriction barrier if acute, or slightly and painlessly beyond the new barrier if chronic, with the patient's assistance.

If chronic, the tissues should be held in slight stretch for at least 10 seconds (longer would be better) in slight stretch to allow a slow lengthening of tissues. (See notes on 'creep' and viscoelasticity in Ch. 2.)

This pattern is repeated until no further gain is achieved (backing off to mid-range for the next contraction, if chronic, and commencing the next contraction from the new resistance barrier if acute).

Alternatively, if there is undue discomfort using the agonists (the muscles being treated) for the contraction, the antagonists to the short muscles can be used by introducing resisted dorsiflexion with the muscle at its barrier or short of it (acute/chronic) followed by painless stretch to the new barrier (acute) or beyond it (chronic), during an exhalation.

Use of antagonists in this way is less effective than use of the agonist but may be a useful strategy if trauma has taken place.

NOTE: Figure 4.2 offers an alternative treatment position for gastrocnemius which can also be used for assessment. Flexion of the knee would allow this position to be used for treating soleus.

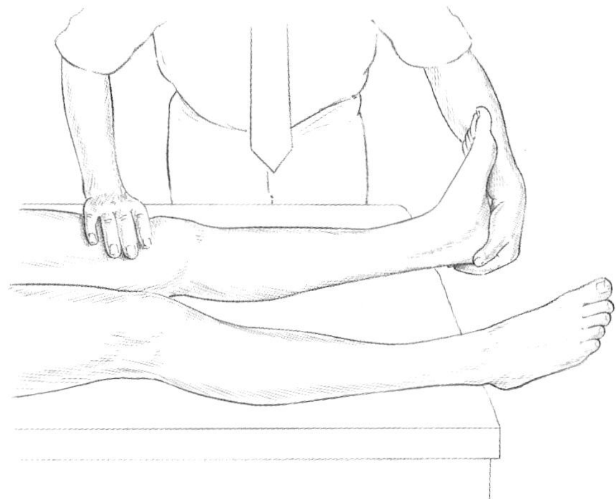

Figure 4.2 MET treatment position for gastrocnemius. If knee were flexed the same position would focus on treatment of soleus only.

2. Assessment and treatment of medial hamstrings and adductors

Assessing for shortness in medial hamstrings (03) (semi-membranosus and semi-tendinosus as well as gracilis) and short adductors (04) (pectineus, adductors brevis, magnus and longus)

Method (a) The patient lies so that the non-tested leg is abducted slightly, heel over the end of the table. The leg to be tested is close to the edge of the bed and the practitioner ensures that the tested leg is in its anatomically correct position, knee in full extension and with no external rotation of the leg, which would negate the test.

The practitioner should effectively stand between patient's leg and the table so that all control of the tested leg is achieved with his lateral (non-table-side) arm/hand, while the table-side hand can rest on and palpate the inner thigh muscles for sensations of bind as it is taken into abduction. Abduction of the tested leg is introduced passively until the first sign of resistance is noted (see Fig. 4.3).

Effectively, there are three indicators of this resistance:

- A sense that the motive hand carrying the leg picks up as an increase in required effort at the moment that the first resistance barrier is passed
- The sense of bind noted by the palpating hand at this same moment
- A visual sign, movement of the pelvis as a whole, laterally towards the tested side, as the barrier is passed.

If abduction produces an angle with the mid-line of 45° or more, then no further test is needed, the abduction is normal, and there is probably no shortness in the short or long adductors (medial hamstrings or, more correctly, gracilis and biceps femoris).

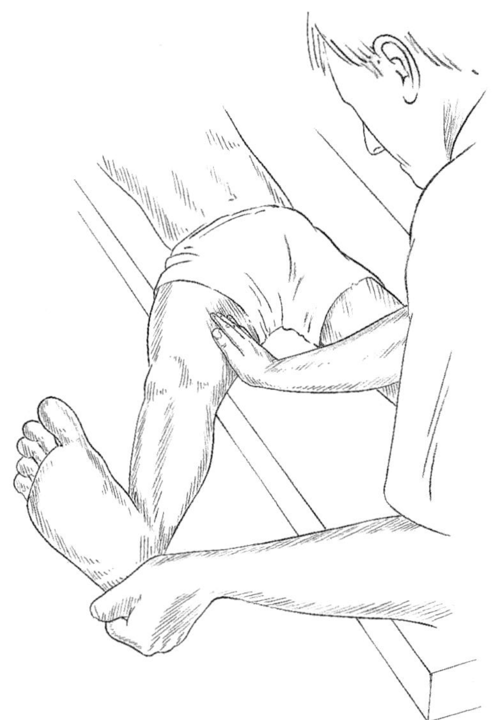

Figure 4.3 Assessment and treatment position for medial hamstrings. Adductor shortness may be evaluated and treated in the same relative position but with the knee of the leg to be treated in flexion.

If, however, abduction ceases before a 45° angle is easily achieved (without effort or a sense of bind in the tissues), then restriction exists in either the medial hamstrings or the short adductors of the thigh.

Screening short adductors (04) from medial hamstrings (03)

As in the tests for gastrocnemius and soleus, it is necessary to screen between shortness of the one and two joint muscles (in this case the short adductors and the medial hamstrings).

This is achieved by abducting the leg to its easy barrier and then introducing flexion of the knee, allowing the lower leg to hang down freely.

If (after knee flexion has been introduced) further abduction is now easily achieved to 45°, this indicates that any previous limitation into abduction was the result of medial hamstring shortness, since this is no longer operating once the knee has been flexed.

If, however, restriction remains (as evidenced by continued 'bind' or obvious restriction in movement towards allowing a 45° excursion once knee flexion has been introduced to the abducted leg), then it is apparent that the short adductors are continuing to prevent movement, and are short.

Assessing for shortness in medial hamstring (03)/short adductors (04)

Method (b) The patient lies at the very end of table (coccyx close to edge), non-tested leg fully flexed at hip and knee and held to chest by patient (or sole of patient's foot resting against practitioner's lateral chest wall) to stabilise pelvis in full rotation, so that the lumbar spine is not in extension.

Tested leg is grasped both above and below the knee and taken into abduction to the first sign of resistance. The practitioner has two free hands in this position, one of which can usefully palpate the inner thigh for bind during the assessment.

If abduction reaches 45°, then the test has revealed no shortness. If a restriction/resistance barrier is noted before 45°, then the knee should be flexed to screen the short adductors from the medial hamstrings as in method (a) above. In all other ways the findings are interpreted as above.

MET treatment of shortness in short and long adductors of the thigh

Precisely the same positions may be adopted for treatment as for testing, whether test method (a) or test method (b) was used.

If the short adductors (pectineus, adductors brevis, magnus and longus) are being treated, then the leg, with knee flexed, is held at the barrier (acute) or a little short of the barrier (chronic).

An isometric contraction is introduced by the patient using around 20% of available strength (longer and somewhat stronger for chronic than acute) employing the agonists (the push is away from the barrier of resistance) or the antagonists (the push is towards the barrier of resistance)

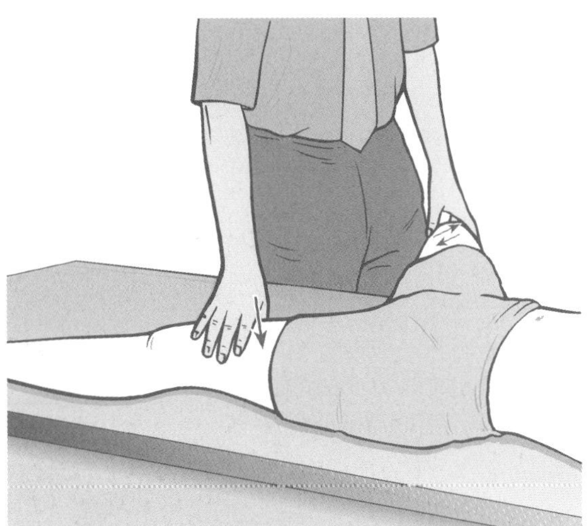

Figure 4.4 Position for treatment of shortness in adductors of the thigh.

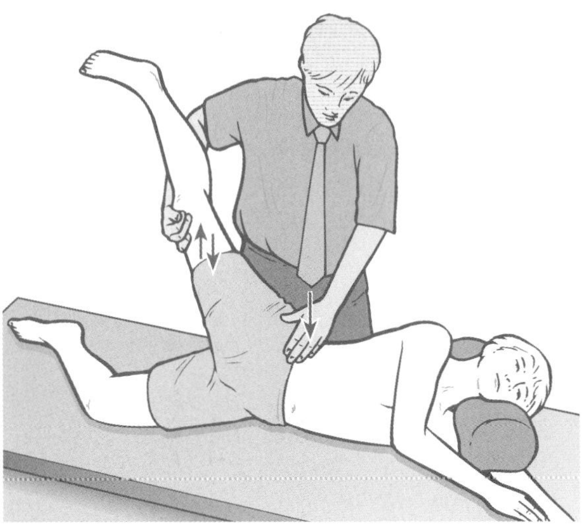

Figure 4.5 Sidelying position for treatment of two-joint adductors of the thigh.

for 7–10 seconds. Appropriate breathing instructions should be given (see notes on breathing in Box 4.2).

After the contraction ceases and the patient has relaxed, the leg is eased to its new barrier (if acute) or painlessly (assisted by the patient) beyond the new barrier and into stretch (if chronic), where it is held for not less than 10 seconds (longer if possible), in order to stretch shortened tissue.

The process is repeated at least once more.

If the medial hamstrings (semi-membranosus, semi-tendinosus as well as gracilis) are being treated, all elements are the same, except that the leg should be held in extension, with no bend of the knee (Fig. 4.4).

Whichever position is used, the subsequent stretch, on an exhalation, is used to (acute) or through (chronic) the barrier to commence normalisation of the short muscles.

Caution and alternative treatment position (Fig. 4.5)

The major error made in treating these particular muscles using MET relates to allowing a pivoting of the pelvis and a low spinal sidebend to occur. Maintenance of the pelvis in a stable position is vital, and this can most easily be achieved via suitable straps or, during treatment, by having the patient side-lying with the affected side uppermost.

Method Patient is side-lying. Practitioner stands behind and uses the caudad arm and hand to control the leg and to palpate for bind, with the treated leg flexed or straight as appropriate. The cephalad hand maintains a firm downwards pressure on the lateral pelvis to ensure stability during stretching. All other elements of treatment are identical to those described for supine treatment above.

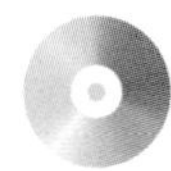

3. Assessment and treatment of hip flexors – rectus femoris, iliopsoas (see also Box 4.4)

Assessment of shortness in hip flexors – rectus femoris (05), iliopsoas (06) (Fig. 4.6A)

Patient lies supine with buttocks (coccyx) as close to end of table as possible, non-tested leg in flexion at hip and knee, held by patient or by having sole of foot of non-tested side placed against the lateral chest wall of the practitioner. Full flexion of the hip helps to maintain the pelvis in full rotation with the lumbar spine flat, which is essential if the test is to be meaningful and stress on the spine is to be avoided.

Box 4.4 Notes on psoas

- Lewit (1985b) mentions that in many ways the psoas behaves as if it were an internal organ. Tension in the psoas may be secondary to kidney disease, and one of its frequent clinical manifestations, when in spasm, is that it reproduces the pain of gall-bladder disease (often after the organ has been removed).
- The definitive signs of psoas problems are not difficult to note, according to Harrison Fryette (1954). He maintains that the distortions produced in inflammation and/or spasm in the psoas are characteristic and cannot be produced by other dysfunction. The origin of the psoas is from 12th thoracic to (and including) the 4th lumbar, but not the 5th lumbar. The insertion is into the lesser trochanter of the femur, and thus, when psoas spasm exists unilaterally, the patient is drawn forwards and sidebent to the involved side. The ilium on the side will rotate backwards on the sacrum, and the thigh will be everted. When both muscles are involved the patient is drawn forward, with the lumbar curve locked in flexion. This is the characteristic reversed lumbar spine. Chronic bilateral psoas contraction creates either a reversed lumbar curve if the erector spinae of the low back are weak, or an increased lordosis if they are hypertonic.
- Lewit says, 'Psoas spasm causes abdominal pain, flexion of the hip and typical antalgesic (stooped) posture. Problems in psoas can profoundly influence thoraco-lumbar stability.'
- The 5th lumbar is not involved directly with psoas, but great mechanical stress is placed upon it when the other lumbar vertebrae are fixed in either a kyphotic or an increased lordotic state. In unilateral psoas spasms, a rotary stress is noted at the level of 5th lumbar. The main mechanical involvement is, however, usually at the lumbodorsal junction. Attempts to treat the resulting pain (frequently located in the region of the 5th lumbar and sacroiliac) by attention to these areas will be of little use. Attention to the muscular component should be a primary focus, ideally using MET.
- Bogduk (Bogduk et al 1992, Bogduk 1997) provides evidence that psoas plays only a small role in the action of the spine, and states that it 'uses the lumbar spine as a base from which to act on the hip'. He goes on to discuss just how much pressure derives from psoas compression on discs: 'Psoas potentially exerts massive compression loads on the lower lumbar discs … upon maximum contraction, in an activity such as sit-ups, the two psoas muscles can be expected to exert a compression on the L5–S1 disc equal to about 100 kg of weight.'
- There exists in all muscles a vital reciprocal agonist–antagonist relationship which is of primary importance in determining their tone and healthy function. Psoas–rectus abdominis have such a relationship and this has important postural implications (see notes on lower crossed syndrome in Ch. 2).
- Observation of the abdomen 'falling back' rather than mounding when the patient flexes indicates normal psoas function. Similarly, if the patient, when lying supine, flexes knees and 'drags' the heels towards the buttocks (keeping them together), the abdomen should remain flat or fall back. If the abdomen mounds or the small of the back arches, psoas is incompetent.
- If the supine patient raises both legs into the air and the belly mounds it shows that the recti and psoas are out of balance. Psoas should be able to raise the legs to at least 30° without any help from the abdominal muscles.
- Psoas fibres merge with (become 'consolidated' with) the diaphragm and it therefore influences respiratory function directly (as does quadratus lumborum).
- Basmajian (1974) informs us that the psoas is the most important of all postural muscles. If it is hypertonic and the abdominals are weak and exercise is prescribed to tone these weak abdominals (such as curl-ups with the dorsum of the foot stabilised), then a disastrous negative effect will ensue in which, far from toning the abdominals, increase of tone in psoas will result, due to the sequence created by the dorsum of the foot being used as a point of support. When this occurs (dorsiflexion), the gait cycle is mimicked and there is a sequence of activation of tibialis anticus, rectus femoris and psoas. If, on the other hand, the feet could be plantarflexed during curl-up exercises, then the opposite chain is activated (triceps surae, hamstrings and gluteals) inhibiting psoas and allowing toning of the abdominals.
- When treating, it is sometimes useful to assess changes in psoas length by periodic comparison of apparent arm length. Patient lies supine, arms extended above head, palms together so that length can be compared. A shortness will commonly be observed in the arm on the side of the shortened psoas, and this should normalise after successful treatment (there may of course be other reasons for apparent difference in arm length, and this method provides an indication only of changes in psoas length).

If the thigh of the tested leg fails to lie in a horizontal position in which it is parallel to the floor/table, then the indication is that iliopsoas is short.

If the lower leg of the tested side fails to achieve an almost 90° angle with the thigh, vertical to the floor, then shortness of the rectus femoris muscle is indicated (Fig. 4.6B). If this is not clearly noted, application of light pressure towards the floor on the lower third of the thigh will produce a compensatory extension of the lower leg only when rectus femoris is short.

A slight degree (10–15°) of hip extension should be possible in this position, by pushing

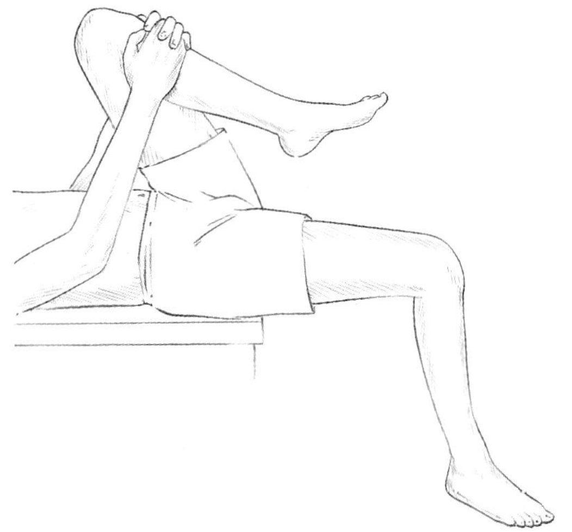

Figure 4.6A Test position for shortness of hip flexors. Note that the hip on the non-tested side must be fully flexed to produce full pelvic rotation. The position shown is normal.

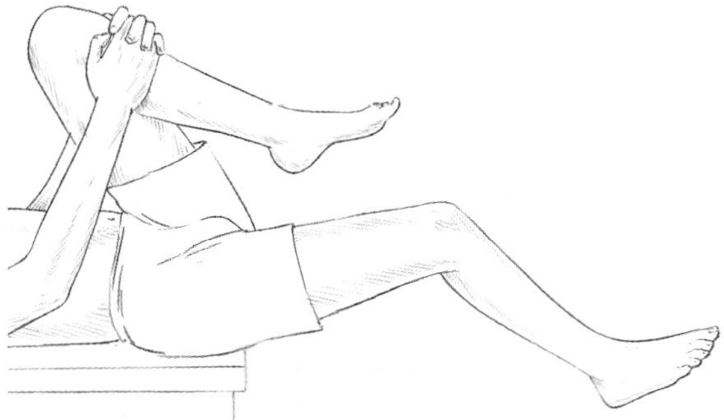

Figure 4.6B In the test position, if the thigh is elevated (i.e. not parallel with the table) probable psoas shortness is indicated. The inability of the lower leg to hang more or less vertically towards the floor indicates probable rectus femoris shortness (TFL shortness can produce a similar effect).

downwards on the thigh, without knee extension occurring. This can subsequently be checked by seeing whether or not the heel on that side can easily flex to touch the buttock of the prone patient (if rectus is short heel will not easily reach the buttock). If effort is required to achieve 10° of hip extension, this confirms iliopsoas shortening on that side. If both psoas and rectus are short, rectus should be treated first.

If the thigh hangs down below a parallel position, this indicates a degree of laxity in iliopsoas (Fig. 4.6C).

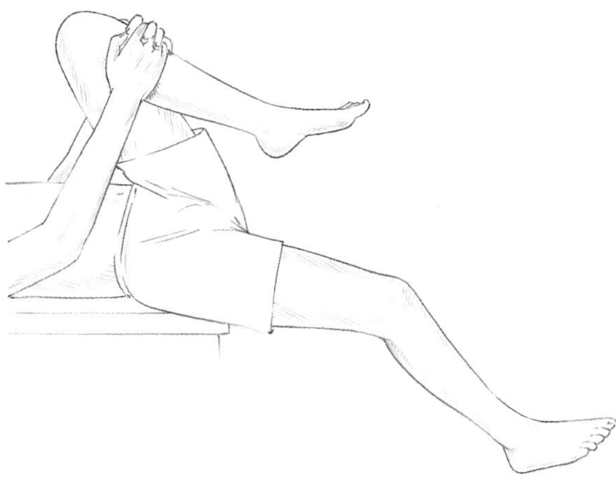

Figure 4.6C The fall of the thigh below the horizontal indicates hypotonic psoas status. Rectus femoris is once again seen to be short, while the relative external rotation of the lower leg (see angle of foot) hints at probable shortened TFL involvement.

A further cause of failure of the thigh to rest parallel to the floor can be due to shortness of tensor fascia lata. If this structure is short (a further test proves it, see later in this chapter) then there should be an obvious groove apparent on the lateral thigh and the patella, and sometimes the whole lower leg will deviate laterally.

A further indication of short psoas is seen if the prone patient's hip is observed to remain in flexion. In this position passive flexion of the knee will result in compensatory lumbar lordosis and increased hip flexion if rectus femoris is also short. (See also functional assessment method for psoas in Ch. 5 and notes on psoas in Box 4.4.)

Mitchell's strength test

Before using MET methods to normalise a short psoas, Mitchell recommends that you have the patient at the end of the table, both legs hanging down and feet turned in so that they can rest on your lateral calf areas as you stand facing the patient.

The patient should press firmly against your calves with her feet as you rest your hands on her thighs and she attempts to lift you from the floor. In this way you assess the relative strength of one leg's effort, as against the other.

Judge which psoas is weaker or stronger than the other. If a psoas has tested short (as in the test described earlier in this chapter) and also tests strong in this test, then it is suitable for MET treatment, according to Mitchell. If it tests short and weak, then other factors such as tight erector spinae muscles should be treated first until psoas tests strong and short, at which time MET should be applied to start the lengthening process.

It is worth recalling Norris's (1999) advice that a slowly performed isotonic eccentric exercise will normally strengthen a weak postural muscle. (Psoas is classified as postural, and a mobiliser, depending on the model being used. Richardson et al (1999) describe psoas as 'an exception' to their deep/superficial rule since, 'it is designed to act exclusively on the hip'. There is therefore universal agreement that psoas will shorten in response to stress.)

NOTE: It has been found to be clinically useful to suggest that before treating a shortened psoas, any shortness in rectus femoris on that side should first be treated.

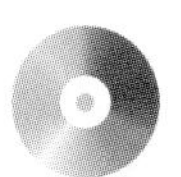

MET treatment for shortness of rectus femoris

Patient lies prone, ideally with a cushion under the abdomen to help avoid hyperlordosis. The practitioner stands on the side of the table of the affected leg so that he can stabilise the patient's pelvis (hand covering sacral area) during the treatment, using the cephalad hand. The affected leg is flexed at hip and knee.

The practitioner can either hold the lower leg at the ankle (as in Fig. 4.7), or the upper leg can be cradled so that the hand curls under the lower thigh and is able to palpate for bind, just above the knee, with the practitioner's upper arm offering resistance to the lower leg.

Either of these holds allows flexion of the knee to the barrier, perceived either as increasing effort, or as palpated bind.

If rectus femoris is short, then the patient's heel will not easily be able to touch the buttock (Fig. 4.7).

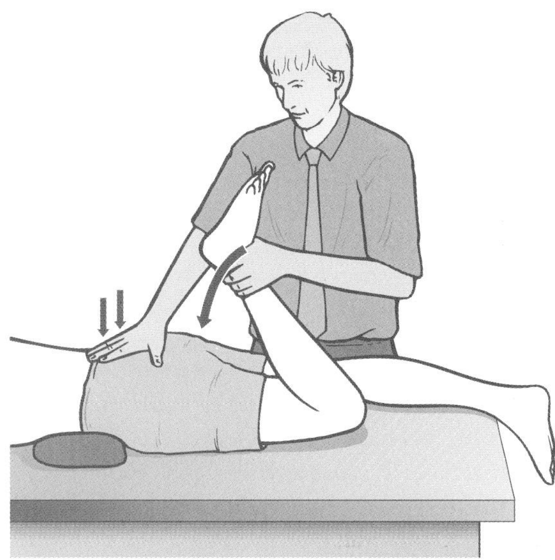

Figure 4.7 MET treatment of left rectus femoris muscle. Note the practitioner's right hand stabilises the sacrum and pelvis to prevent undue stress during the stretching phase of the treatment.

Once the restriction barrier has been established (how close can the heel get to the buttock before the barrier is noted?) the decision will have been made as to whether to treat this as an acute problem (from the barrier), or as a chronic problem (short of the barrier).

Appropriate degrees of resisted isometric effort are then introduced. For an acute problem a mild 15% of MVC (maximum voluntary contraction), or a longer, stronger (up to 25% of MVC) effort for a chronic problem, is used as the patient tries to both straighten the leg and take the thigh towards the table (this activates both ends of rectus).

Appropriate breathing instructions should be given (see notes on breathing earlier in this chapter, Box 4.2).

The contraction is followed, on an exhalation, by taking of the muscle to, or stretching through, the new barrier, by taking the heel towards the buttock with the patient's help. Remember to increase slight hip extension before the next contraction (using a cushion to support the thigh) as this removes slack from the cephalad end of rectus femoris.

Repeat once or twice using agonists or antagonists.

Once a reasonable degree of increased range has been gained in rectus femoris it is appropriate to treat psoas, if this has tested as short.

MET treatment of psoas

Method (a) (Fig. 4.8) Psoas can be treated in the prone position described for rectus above, in which case the stretch following the patient's isometric effort to bring the thigh to the table against resistance would be concentrated on extension of the thigh, either to the new barrier of resistance if acute or past the barrier, placing stretch on psoas, if chronic.

The patient is prone with a pillow under the abdomen to reduce the lumbar curve. The practitioner stands on the side opposite the side of psoas to be treated, with the table-side hand supporting the thigh. The non-table-side hand is placed so that the heel of that hand is on the sacrum, applying pressure towards the floor, to maintain pelvic stability (see also Fig. 4.11A).

The fingers of that hand are placed so that the middle, ring and small fingers are on one side of L2/3 segment and the index finger on the other. This allows these fingers to sense a forwards (anteriorly directed) 'tug' of the vertebrae when psoas is stretched past its barrier. (An alternative hand position is offered by Greenman (1996) who suggests that the stabilising contact on the pelvis should apply pressure towards the table, on the ischial tuberosity, as thigh extension is introduced. The author agrees that this is a more comfortable contact than the sacrum. However, it fails to allow access to palpation of the lumbar spine during the procedure.)

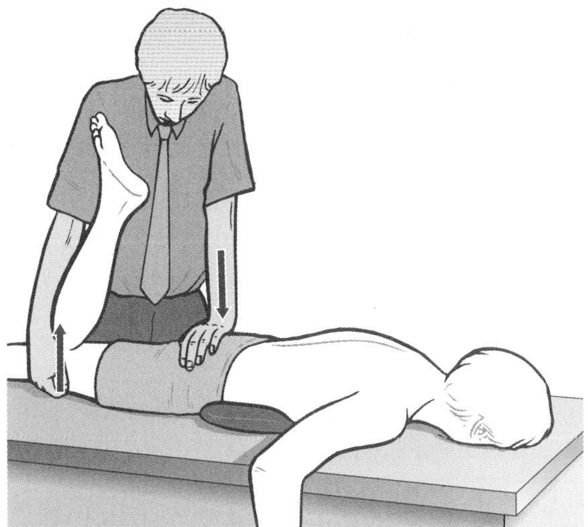

Figure 4.8 MET treatment of psoas with stabilising contact on ischial tuberosity as described by Greenman (1996).

The practitioner eases the thigh (knee is flexed) off the table surface and senses for ease of movement into extension of the hip. If there is a strong sense of resistance there should be an almost simultaneous awareness of the palpated vertebral segment moving anteriorly.

It should – if psoas is normal – be possible to achieve approximately 10° of hip extension before that barrier is reached, without force. Greenman (1996) suggests that 'Normally the knee can be lifted 6 inches [15 cm] off the table. If less, tightness and shortness of psoas is present.'

Having identified the barrier, the practitioner either works from this (in an acute setting) or short of it (in a chronic setting) as the patient is asked to bring the thigh towards the table against resistance, using 15–25% of their maximal voluntary contraction potential, for 7–10 seconds.

Following release of the effort (with appropriate breathing assistance if warranted), the thigh is eased to its new barrier if acute, or past that barrier, into stretch (with patient's assistance, 'gently push your foot towards the ceiling').

If stretch is introduced, this is held for not less than 10 seconds and ideally up to 30 seconds.

It is important that as stretch is introduced no hyperextension occurs of the lumbar spine. Pressure from the heel of hand on the sacrum can usually ensure that spinal stability is maintained.

The process is then repeated.

Method (b) (Fig. 4.9A) Grieve's method involves using the supine test position, in which the patient lies with the buttocks at the very end of the table, non-treated leg fully flexed at hip and knee and either held in that state by the patient, or by placement of the patient's foot against the practitioner's lateral chest wall. The leg on the affected side is allowed to hang freely with the medioplantar aspect resting on the practitioner's far knee or shin.

The practitioner stands sideways on to the patient, at the foot of the table, with both hands

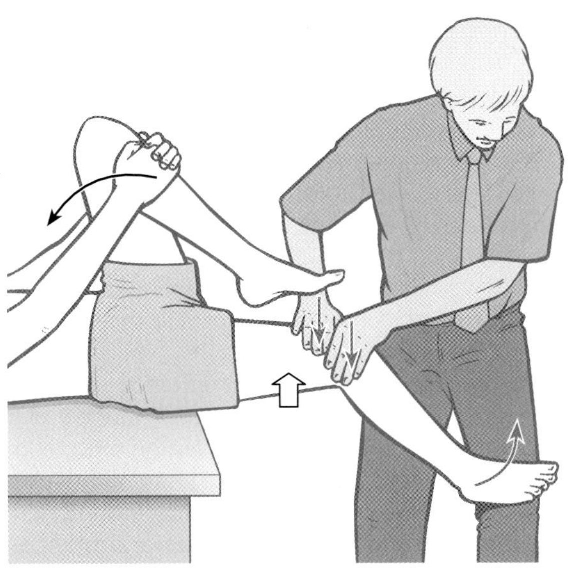

Figure 4.9A MET treatment of psoas using Grieve's method, in which there is placement of the patient's foot, inverted, against the practitioner's thigh. This allows a more precise focus of contraction into psoas when the hip is flexed against resistance.

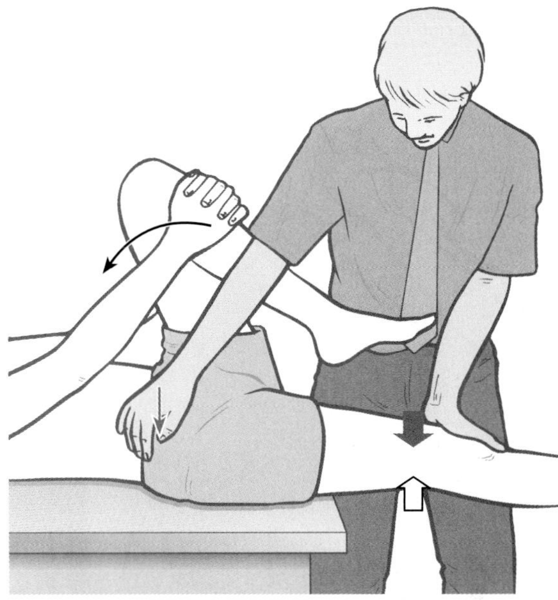

Figure 4.9B Psoas treatment variation, with the leg held straight and the pelvis stabilised.

holding the thigh of the extended leg. The practitioner's far leg should be flexed slightly at the knee so that the patient's foot can rest as described. This is used as a contact which, with the hands, resists the attempt of the patient to *externally rotate the leg* and, at the same time, *flex the hip*.

The practitioner resists both efforts, and an isometric contraction of the psoas and associated muscles therefore takes place.

This combination of forces focuses the contraction effort into psoas very precisely.

Appropriate breathing instructions should be given (see notes on breathing, Box 4.2).

If the condition is acute, the treatment of the patient's leg commences from the restriction barrier, whereas if the condition is chronic, the leg is elevated into a somewhat more flexed position.

After the isometric contraction, using an appropriate degree of effort (i.e. is this acute or chronic?), the thigh should, on an exhalation, either be taken to the new restriction barrier, without force (acute), or through that barrier with slight, painless pressure towards the floor on the anterior aspect of the thigh (chronic), and held there for 10–30 seconds (see Fig 4.10B; see also variation Fig. 4.9B).

Repeat until no further gain is achieved.[3]

Method (c) (Figs. 4.10A, B) This method is appropriate for chronic psoas problems only. The supine test position is used in which the patient lies with the buttocks at the very end of the table, non-treated leg fully flexed at hip and knee and either held in that state by the patient (Fig 4.10A), or by the practitioner's hand (Fig 4.7B), or by placement of the patient's foot against the practitioner's lateral chest wall. The leg on the affected side is allowed to hang freely.

The practitioner resists (for 7–10 seconds) a light attempt of the patient to flex the hip.

Appropriate breathing instructions should be given (see notes on breathing, Box 4.2).

After the isometric contraction, using an appropriate degree of effort, the thigh should, on an exhalation, be taken very slightly beyond the restriction barrier, with a light degree of painless pressure towards the floor, and held there for 10–30 seconds (Fig. 4.10B).

Repeat until no further gain is achieved.[3]

[3] Direct inhibitory pressure techniques applied the vertebral attachments of psoas through the mid-line is an effective alternative approach, especially in acute psoas conditions. This is not usually applicable in overweight individuals.

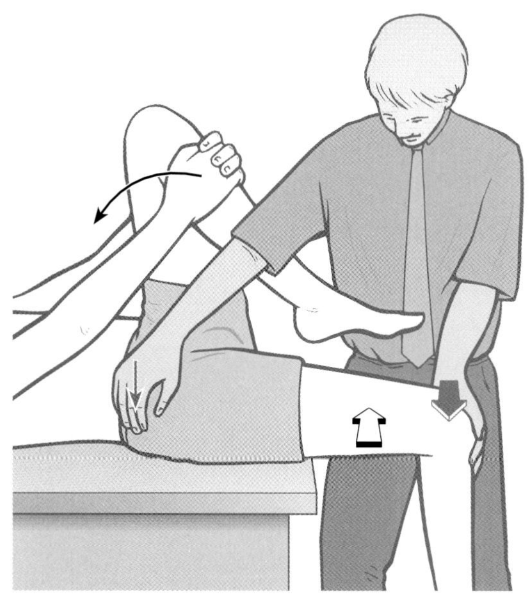

Figure 4.10A MET treatment involves the patient's effort to flex the hip against resistance.

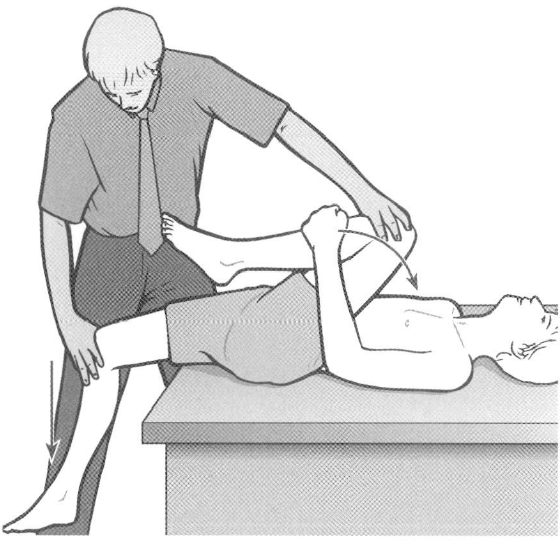

Figure 4.10B Stretch of psoas, which follows the isometric contraction (Fig. 4.10A) and is achieved by means of gravity plus additional practitioner effort.

Self-treatment of psoas

Method (a) Lewit suggests self-treatment in a position as above in which the patient lies close to the end of a bed (Fig 4.10A without the practitioner) with one leg fully flexed at the hip and knee and held in this position throughout, while the other leg is allowed to reach the limit of its stretch, as gravity pulls it towards the floor.

The patient then lifts this leg slightly (say 2 cm) to contract psoas, holding this for 7–10 seconds, before slowly allowing the leg to ease towards the floor.

This stretch position is held for a further 30 seconds, and the process is repeated three to five times.

The counterpressure in this effort is achieved by gravity.

Method (b) Patient kneels on leg on side to be self-stretched so that the knee is behind the trunk, which remains vertical throughout. The non-treated side leg is placed anteriorly, knee flexed to 90°, foot flat on floor. The patient maintains a slight lumbar lordosis throughout the procedure as she lightly contracts psoas by drawing the treated side knee anteriorly (i.e. flexing the hip) without actually moving it.

Resistance to this isometric movement is provided by the knee contact with the (carpeted) floor.

After 7–10 seconds the patient releases this effort, and while maintaining a lumbar lordosis and vertical trunk, eases her pelvis and trunk anteriorly to initiate a sense of stretch on the anterior thigh and hip area.

This is maintained for not less than 30 seconds before a further movement anteriorly of the pelvis and trunk introduces additional psoas stretch (see also Fig. 4.11B).

4. Assessment and treatment of hamstrings

Should obviously tight hamstrings always be treated? Van Wingerden (1997), reporting on the earlier work of Vleeming (Vleeming et al 1989), states that both intrinsic and extrinsic support for the sacroiliac joint derives in part from hamstring (biceps femoris) status. Intrinsically the influence is via the close anatomical and physiological relationship between biceps femoris and the sacrotuberous ligament (they frequently attach via a strong tendinous link): 'Force from the biceps

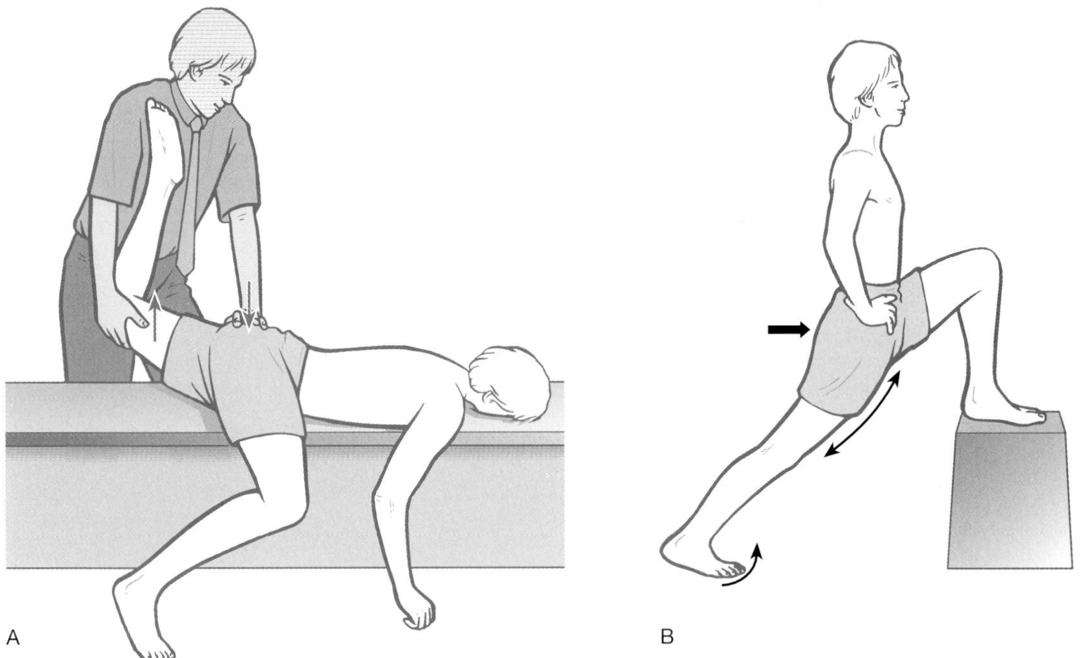

Figure 4.11 **A** Alternative prone treatment position, not described in text (see also Fig. 4.8). **B** Psoas self-stretch, not described in text.

femoris muscle can lead to increased tension of the sacrotuberous ligament in various ways. Since increased tension of the sacrotuberous ligament diminishes the range of sacroiliac joint motion, the biceps femoris can play a role in stabilisation of the SIJ.'

He also notes that in low back patients, forward flexion is often painful as the load on the spine increases. This happens whether flexion occurs in the spine or via the hip joints (tilting of the pelvis). If the hamstrings are tight and short they effectively prevent pelvic tilting. 'In this respect, an increase in hamstring tension might well be part of a defensive arthrokinematic reflex mechanism of the body to diminish spinal load.' If such a state of affairs is long-standing, the hamstrings (biceps femoris) will shorten, possibly influencing sacroiliac and lumbar spine dysfunction.

The decision to treat tight ('tethered') hamstrings should therefore take account of *why it is tight*, and consider that in some circumstances it might be offering beneficial support to the SIJ or be reducing low back stress.

Assessment for shortness in hamstrings (07) (Fig. 4.12A, B)

If the hip flexors (psoas, etc.) have previously tested as short, then the test position for the hamstrings needs to commence with the non-tested leg flexed at knee and hip, foot resting flat on the treatment surface to ensure full pelvic rotation into neutral (as in Fig 4.12B). If no hip flexor shortness was observed, then the non-tested leg should lie flat on the surface of the table.

Hamstring test (a) The patient lies supine with non-tested leg either flexed or straight, depending on previous test results for hip flexors.

The tested leg is taken into a straight leg raised (SLR) position, no flexion of the knee being allowed, with minimal force employed. The first sign of resistance (or palpated bind) is assessed as the barrier of restriction.

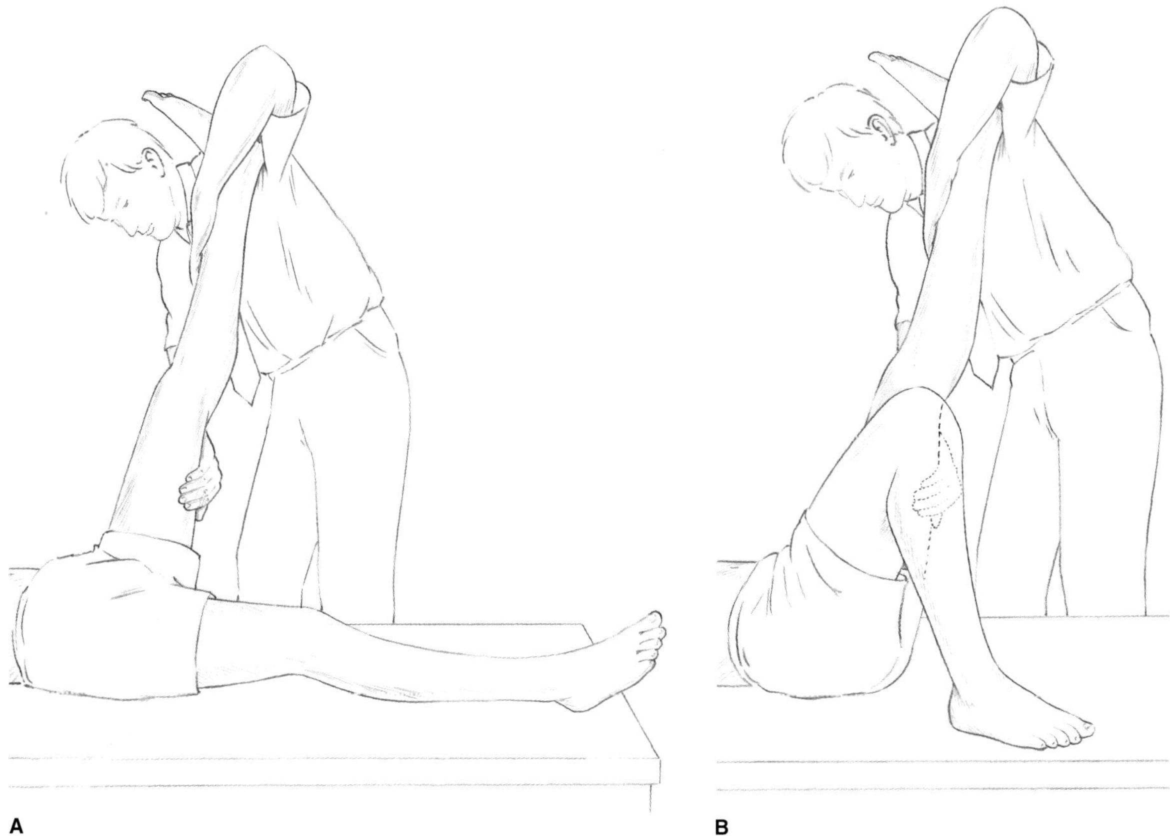

Figure 4.12 (**A**) Assessment for shortness in hamstring muscles. The practitioner's right hand palpates for bind/the first sign of resistance, while the left hand maintains the patient's knee in extension. (**B**) MET treatment of shortened hamstrings. Following an isometric contraction, the leg is taken to or through the resistance barrier (depending on whether the problem is acute or chronic).

If straight leg raising to 80° is not easily possible, then there exists some shortening of the hamstrings and the muscles can be treated in the leg straight position (see below).

Hamstring test (b) (Fig. 4.13) Whether or not an 80° elevation is easily achieved, a variation in testing is also needed to evaluate the lower fibres. To make this assessment the tested leg is taken into *full* hip flexion (helped by patient holding upper thigh with both hands (see Fig. 4.13). The knee is then straightened until resistance is felt or bind is noted by palpation of the lower hamstrings.

If the knee cannot straighten with the hip flexed, this indicates shortness in the lower hamstring fibres and the patient will report a degree of pull behind the knee and lower thigh. Treatment of this is carried out in the test position.

If, however, the knee is capable of being straightened with the hip flexed, having previously not been capable of achieving an 80° straight leg raise, then the lower fibres are cleared of shortness and it is the upper fibres of hamstrings which require attention using MET, working from the SLR test position.

Hamstring test (c) Lewit (1999) describes a functional test (see also Fig. 5.10B) which helps to screen for overactivity in the erector spinae and/or hamstrings, indicating also weakness of gluteus maximus.

The patient is prone and the practitioner places palpating hands on the lower buttock/upper

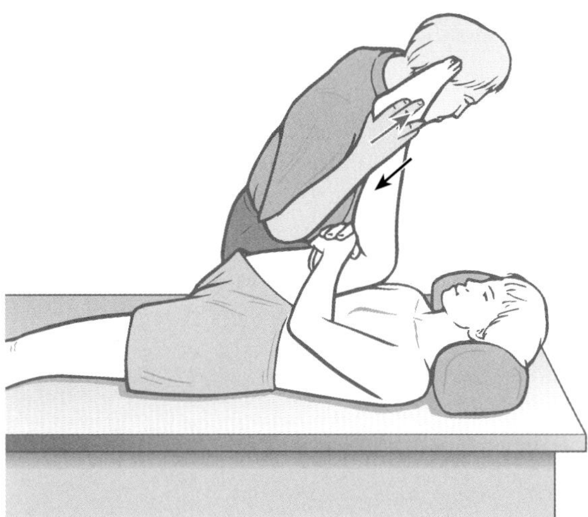

Figure 4.13 Assessment and treatment position for lower hamstring fibres.

thigh (gluteal/hamstring contact) and the low back (erector spinae contact) as the patient is asked to extend the hip, leg kept straight.

The normal sequence is for the hamstrings to commence the elevation of the thigh with almost instant gluteal involvement, followed by the erectors. If gluteus maximus is weak (see lower crossed syndrome notes in Ch. 2) there may still be strong extension of the thigh, but with the hamstrings and erectors doing most of the work. This is an indication of overactivity (i.e. stress) in these postural muscles and therefore suggests shortness.

In extreme cases the movement of thigh/hip extension is initiated by the erector spinae themselves, and these are then almost certainly short.[4]

MET for shortness of lower hamstrings

If the lower hamstring fibres are implicated as being short (see hamstring test (b) above), then the treatment position is identical to the test position.

This means that the non-treated leg needs to be either flexed or straight on the table, depending upon whether hip flexors have previously been shown to be short or not (see above), and the treated leg needs to be flexed at both the hip and knee, and then straightened by the practitioner until the restriction barrier is identified (one hand should palpate the tissues behind the knee for sensations of bind as the lower leg is straightened).

Depending upon whether it is an acute situation or a chronic problem, the isometric contraction against resistance is introduced at this 'bind' barrier (if acute) or a little short of it (if chronic). The instruction might be something such as 'try to gently bend your knee, against my resistance, starting slowly and using only a quarter of your strength'. (It is particularly important with the hamstrings to take care regarding cramp, and so it is suggested that no more than 25% of patients' effort should ever be used during isometric contractions in this region.)

Following the 7–10 seconds of contraction (holding the breath if possible, see Box 4.2) followed by complete relaxation, the leg should, on an exhalation, be straightened at the knee towards its new barrier (in acute problems) and through that barrier, with a degree of stretch (if chronic), with the patient's assistance. This slight stretch should be held for not less than 10 (and up to 30) seconds.

Repeat the process until no further gain is possible (usually one or two repetitions achieve the maximum degree of lengthening available at any one session).

Antagonist muscles can also be used isometrically by having the patient try to extend the knee during the contraction rather than bending it, followed by the same stretch as would be adopted if the agonist (affected muscle) had been employed.

MET for shortness of upper hamstrings

If the upper fibres are involved (i.e. hamstring test (a) above), then treatment is performed in the straight leg raised (SLR) position, with the knee maintained in extension at all times. The other leg should be flexed at hip and knee or straight,

[4] Extension of the hip is a normal part of the gait cycle and therefore a movement which is usually made thousands of times daily. It is easy to imagine the degree of overuse stress (and therefore ultimately shortness) in hamstrings which are compensating for the weakness in the gluteal muscles. If this pattern exists the hamstrings can be assumed to be short and out of balance with their synergists and likely to benefit from MET.

depending on the hip flexor findings as explained above. In all other details the procedures are the same as for treatment of lower hamstring fibres except that the leg is kept straight.

Alternative methods

An alternative position for treatment of hamstrings is for the supine patient to flex the affected hip fully. The flexed knee is extended by the practitioner to the point of resistance (identifying the barrier). The calf of the lower leg is placed on the shoulder of the practitioner, who stands facing the head of the table on the side of the treated leg.

If the right leg of the patient is being treated, the calf will rest on the practitioner's right shoulder, and the practitioner's right hand stabilises the patient's extended unaffected leg against the table. The practitioner's left hand holds the treated leg thigh to both maintain stability and to palpate for bind when the barrier is being assessed.

The patient is asked to attempt to straighten the lower leg (i.e. extend the knee) utilising the antagonists to the hamstrings, employing 20% of the strength in the quadriceps. This is resisted by the practitioner for 7–10 seconds.

Appropriate breathing instructions should be given (see notes on breathing, Box 4.2).

The leg is then extended at the knee to its new hamstring limit if the problem is acute (or stretched slightly if chronic) after relaxation and the procedure is then repeated.

Or

In this same position, the patient may attempt to flex the knee against resistance, thus employing the hamstrings isometrically for 7–10 seconds (with appropriate breathing, see Box 4.2).

After relaxation, the muscles are taken further to or through their new barrier (depending upon whether the problem is acute or chronic).

Or

Starting from the same position, a combined contraction may be introduced (Moore et al 1980). The instruction to the patient would be to pull the thigh towards her own face (i.e. to flex the hip) and to push the lower leg downward onto the practitioner's shoulder (i.e. flexing the knee).

This effectively contracts both the quadriceps and the hamstrings, thus inducing both postisometric relaxation and reciprocal inhibition, which facilitates, on an exhalation, subsequent easing to, or stretching through, the restriction barrier of the tight hamstrings.

5. Assessment and treatment of tensor fascia lata (see also Box 4.5)

Assessment of shortness in tensor fascia lata (TFL) (08)

The test recommended is a modified form of Ober's test (see Fig. 4.14).

Patient is side-lying with back close to the edge of the table. The practitioner stands behind the patient, whose lower leg is flexed at hip and knee and held in this position, by the patient, for stability. The tested leg is supported by the practitioner, who must ensure that there is *no hip flexion*, which would nullify the test.

The leg is extended only to the point where the iliotibial band lies over the greater trochanter. The tested leg is held by the practitioner at ankle and knee, with the whole leg in its anatomical position, neither abducted nor adducted and not forward or backward of the body.

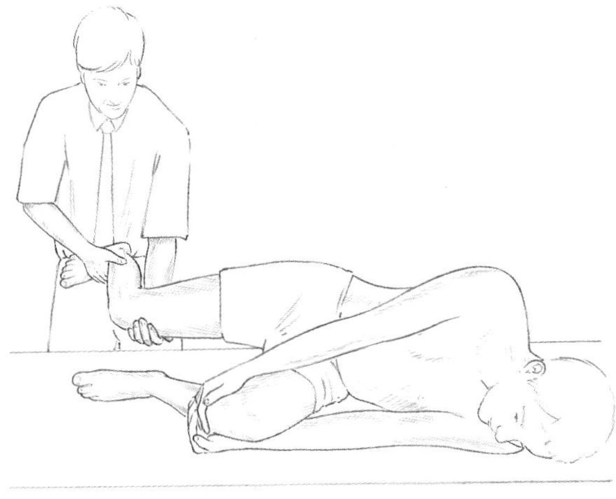

Figure 4.14 Assessment for shortness of TFL – modified Ober's test. When the hand supporting the flexed knee is removed the thigh should fall to the table if TFL is not short.

Box 4.5 Notes on TFL

- Mennell (1964) and Liebenson (1996) say that TFL shortness can produce all the symptoms of acute and chronic sacroiliac problems.
- Pain from TFL shortness can be localised to the posterior superior iliac spine (PSIS), radiating to the groin or down any aspect of the thigh to the knee.
- Although the pain may arise in the sacroiliac (SI) joint, dysfunction in the joint may be caused and maintained by taut TFL structures.
- Pain from the band itself can be felt in the lateral thigh, with referral to hip or knee.
- TFL can be 'riddled' with sensitive fibrotic deposits and trigger point activity.
- There is commonly a posteriority of the ilium associated with short TFL.
- TFL's prime phasic activity (all postural structures also have some phasic function) is to assist the gluteals in abduction of the thigh.
- If TFL and psoas are short they may, according to Janda, 'dominate' the gluteals on abduction of the thigh, so that a degree of lateral rotation and flexion of the hip will be produced, rotating the pelvis backwards.
- Rolf (1977) points out that persistent exercise such as cycling will shorten and toughen the fascial iliotibial band 'until it becomes reminiscent of a steel cable'. This band crosses both hip and knee, and spatial compression allows it to squeeze and compress cartilaginous elements such as the menisci. Ultimately, it will no longer be able to compress, and rotational displacement at knee and hip will take place.

The practitioner carefully introduces flexion at the knee to 90°, without allowing the hip to flex, and then, holding just the ankle, allows the knee to fall towards the table.

If TFL is normal, the thigh and knee will fall easily, with the knee contacting the table surface (unless unusual hip width, or thigh length prevent this). If the upper leg remains aloft, with little sign of 'falling' towards the table, then either the patient is not letting go or the TFL is short and does not allow it to fall. As a rule the band will palpate as tender under such conditions.

Lewit's TFL palpation (Lewit 1999; see also functional assessment method in Ch. 5)

Patient is side-lying and practitioner stands facing the patient's front, at hip level. The practitioner's cephalad hand rests over the anterior superior iliac spine (ASIS) so that it can also palpate over the trochanter. It should be placed so that the fingers rest on the TFL and trochanter with the thumb on gluteus medius. The caudad hand rests on the mid-thigh to apply slight resistance to the patient's effort to abduct the leg.

The patient's table-side leg is slightly flexed to provide stability, and there should be a vertical line to the table between one ASIS and the other (i.e. no forwards or backwards 'roll' of the pelvis).

The patient abducts the upper leg (which should be extended at the knee and slightly hyperextended at the hip) and the practitioner should feel the trochanter 'slip away' as this is done.

If, however, the whole pelvis is felt to move rather than just the trochanter, there is inappropriate muscular imbalance. (In balanced abduction gluteus comes into action at the beginning of the movement, with TFL operating later in the pure abduction of the leg. If there is an overactivity (and therefore shortness) of TFL, then there will be pelvic movement on the abduction, and TFL will be felt to come into play before gluteus.) The abduction of the thigh movement will then be modified to include external rotation and flexion of the thigh (Janda 1996). This confirms a stressed postural structure (TFL), which implies shortness.

It is possible to increase the number of palpation elements involved by having the cephalad hand also palpate (with an extended small finger) quadratus lumborum during leg abduction.

In a balanced muscular effort to lift the leg sideways, quadratus should not become active until the leg has been abducted to around 25–30°. When quadratus is overactive it will often start the abduction along with TFL, thus producing a pelvic tilt.[5] (See also Fig. 5.11A and B.)

[5] Remember that a lateral 'corset' of muscles exists to stabilise the pelvic and low back structures and that if TFL and quadratus (and/or psoas) shorten and tighten, the gluteal muscles will weaken. This test gives the proof of such imbalance existing. (See notes on lower crossed syndrome in Ch. 2.)

Method (a) Supine MET treatment of shortened TFL (Fig. 4.15) The patient lies supine with the unaffected leg flexed at hip and knee. The affected side leg is adducted to its barrier which necessitates it being brought under the opposite leg/foot.

Using guidelines for acute and chronic problems, the structure will either be treated at, or short of, the barrier of resistance, using light or fairly strong isometric contractions for short (7 second) or long (up to 20 seconds) durations, using appropriate breathing patterns as described earlier in this chapter (Box 4.2).

The practitioner uses his trunk to stabilise the patient's pelvis by leaning against the flexed (non-affected side) knee. The practitioner's caudad arm supports the affected leg so that the knee is stabilised by the hand. The other hand maintains a stabilising contact on the affected side ASIS.

The patient is asked to abduct the leg against resistance using minimal force. After the contraction ceases and the patient has relaxed using appropriate breathing patterns, the leg is taken to or through the new restriction barrier (into adduction past the barrier) to stretch the muscular fibres of TFL (the upper third of the structure).

Care should be taken to ensure that the pelvis is not tilted during the stretch. Stability is achieved by the practitioner increasing pressure against the flexed knee/thigh.

This whole process is repeated until no further gain is possible.

Method (b) Alternative supine MET treatment of shortened TFL (Fig. 4.16) The patient adopts the same position as for psoas assessment, lying at the end of the table with non-tested side leg in full hip flexion and held by the patient, with the tested leg hanging freely, knee flexed.

The practitioner stands at the end of the table facing the patient so that his left lower leg (for a right-sided TFL treatment) can contact the patient's foot. The practitioner's left hand is placed on the patient's distal femur and with this he introduces internal rotation of the thigh, and external rotation of the tibia (by means of light pressure on the distal foot from his lower leg).

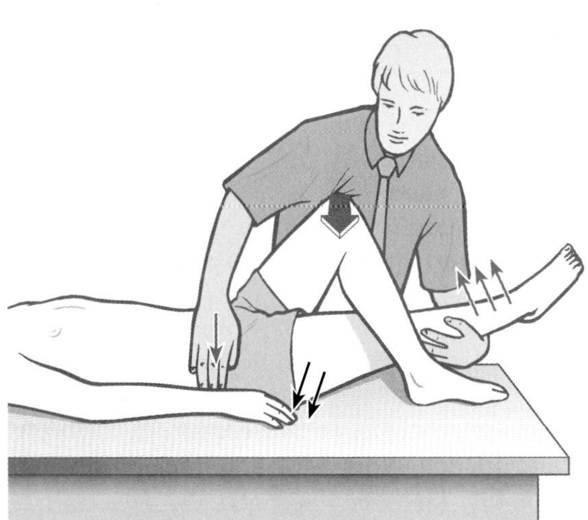

Figure 4.15 MET treatment of TFL (see Fig. 1.4 for description of isolytic variation). If a standard MET method is being used, the stretch will follow the isometric contraction in which the patient will attempt to move the right leg to the right against sustained resistance. It is important for the practitioner to maintain stability of the pelvis during the procedure. Note: the hand positions in this figure are a variation of those described in the text.

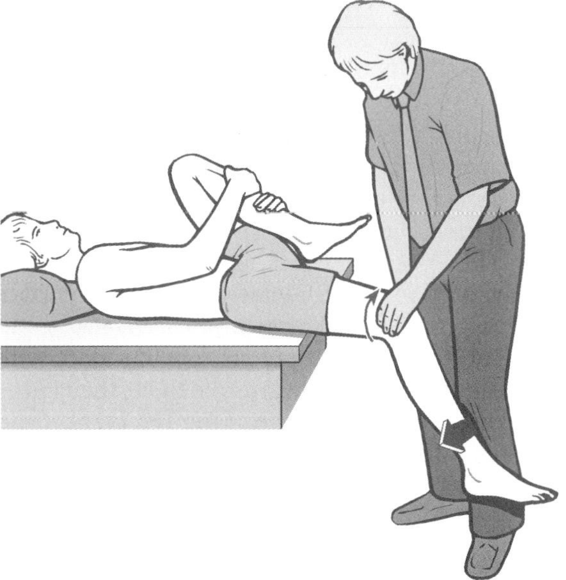

Figure 4.16 MET treatment of psoas using Grieve's method, in which there is placement of the patient's foot, inverted, against the operator's thigh. This allows a more precise focus of contraction into psoas when the hip is flexed against resistance.

During this process the practitioner senses for resistance (the movement should have an easy 'springy' feel, not wooden or harsh) and observes for a characteristic depression or groove on the lateral thigh, indicating shortness of TFL.

This resistance barrier is identified and the leg held just short of it for a chronic problem, as the patient is asked to externally rotate the tibia, and to adduct the femur, against resistance, for 7–10 seconds.

Following this the practitioner eases the leg into a greater degree of internal hip rotation and external tibial rotation, and holds this stretch for 10–30 seconds.

Method (c) Isolytic variation If an isolytic contraction is introduced in order to stretch actively the interface between elastic and non-elastic tissues, then there is a need to stabilise the pelvis more efficiently, either by use of wide straps or another pair of hands holding the ASIS downwards towards the table during the stretch.

The procedure consists of the patient attempting to abduct the leg as the practitioner overcomes the muscular effort, forcing the leg into adduction. The contraction/stretch should be rapid (2–3 seconds at most to complete).

Repeat several times.

Method (d) Side-lying MET treatment of TFL The patient lies on the affected TFL side with the upper leg flexed at hip and knee and resting forward of the affected leg. The practitioner stands behind patient and uses caudad hand and arm to raise the affected leg (which is on the table) while stabilising the pelvis with the cephalad hand, or uses both hands to raise the affected leg into slight adduction (appropriate if strapping used to hold pelvis to table).

The patient contracts the muscle against resistance by trying to take the leg into abduction (towards the table) using breathing assistance as appropriate (see notes on breathing, Box 4.2).

After the effort, on an exhalation, the practitioner lifts the leg into adduction beyond the barrier to stretch the interface between elastic and non-elastic tissues.

Repeat as appropriate or modify to use as an isolytic contraction by stretching the structure past the barrier during the contraction.

Additional TFL methods

Mennell has described superb soft tissue stretching techniques for releasing TFL. These involve a series of snapping actions applied by thumbs to the anterior fibres with patient side-lying, followed by a series of heel of hand thrusts across the long axis of the posterior TFL fibres.

Additional release of TFL contractions is possible by use of elbow or heel of hand 'stripping' of the structure, neuromuscular deep tissue approaches (using thumb or a rubber-tipped T-bar) applied to the upper fibres and those around the knee, and specific deep tissue release methods. Most of these are distinctly uncomfortable and all require expert tuition.[6]

Self-treatment and maintenance

The patient lies on her side, on a bed or table, with the affected leg uppermost and hanging over the edge (lower leg comfortably flexed). The patient may then introduce an isometric contraction by slightly lifting the hanging leg a few centimeters, and holding this position for 10 seconds, before slowly releasing and allowing gravity to take the leg towards the floor, so introducing a greater degree of stretch. This is held for up to 30 seconds and the process is then repeated several times in order to achieve the maximum available stretch in the tight soft tissues. The counterforce in this isometric exercise is gravity.

6. Assessment and treatment of piriformis (see also Boxes 4.6 and 4.7)

Assessment of shortened piriformis (09)

Test (a) Stretch test When short, piriformis will cause the affected side leg of the supine patient to appear to be short and externally rotated.

With the patient supine, the tested leg is placed into flexion at the hip and knee so that the foot rests on the table lateral to the contralateral knee

---

[6] Many of these methods are described and illustrated in *Modern Neuromuscular Techniques* (1996) by the author, published by Churchill Livingstone, Edinburgh.

(the tested leg is crossed over the straight non-tested leg, in other words as shown in Fig. 4.17). The angle of hip flexion should not exceed 60° (see notes on piriformis in Box 4.6).

The non-tested side ASIS is stabilised to prevent pelvic motion during the test and the knee of the tested side is pushed into adduction to place a stretch on piriformis.

If there is a short piriformis the degree of adduction will be limited and the patient will report discomfort behind the trochanter.

Test (b) Palpation test (Fig. 4.18) The patient is side-lying, tested side uppermost. The practitioner stands at the level of the pelvis in front of and facing the patient, and, in order to contact the insertion of piriformis, draws imaginary lines between:

- ASIS and ischial tuberosity, and
- PSIS and the most prominent point of trochanter.

Where these reference lines cross, just posterior to the trochanter, is the insertion of the muscle, and pressure here will produce marked discomfort if the structure is short or irritated.

If the most common trigger point site in the belly of the muscle is sought, then the line from the ASIS should be taken to the tip of the coccyx rather than to the ischial tuberosity. Pressure where this line crosses the other will access the mid-point of the belly of piriformis where triggers are common. Light compression here which produces a painful response is indicative of a stressed muscle and possibly an active myofascial trigger point.

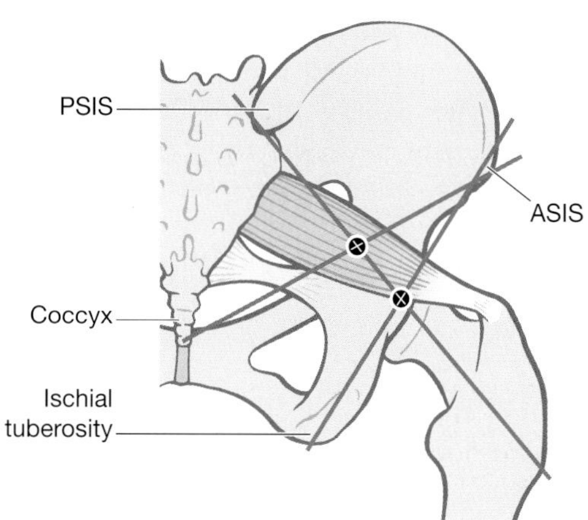

Figure 4.18 Using bony landmarks as coordinates the commonest tender areas are located in piriformis, in the belly and at the attachment of the muscle.

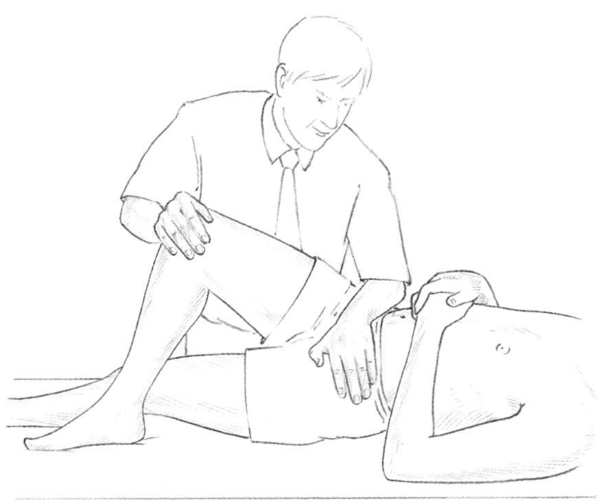

Figure 4.17 MET treatment of piriformis muscle with patient supine. The pelvis must be maintained in a stable position as the knee (right in this example) is adducted to stretch piriformis following an isometric contraction.

Piriformis strength test

The patient lies prone, both knees flexed to 90°, with practitioner at foot of table grasping lower legs at the limit of their separation (which internally rotates the hip and therefore allows comparison of range of movement permitted by shortened external rotators such as the piriformis).

The patient attempts to bring the ankles together as the practitioner assesses the relative strength of the two legs. Mitchell et al (1979) suggest that if there is relative shortness (as evidenced by the lower leg not being able to travel as far from the mid-line as its pair in this position), and if that same side also tests strong, then MET is called for. If there is shortness but also weakness then the reasons for the weakness need to be dealt with prior to stretching using MET.

Box 4.6 Notes on piriformis

- Piriformis paradox. The performance of external rotation of the hip by piriformis occurs when the angle of hip flexion is 60° or less. Once the angle of hip flexion is greater than 60° piriformis function changes, so that it becomes an internal rotator of the hip (Gluck & Liebenson 1997, Lehmkuhl & Smith 1983). The implications of this are illustrated in Figures 4.17 and 4.19.
- This postural muscle, like all others which have a predominence of type I fibres, will shorten if stressed. In the case of piriformis, the effect of shortening is to increase its diameter and because of its location this allows for direct pressure to be exerted on the sciatic nerve, which passes under it in 80% of people. In the other 20% the nerve passes through the muscle so that contraction will produce veritable strangulation of the sciatic nerve.
- In addition, the pudendal nerve and the blood vessels of the internal iliac artery, as well as common perineal nerves, posterior femoral cutaneous nerve and nerves of the hip rotators, can all be affected.
- If there is sciatic pain associated with piriformis shortness, then on straight leg raising, which reproduces the pain, external rotation of the hip should relieve it, since this slackens piriformis. (This clue may, however, only apply to any degree if the individual is one of those in whom the nerve actually passes through the muscle.)
- The effects can be circulatory, neurological and functional, inducing pain and paraesthesia of the affected limb as well as alterations to pelvic and lumbar function. Diagnosis usually hinges on the absence of spinal causative factors and the distributions of symptoms from the sacrum to the hip joint, over the gluteal region and down to the popliteal space. Palpation of the affected piriformis tendon, near the head of the trochanter, will elicit pain and the affected leg will probably be externally rotated.
- The piriformis muscle syndrome is frequently characterised by such bizarre symptoms that they may seem unrelated. One characteristic complaint is a persistent, severe, radiating low back pain extending from the sacrum to the hip joint, over the gluteal region and the posterior portion of the upper leg, to the popliteal space. In the most severe cases the patient will be unable to lie or stand comfortably, and changes in position will not relieve the pain. Intense pain will occur when the patient sits or squats since this type of movement requires external rotation of the upper leg and flexion at the knee.
- Compression of the pudendal nerve and blood vessels which pass through the greater sciatic foramen and re-enter the pelvis via the lesser sciatic foramen is possible because of piriformis contracture. Any compression would result in impaired circulation to the genitalia in both sexes. Since external rotation of the hips is required for coitus by women, pain noted during this act could relate to impaired circulation induced by piriformis dysfunction. This could also be a basis for impotency in men. (See also Box 4.7.)
- Piriformis involvement often relates to a pattern of pain which includes:
  - pain near the trochanter
  - pain in the inguinal area
  - local tenderness over the insertion behind trochanter
  - SI joint pain on the opposite side
  - externally rotated foot on the same side
  - pain unrelieved by most positions with standing and walking being the easiest
  - limitation of internal rotation of the leg which produces pain near the hip
  - short leg on the affected side.
- The pain itself will be persistent and radiating, covering anywhere from the sacrum to the buttock, hip and leg including inguinal and perineal areas.
- Bourdillon (1982) suggests that piriformis syndrome and SI joint dysfunction are intimately connected and that recurrent SI problems will not stabilise until hypertonic piriformis is corrected.
- Janda (1996) points to the vast amount of pelvic organ dysfunction to which piriformis can contribute due to its relationship with circulation to the area.
- Mitchell et al (1979) suggest that (as in psoas example above) piriformis shortness should only be treated if it is tested to be short and stronger than its pair. If it is short and weak (see p. 110 for strength test), then whatever is hypertonic and influencing it should be released and stretched first (Mitchell et al 1979). When it tests strong and short, piriformis should receive MET treatment.
- Since piriformis is an external rotator of the hip it can be inhibited (made to test weak) if an internal rotator such as TFL is hypertonic or if its pair is hypertonic, since one piriformis will inhibit the other.

Box 4.7 Working and resting muscles

Richard (1978) reminds us that a working muscle will mobilise up to 10 times the quantity of blood mobilised by a resting muscle. He points out the link between pelvic circulation and lumbar, ischiatic and gluteal arteries and the chance this allows to engineer the involvement of 2400 square metres of capillaries by using repetitive pumping of these muscles (including piriformis).

The therapeutic use of this knowledge involves the patient being asked to repetitively contract both piriformis muscles against resistance. The patient is supine, knees bent, feet on the table; the practitioner resists their effort to abduct their flexed knees, using pulsed muscle energy approach (Ruddy's method) in which two isometrically resisted pulsation/contractions per second are introduced for as long as possible (a minute seems a long time doing this).

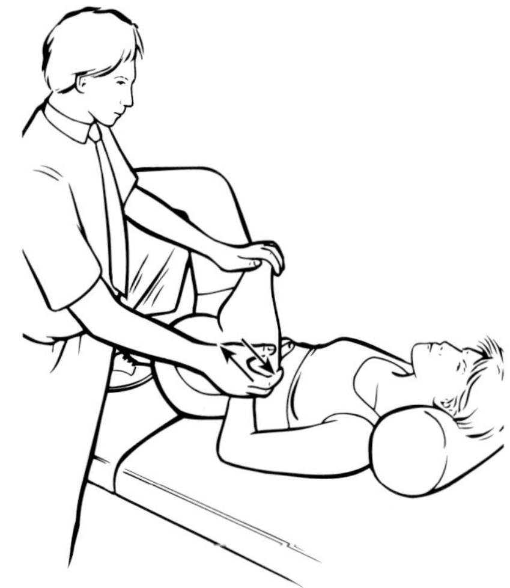

Figure 4.19 MET treatment of piriformis with hip fully flexed and externally rotated (see Box 4.6, first bullet point).

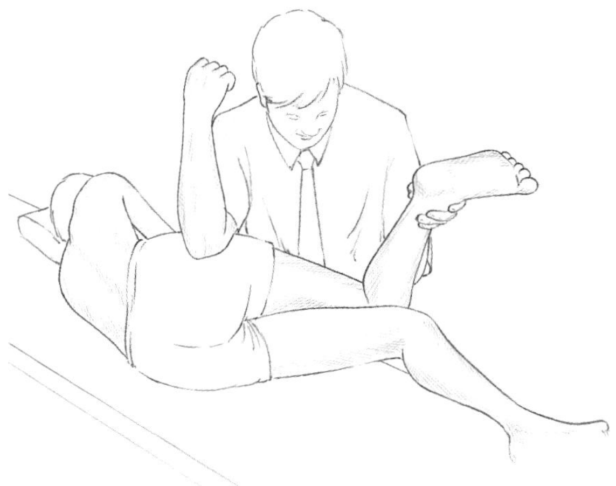

Figure 4.20 A combined ischaemic compression (elbow pressure) and MET side-lying treatment of piriformis. The pressure is alternated with isometric contractions/stretching of the muscle until no further gain is achieved.

MET treatment of piriformis

Piriformis method (a) Side-lying The patient is side-lying, close to the edge of the table, affected side uppermost, both legs flexed at hip and knee. The practitioner stands facing the patient at hip level.

The practitioner places his cephalad elbow tip *gently* over the point behind trochanter, where piriformis inserts. The patient should be close enough to the edge of the table for the practitioner to stabilise the pelvis against his trunk (Fig. 4.20). At the same time, the practitioner's caudad hand grasps the ankle and uses this to bring the upper leg/hip into internal rotation, taking out all the slack in piriformis.

A degree of inhibitory pressure (sufficient to cause discomfort but not pain) is applied via the elbow for 5–7 seconds while the muscle is kept at a reasonable but not excessive degree of stretch. The practitioner maintains contact on the point, but eases pressure, and asks the patient to introduce an isometric contraction (25% of strength for 5–7 seconds) to piriformis by bringing the lower leg towards the table against resistance. (The same acute and chronic rules as discussed previously are employed, together with cooperative breathing if appropriate, see Box 4.2.)

After the contraction ceases and the patient relaxes, the lower limb is taken to its new resistance barrier and elbow pressure is reapplied.

This process is repeated until no further gain is achieved.

Piriformis method (b)1 This method is a variation on the method advocated by TePoorten (1960) which calls for longer and heavier compression, and no intermediate isometric contractions.

In the first stage of TePoorten's method the patient lies on the non-affected side with knees flexed and hip joints flexed to 90°.The practitioner places his elbow on the piriformis musculotendinous junction and a steady pressure of 20–30 lb (9–13 kg) is applied. With his other hand he abducts the foot so that it will force an internal rotation of the upper leg.

The leg is held in this rotated position for periods of up to 2 minutes.

This procedure is repeated two or three times.

The patient is then placed in the supine position and the affected leg is tested for freedom of both external and internal rotation.

Piriformis method (b)2 The second stage of TePoorten's treatment is performed with the patient supine with both legs extended. The foot of the affected leg is grasped and the leg is flexed at both the knee and the hip. As knee and hip flexion is performed the practitioner turns the foot inward, so inducing an external rotation of the upper leg. The practitioner then extends the knee, and simultaneously turns the foot outward, resulting in an internal rotation of the upper leg.

During these procedures the patient is instructed to *partially* resist the movements introduced by the practitioner (i.e. the procedure becomes an isokinetic activity).

This treatment method, repeated two or three times, serves to relieve the contracture of the muscles of external and internal hip rotation.

Piriformis method (c) A series of MET isometric contractions and stretches can be applied with the patient prone and the affected side knee flexed. The hip is rotated internally by the practitioner using the foot as a lever to ease it laterally, so putting piriformis at stretch. Acute and chronic guidelines described earlier are used to determine the appropriate starting point for the contraction (at the barrier for acute and short of it for chronic).

The patient attempts to lightly bring the heel back towards the midline against resistance (avoiding strong contractions to avoid knee strain in this position) and this is held for 7–10 seconds.

After release of the contraction the hip is rotated further to move piriformis to or through the barrier, as appropriate.

Application of inhibitory pressure to the attachment or belly of piriformis is possible via thumb, if deemed necessary.

Piriformis method (d) A general approach which balances muscles of the region, as well as the pelvic diaphragm, is achieved by having the patient squat while the practitioner stands and stabilises both shoulders, preventing the patient from rising as this is attempted, while the breath is held.

After 7–10 seconds the effort is released; a deeper squat is performed, and the procedure is repeated several times.

Piriformis method (e) This method is based on the test position (see Fig. 4.17) and is described by Lewit (1992).

With the patient supine, the treated leg is placed into flexion at the hip and knee, so that the foot rests on the table lateral to the contralateral knee (the leg on the side to be treated is crossed over the other, straight, leg). The angle of hip flexion should not exceed 60° (see notes on piriformis, Box 4.6, for explanation).

The practitioner places one hand on the contralateral ASIS to prevent pelvic motion, while the other hand is placed against the lateral flexed knee as this is pushed into resisted abduction to contract piriformis for 7–10 seconds.

Following the contraction the practitioner eases the treated side leg into adduction until a sense of resistance is noted; this is held for 10–30 seconds.

Piriformis method (f) Since contraction of one piriformis inhibits its pair, it is possible to self-treat an affected short piriformis by having the patient lie up against a wall with the *non-affected* side touching it, both knees flexed (modified from Retzlaff 1974).

The patient monitors the affected side by palpating behind the trochanter, ensuring that no contraction takes place on that side.

After a contraction lasting 10 seconds or so of the non-affected side (the patient presses the knee against the wall), the patient moves away from the wall and the position described for piriformis test (see Fig. 4.17) above is adopted, and the patient pushes the affected side knee into adduction, stretching piriformis on that side.

This is repeated several times.

7. Assessment and treatment of quadratus lumborum (see also Box 4.8)

Assessment of shortness in quadratus lumborum (10) (Fig. 4.21)

Review Lewit's functional palpation test described under the heading assessment and treatment of tensor fascia lata (p. 106).

When the leg of the side-lying patient is abducted, and the practitioner's palpating hand senses that quadratus becomes involved in this process before the leg has reached at least 25° of elevation, then it is clear that quadratus is overactive. If it has been overactive for any length of time then it is almost certainly hypertonic and short, and a need for MET can be assumed.

Quadratus lumborum test (a) (See also Fig. 5.11A, B.) The patient is side-lying and is asked to take the upper arm over the head to grasp the top

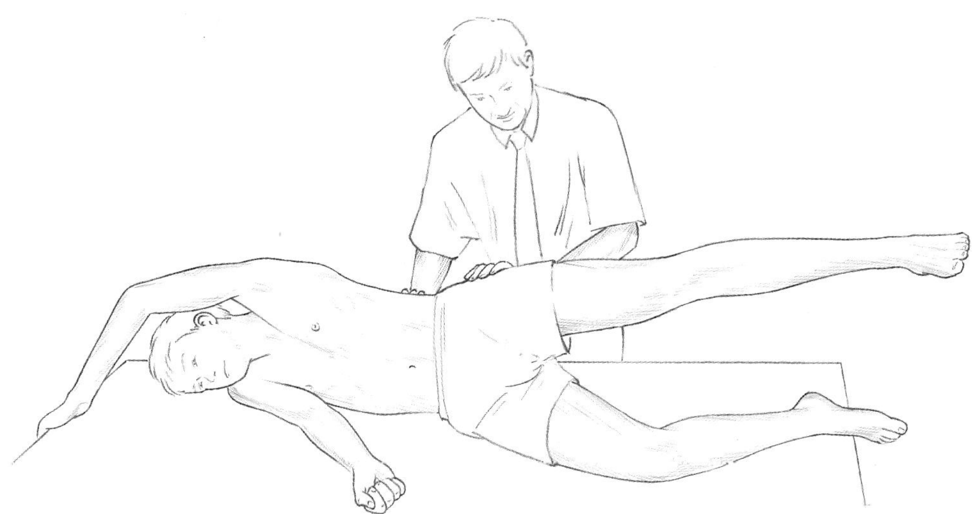

Figure 4.21 Palpation assessment for quadratus lumborum overactivity. The muscle is palpated, as is gluteus medius, during abduction of the leg. The correct firing sequence should be gluteus, followed at around 25° elevation by quadratus. If there is an immediate 'grabbing' action by quadratus it indicates overactivity, and therefore stress, so shortness can be assumed (see details of similar functional assessments in Ch. 5).

edge of the table, 'opening out' the lumbar area. The practitioner stands facing the back of the patient, and has easy access for palpation of quadratus lumborum's lateral border – a major trigger point site (Travell & Simons 1992) – with the cephalad hand.

Activity of quadratus is tested (palpated for) with the cephalad hand as the leg is abducted, while also palpating gluteus medius with the caudad hand.

If the muscles act simultaneously, or if quadratus fires first, then it is stressed, probably short, and will benefit from stretching.

Quadratus lumborum test (b) The patient stands, back towards crouching practitioner. Any leg length disparity (based on pelvic crest height) is equalised by using a book or pad under the short leg side heel. With the patient's feet shoulder-width apart, a pure sidebending is requested, so that the patient runs a hand down the lateral thigh/calf. (Normal level of sidebending excursion allows the fingertips to reach to just below the knee.) (See Fig. 3.2A, B, C.)

The side to which the fingertips travel furthest is assessed.

If sidebending to one side is limited then quadratus on the opposite side is probably short.

Combined evidence from palpation (test a) and this sidebending test indicate whether or not it is necessary to treat quadratus.

MET for shortness in quadratus lumborum ('banana')

Quadratus lumborum MET method (a) (Fig. 4.22) The patient lies supine with the feet crossed (the side to be treated crossed under the non-treated side leg) at the ankle. The patient is arranged in a light sidebend, away from the side to be treated, so that the pelvis is towards that side, and the feet and head away from that side ('banana shaped'). As this sidebend is being achieved the affected quadratus can be palpated for bind so that the barrier is correctly identified.

The patient's heels are placed just off the side of the table, anchoring the lower extremities and pelvis. The patient places the arm of the side to be treated behind her neck as the practitioner, standing on the side opposite that to be treated, slides his cephalad hand under the patient's shoulders to grasp the treated side axilla. The patient grasps the practitioner's cephalad arm at the elbow, with the treated side hand, making the contact more secure.

Box 4.8 Notes on quadratus lumborum

- Norris (2000) describes the divided roles in which quadratus is involved:

> The quadratus lumborum has been shown to be significant as a stabiliser in lumbar spine movements (McGill et al 1996) while tightening has also been described (Janda 1983). It seems likely that the muscle may act functionally differently in its medial and lateral portions, with the medial portion being more active as a stabiliser of the lumbar spine, and the lateral more active as a mobiliser [see stabiliser/mobiliser discussion Ch. 2]. Such sub-division is seen in a number of other muscles for example the gluteus medius where the posterior fibres are more posturally involved (Jull 1994) the internal oblique where the posterior fibres attaching to the lateral raphe are considered stabilisers (Bergmark 1989) the external oblique where the lateral fibres work during flexion in parallel with the rectus abdominis (Kendall et al 1993).

- Janda (1983) observes that, when the patient is sidebending (as in method (b)) 'when the lumbar spine appears straight, with compensatory motion occurring only from the thoraco-lumbar region upwards, tightness of quadratus lumborum may be suspected'. This 'whole lumbar spine' involvement differs from a segmental restriction which would probably involve only a part of the lumbar spine.
- Quadratus fibres merge with the diaphragm (as do those of psoas), which makes involvement in respiratory dysfunction a possibility since it plays a role in exhalation, both via this merging and by its attachment to the 12th rib.
- Shortness of quadratus, or the presence of trigger points, can result in pain in the lower ribs and along the iliac crest if the lateral fibres are affected.
- Shortness of the medial fibres, or the presence of trigger points, can produce pain in the sacroiliac joint and the buttock.
- Bilateral contraction produces extension and unilateral contraction produces extension and sidebending to the same side.
- The important transition region, the lumbodorsal junction (LDJ), is the only one in the spine in which two mobile structures meet, and dysfunction results in alteration of the quality of motion between these structures (upper and lower trunk/dorsal and lumbar spines). In dysfunction there is often a degree of spasm or tightness in the muscles which stabilise the region, notably: psoas and erector spinae of the thoracolumbar region, as well as quadratus lumborum and rectus abdominis.
- Symptomatic differential diagnosis of muscle involvement at the LDJ is possible as follows:
  - — psoas involvement usually triggers abdominal pain if severe and produces flexion of the hip and the typical antalgesic posture of lumbago
  - — erector spinae involvement produces low back pain at its caudad end of attachment and interscapular pain at its thoracic attachment (as far up as the mid-thoracic level)
  - — quadratus lumborum involvement causes lumbar pain and pain at the attachment of the iliac crest and lower ribs
  - — rectus abdominis contraction may mimic abdominal pain and result in pain at the attachments at the pubic symphysis and the xiphoid process, as well as forward-bending of the trunk and restricted ability to extend the spine.

There is seldom pain at the site of the lesion in LDJ dysfunction. Lewit (1992) points out that even if a number of these muscles are implicated, it is seldom necessary, using PIR methods, to treat them all since, as the muscles most involved (discovered by tests for shortness, overactivity, sensitivity and direct palpation) are stretched and normalised, so will others begin automatically to normalise.

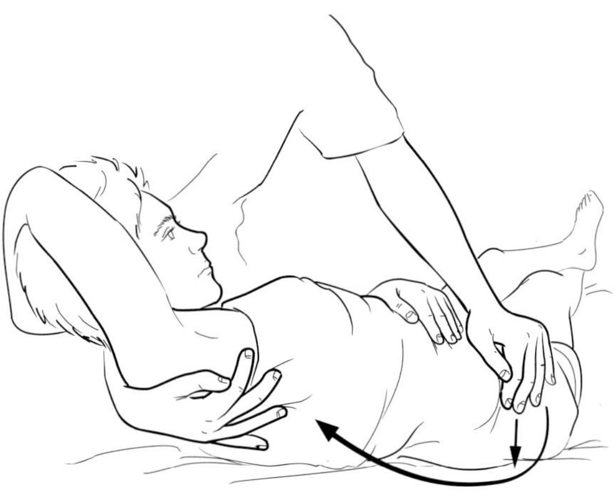

Figure 4.22 MET treatment of quadratus lumborum utilising 'banana' position.

The patient's treated side elbow should, at this stage, be pointing superiorly. The practitioner's caudad hand is placed firmly but carefully on the anterior superior iliac spine, on the side to be treated.

The patient is instructed to very lightly sidebend towards the treated side. This should produce an isometric contraction in quadratus lumborum on the side to be treated.

After 7 seconds the patient is asked to relax completely, and then to sidebend towards the non-treated side, as the practitioner simultaneously transfers his bodyweight from the cephalad leg to the caudad leg and leans backwards slightly, in order to sidebend the patient.

This effectively stretches quadratus lumborum. The stretch is held for 15–20 seconds, allowing a lengthening of shortened musculature in the region.

Repeat as necessary.

Quadratus lumborum MET method (b) (Fig 4.23) The practitioner stands behind the side-lying patient, at waist level. The patient has the uppermost arm extended over the head to firmly grasp the top end of the table and, on an inhalation, abducts the uppermost leg until the practitioner palpates strong quadratus activity (elevation of around 30° usually).

The patient holds the leg (and, if appropriate, the breath, see Box 4.2) isometrically in this manner, allowing gravity to provide resistance.

After the 10-second (or so) contraction, the patient allows the leg to hang slightly behind him over the back of the table. The practitioner straddles this and, cradling the pelvis with both hands (fingers interlocked over crest of pelvis), leans back to take out all slack and to 'ease the pelvis away from the lower ribs' during an exhalation.

The stretch should be held for between 10 and 30 seconds. (The method will only be successful if the patient is grasping the top edge of the table, so providing a fixed point from which the practitioner can induce stretch.)

Contraction followed by stretch is repeated once or twice more with raised leg in front of, and once or twice with raised leg behind the trunk in order to activate different fibres.

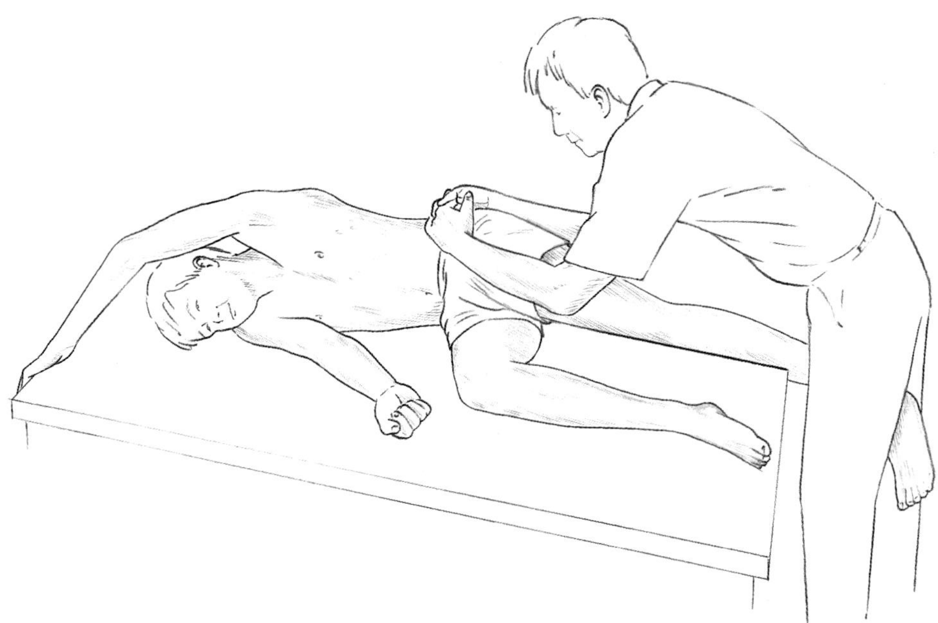

Figure 4.23 MET treatment of quadratus lumborum. Note that it is important after the isometric contraction (sustained raised/abducted leg) that the muscle be eased into stretch, avoiding any defensive or protective resistance which sudden movement might produce. For this reason, body weight rather than arm strength should be used to apply traction.

The direction of stretch should be varied so that it is always in the same direction as the long axis of the abducted leg. This calls for the practitioner changing from the back to the front of the table for the best results.

When the leg hangs to the back of the trunk the long fibres of the muscle are mainly affected; and when the leg hangs forward of the body the diagonal fibres are mainly involved.

Quadratus lumborum MET method (c) Gravity-induced postisometric relaxation of quadratus lumborum – self-treatment (See Fig. 3.2A–C and captions, p. 80) The patient stands, legs apart, bending sideways. The patient inhales and slightly raises the trunk (a few centimetres) at the same time as looking (with the eyes only) away from the side to which side-flexion is taking place. On exhalation, the sidebend is allowed to slowly go further to its elastic limit, while the patient looks towards the floor, in the direction of the side-flexion. (Care is needed that very little, if any, forward or backward bending is taking place at this time.) This sequence is repeated a number of times.

Eye positions influence the tendency to flex and sidebend (eyes look down) and extend (eyes look up) (Lewit 1999).

Gravity-induced stretches of this sort require holding the stretch position for at least as long as the contraction, and ideally longer. More repetitions may be needed with a large muscle such as quadratus, and home stretches should be advised several times daily.

Quadratus lumborum MET method (d) The side-lying treatment of latissimus dorsi described below (p. 122) also provides an effective quadratus stretch when the stabilising hand rests on the pelvic crest (see Fig. 4.29).

8. Assessment and treatment of pectoralis major and latissimus dorsi

Assessment of shortened pectoralis major (11) and latissimus dorsi (12)

Latissimus and pectoral test (a) Observation is as accurate as most palpation for evidence of pectoralis major shortening. The patient will have a rounded shoulder posture – especially if the clavicular aspect is involved.

Or

The patient lies supine with upper arms on the table, hands resting palm down on the lower abdomen. The practitioner observes from the head and notes whether either shoulder is held in an anterior position in relation to the thoracic cage. If one or both shoulders are forward of the thorax, pectoralis muscles are short (Fig. 4.24).

Latissimus and pectoral test (b) The patient lies supine with the head several feet from the top edge of the table, and is asked to rest the arms, extended above the head, on the treatment surface, palms upwards (Fig. 4.25).

If these muscles are normal, the arms should be able to easily reach the horizontal when directly above the shoulders, and also to be in contact with the surface for almost all of the length of the upper arms, with no arching of the back or twisting of the thorax.

If either arm cannot reach the vertical above the shoulder, but is held laterally, elbow pulled outwards, then latissimus dorsi is probably short on that side. If an arm cannot rest with the

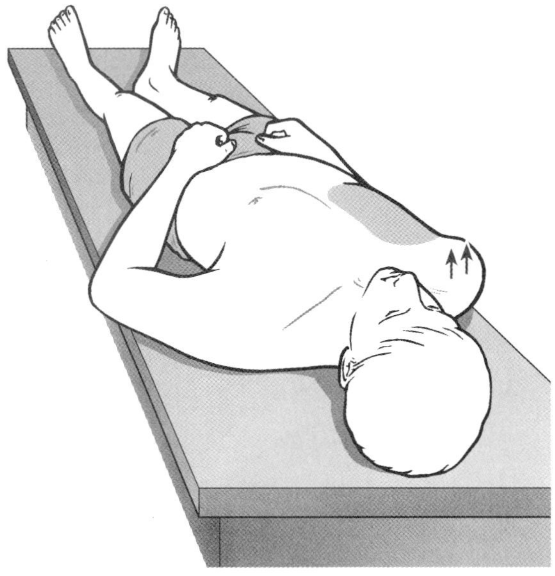

Figure 4.24 Observation assessment in which pectoral shortness on the right is suggested by the inability of the shoulder to rest on the table.

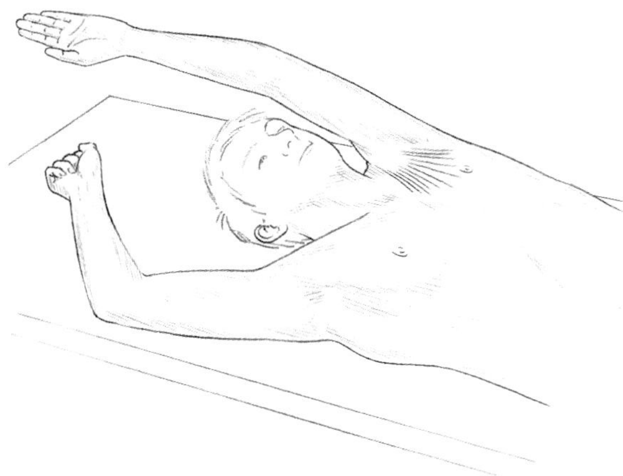

Figure 4.25 Assessment of shortness in pectoralis major and latissimus dorsi. Visual assessment is used: if the arm on the tested side is unable to rest along its full length, shortness of pectoralis major is probable; if there is obvious deviation of the elbow laterally, probable latissimus shortening is indicated.

dorsum of the upper arm in contact with the table surface without effort, then pectoral fibres are almost certainly short.

Pectoralis major test. Assessment of shortness in pectoralis major (Fig. 4.26) Assessment of the subclavicular portion of pectoralis major involves abduction of the arm to 90° (Lewit 1985b). In this position the tendon of pectoralis major at the sternum should not be found to be unduly tense, even with maximum abduction of the arm, unless the muscle is short.

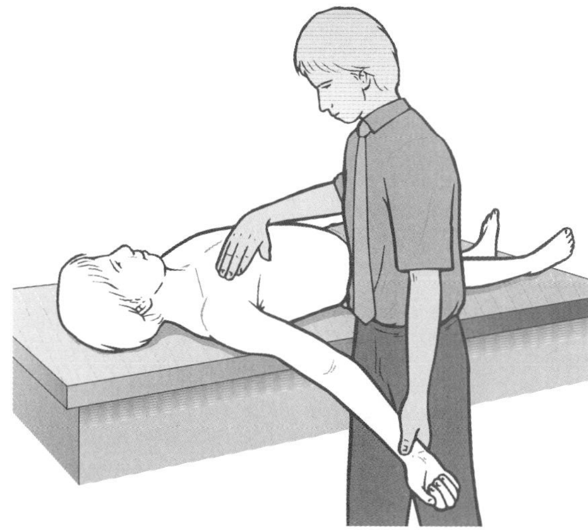

Figure 4.26 Palpation assessment for shortness of subclavicular portion of pectoralis major.

For assessment of sternal attachment the arm is brought into elevation and abduction as the muscle, as well as the tendon on the greater tubercle of the humerus, is palpated. If the sternal fibres have shortened, tautness will be visible and tenderness of the tissues under palpation will be reported.

Pectoralis major test. Assessment for strength of pectoralis major Patient is supine with arm in abduction at the shoulder joint and medially rotated (palm is facing down) with the elbow extended. The practitioner stands at the head and secures the opposite shoulder with one hand to prevent any trunk torsion and contacts the dorsum of the distal humerus, on the tested side, with the other.

The patient attempts to lift the arm and to adduct it across the chest, against resistance, as strength is assessed in the sternal fibres.

Different arm positions can be used to assess clavicular and costal fibres: for example with an angle of abduction/elevation of 135° costal and abdominal fibres will be involved; with abduction/elevation of 45° the clavicular fibres will be assessed. The practitioner should palpate to ensure that the 'correct' fibres contract when assessments are being made.

If this postural muscle tests as weak it may be useful to use Norris's (1999) approach of strengthening it by means of a slowly applied isotonic eccentric (isolytic) contraction, before proceeding to an MET stretching procedure.

MET treatment of short pectoralis major

Pectoralis major MET method (a) (Fig. 4.27A, B) The patient lies supine with the arm abducted in a direction which produces the most marked evidence of pectoral shortness (assessed by palpation and visual evidence of the particular fibres involved as described in tests above). The more elevated the arm (i.e. the closer to the head), the more focus there will be on costal and abdominal fibres. With a lesser degree of abduction (to around 45°), the focus is more on the clavicular fibres. Between

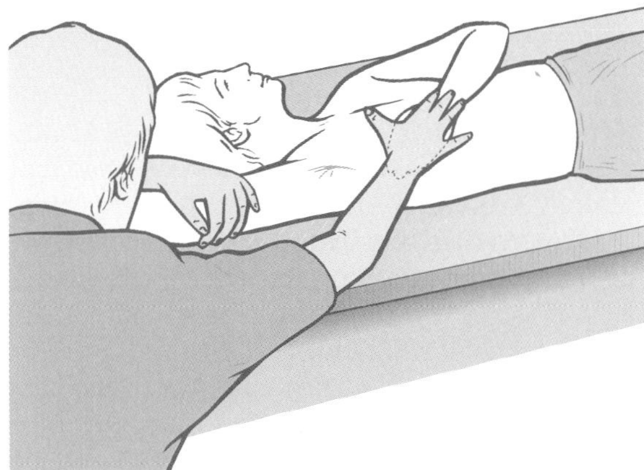

Figure 4.27A MET treatment of pectoral muscle – abdominal attachment. Note that the fibres being treated are those which lie in line with the long axis of the humerus.

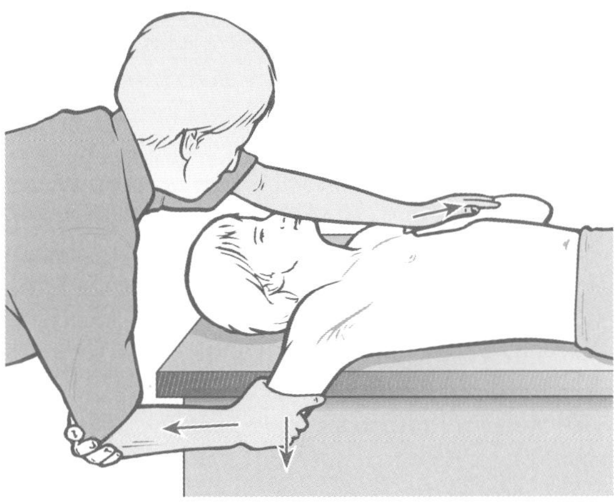

Figure 4.27B An alternative hold for application of MET to pectoral muscle – sternal attachment. Note that the patient needs to be close to the edge of the table in order to allow the arm to be taken towards the floor once the slack has been removed, during the stretching phase after the isometric contraction.

these two extremes lies the position which influences the sternal fibres most directly.

The patient lies as close to the side of the table as possible so that the abducted arm can be brought below the horizontal level in order to apply gravitational pull and passive stretch to the fibres, as appropriate. The practitioner stands on the side to be treated and grasps the humerus.

A useful arm hold, which depends upon the relative size of the patient and the practitioner, involves the practitioner grasping the anterior aspect of the patient's flexed upper arm just above the elbow, while the patient cups the practitioner's elbow and holds this contact throughout the procedure (see Fig. 4.27B).

The patient's hand is placed on the contact (attachments of shortened fibres) area on the thorax so that the hand acts as a 'cushion'. This is both more physically comfortable and also prevents physical contact with emotionally sensitive areas such as breast tissue. The practitioner's thenar or hyperthenar eminence is placed over the patient's 'cushion' hand in order to stabilise the area during the contraction and stretch, preventing movement of it.

Commencing with the patient's arm in a position which takes the affected fibres to just short of their restriction barrier (for a chronic problem), the patient introduces a light contraction (20% of strength) involving adduction against resistance from the practitioner, for 7–10 seconds.

As a rule the long axis of the patient's upper arm should be in a straight line with the fibres being treated. If a trigger point has previously been identified in pectoralis, the practitioner should ensure – by means of palpation if necessary, or by observation – that the fibres housing the triggers are involved in the contraction.

As the patient exhales following complete relaxation of the area, a stretch through the new barrier is activated by the patient and maintained by the practitioner. Stretch is achieved via the positioning and leverage of the arm as the contact hand on the thorax acts as a stabilising point only.

The stretch needs to be one in which the arm is first pulled away (distracted) from the thorax, with the patient's assistance ('ease your arm away from your shoulder'), before the stretch is introduced which involves the humerus being taken below the horizontal ('ease your arm towards the floor').

During the stretching phase it is important for the entire thorax to be stabilised. No rolling or twisting of the thorax in the direction of the stretch should be permitted. The stretching procedure should be thought of as having two phases: first the slack being removed by distracting the arm away from the contact/stabilising hand on the thorax; second, movement of the arm towards the floor, initiated by the practitioner bending his knees.

Stretching (after an isometric contraction) should be repeated two or three times in each position. All attachments should be treated, which calls for the use of different arm positions, as discussed above, each with different stabilising ('cushion') contacts as the various fibre directions and attachments are isolated.

Pectoralis major MET method (b) (Fig. 4.28) The patient is prone with face in a face hole or cradle. Her right arm is abducted to 90° and the elbow flexed to 90° palm towards the floor, with the upper arm supported by the table. The practitioner stands at waist level, facing cephalad, and places his non-table-side hand palm to palm with the patient's so that the patient's forearm is in contact with the ventral surface of the practitioner's forearm. The practitioner's table-side hand rests on the patient's right scapula area, ensuring that no trunk rotation occurs.

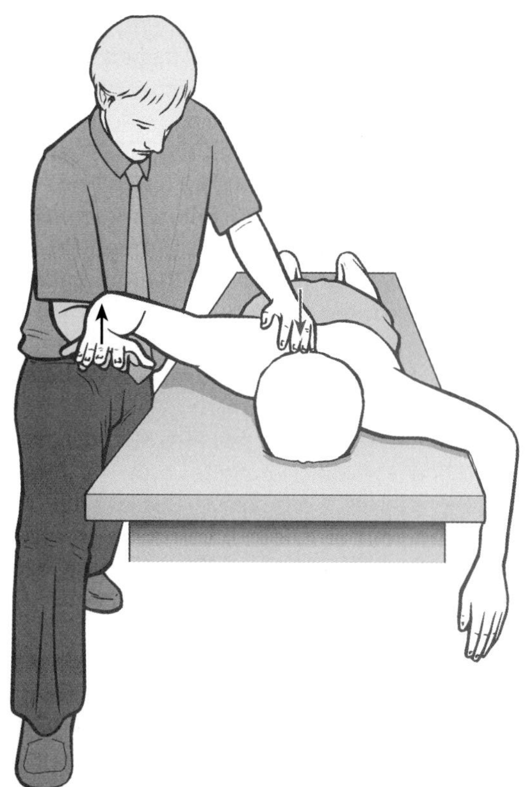

Figure 4.28 MET for pectoralis major in prone position.

The practitioner eases the patient's arm into extension at the shoulder until he senses the first sign of resistance from pectoralis. It is important when extending the arm in this way to ensure that no trunk rotation occurs and that the anterior surface of the shoulder remains in contact with the table throughout.

The patient is asked, using no more than 20% of strength, to bring her arm towards the floor and across her chest, with the elbow taking the lead in this attempted movement, which is completely resisted by the practitioner. The practitioner ensures that the patient's arm remains parallel with the floor throughout the isometric contraction.

Following release of the contraction effort, and on an exhalation, the arm is taken into greater extension, with the patient's assistance, and held at stretch for not less than 20 seconds.

This procedure is repeated two or three times, slackening the muscle slightly from its end-range before each subsequent contraction to reduce discomfort and for ease of application of the contraction.

Variations in pectoralis fibre involvement can be achieved by altering the angle of abduction – with a more superior angle (around 140°) the lower sternal and costal fibres, and with a lesser angle (around 45°) the clavicular fibres will be committed.

Pectoralis major MET method (c) Bilateral MET stretching of pectoralis major (sternocostal aspects) involves having the patient supine, knees and hips flexed, in order to provide stability to the spinal regions, preventing lumbar lordosis. A shallow but firm cushion should be placed between the scapulae, allowing a better excursion of the shoulders during this stretch. The chin should be tucked in and, if more comfortable, a small cushion placed under the neck. Ideally a strap/belt should be used to fix the thorax to the table, but this is not essential.

The practitioner stands at the head of the table and grasps the patient's elbows or forearms, which are flexed, laterally rotated and held in a position to induce the most taut aspects of the muscles to become prominent.

Starting from such a barrier or short of it (acute/chronic), the patient is asked to contract the muscles by bringing the arms upwards and towards the table for 10 seconds or so during a held breath.

Following the contraction and complete relaxation, the arms are taken to a new or through the restriction barrier, as appropriate, during an exhalation.

Repeat as necessary several times more.[7]

Pectoralis major MET method (d) By adopting the same positions – but with the arms of the patient more laterally placed so that they are laterally rotated and in 90° abduction from the shoulder (upper arms are straight out sideways from the shoulder) and there is 90° flexion at the elbows, with the practitioner contacting the area just proximal to the flexed elbows – a more direct stretch of the clavicular insertions of the muscle can be achieved, using all the same contraction and stretch elements as in (b) above.[8]

Latissimus dorsi test for shortness

To screen latissimus dorsi (12), the standing patient is asked to bend forwards and allow the arms to hang freely from the shoulders as she holds a half-bend position, trunk parallel with the floor.

If the arms are hanging other than perpendicular to the floor there is probably some muscular restriction involved, and if this involves latissimus the arms will be held closer to the legs than perpendicular (if they hang markedly forward of such a position then trapezius shortening is probable, see below).

To screen latissimus in this position, one side at a time, the practitioner stands in front of the patient (who remains in this half-bend position) and, stabilising the scapula area with one hand, grasps the arm at elbow level and gently draws the tested side (straight) arm forwards. It should, without undue effort or excessive bind in the tissues being held, allow itself to be taken to a position where the elbow is higher than the level of the back of the head. If this is not possible, then latissimus is short.

MET treatment of short latissimus dorsi

Short latissimus dorsi MET method (a) The patient lies supine with the feet crossed (the side to be treated crossed under the non-treated side leg at the ankle). The patient is arranged in a light sidebend away from the side to be treated so that the pelvis is towards that side, and the feet and head away from that side. The heels are placed just off the edge of the table, so anchoring the lower extremities.

The patient places her arm on the side to be treated behind her neck, as the practitioner, standing on the side opposite that to be treated, slides his cephalad hand under the patient's shoulders to grasp the treated side axilla. The patient grasps the practitioner's cephalad arm at the elbow, making this contact more secure. The patients treated side elbow should point superiorly. The practitioner's caudad hand is placed on the anterior superior iliac spine on the side being treated.

The patient is instructed to very lightly take the pointed elbow towards the sacrum and also to lightly try to bend backwards and towards the treated side. This should produce a light isometric contraction in latissimus dorsi on the side to be treated. After 7 seconds they are asked to relax completely as the practitioner transfers his body weight from the cephalad leg to the caudad leg, to sidebend the patient. Simultaneously the practitioner stands more erect and leans in a caudad direction.

This effectively lifts the patient's thorax from the table surface and introduces a stretch into latissimus (especially if the patient has maintained a grasp on the practitioner's elbow and the practitioner has a firm hold on the patient's axilla).

This stretch is held for 15–30 seconds allowing a lengthening of shortened musculature in the region. (Note: starting position is as for Fig. 4.22.)

---

[7] Methods (c) and (d) can be adapted to a seated position if the back is well supported (on a chair back with a cushion for example). All other elements stay the same.

[8] Serratus anterior will also be stretched by many of these pectoral treatment procedures. There is no specific assessment test for serratus but its shortness will be noted by sensitive attachment sites on the anterior axillary line.

Repeat as necessary.

Short latissimus dorsi MET method (b) The patient is side-lying, affected side up. The arm is taken into abduction to the point of resistance, so that it is possible to visualise, or palpate, the insertion of the shortened fibres on the lateral chest wall.

The condition is treated in either the acute or chronic mode of MET, at or short of the barrier, as appropriate.

As shown in Figure 4.29, the practitioner stands near the head of the patient, slightly behind, and holds the upper arm in the chosen position while applying the other hand to stabilise the posterior thorax area, or the pelvic crest, from where the stretch will be made.[9]

A build-up of tension should be palpated under the stabilising hand as the patient introduces an isometric contraction by attempting to bring the arm towards the ceiling, backwards and down (towards their own lower spine) against firm resistance, using only a modest amount of effort (20%) and holding the breath if appropriate (see notes on breathing, Box 4.2).

After 7–10 seconds, both the effort and breath are released and the patient relaxes completely, at which time the practitioner introduces stretch to or through the barrier (acute/chronic), bringing the humerus into greater adduction while applying a stretching/stabilising contact on the trunk (with separate contractions and stretches for each contact) anywhere between the lateral chest wall and the crest of the pelvis.

A downward movement of the humerus, towards the floor, assists the stretch following a separation of the practitioner's two contact hands to remove all slack. As in the stretch of pectoralis major, there should be two phases – a distraction, taking out the slack, and a movement towards the floor of the practitioner, by flexing the knees – to induce a safe stretch.

Repeat as necessary.

Ultimately, it should be possible to achieve complete elevation of the arm without stress or obvious shortness in latissimus fibres so that the upper arm can rest alongside the ear of the supine patient.

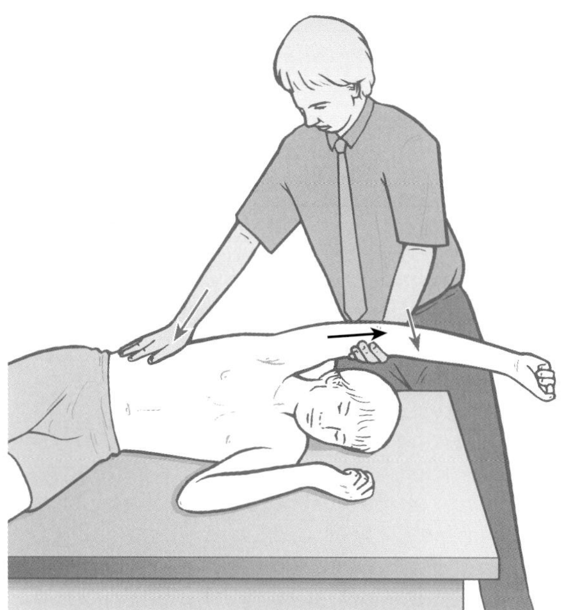

Figure 4.29 Treatment of latissimus dorsi. A variety of different positions are required for the stabilising hand (on the chest wall as well as on the crest of the pelvis) to allow for precise application of stretches of fibres with different attachments, following the sequence of isometric contractions.

9. Assessment and treatment of upper trapezius

Lewit (1999) simplifies the need to assess for shortness by stating, 'The upper trapezius should be treated if tender and taut.' Since this is an almost universal state in modern life, it seems that everyone requires MET application to this muscle. Lewit also notes that a characteristic mounding of the muscle can often be observed when it is very short, producing the effect of 'Gothic shoulders', similar to the architectural supports of a Gothic church tower (see Fig. 2.13).

Assessment for shortness of upper trapezius (13) (Fig. 4.30)

Test for upper trapezius for shortness (a) See scapulohumeral rhythm test (Ch. 5) which helps

[9] When the contact/stabilising hand is on the crest of the pelvis, the stretch using the arm as a lever will effectively also stretch quadratus lumborum.

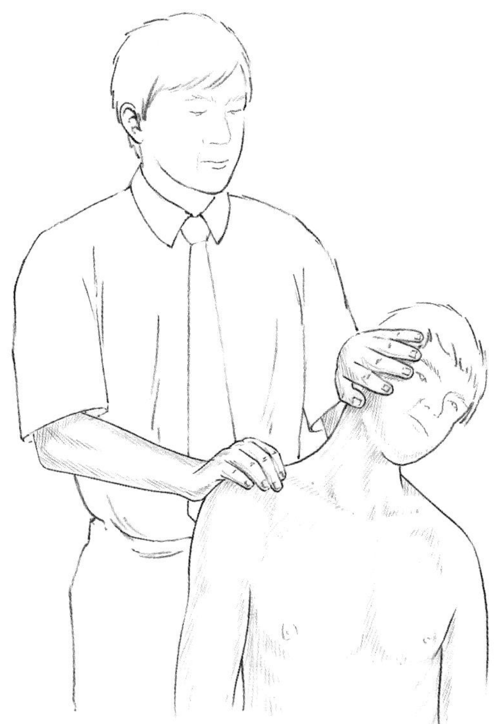

Figure 4.30 Assessment of the relative shortness of the right side upper trapezius. One side is compared with the other (for both the range of unforced motion and the nature of the end-feel of motion) to ascertain the side most in need of MET attention.

identify excessive activity or inappropriate tone in levator scapula and upper trapezius, which, because they are postural muscles, indicates shortness (Fig 5.13A, B).

Greenman (1996) describes a functional 'firing sequence' assessment which identifies general imbalance and dysfunction involving the upper and lower fixators of the shoulder (Fig. 4.31).

The patient is seated and the practitioner stands behind. The practitioner rests his right hand over the right shoulder area to assess firing sequence of muscles. The other hand can be placed either on the mid-thoracic region, mainly on the side being assessed, or spanning the lower back to palpate quadratus firing. The assessment should be performed at least twice so that various hand positions are used for different muscles (as in Fig. 4.31).

Greenman bases his description on Janda (1983), who notes the 'correct' sequence for shoulder abduction, when seated, as involving: *supraspinatus, deltoid, infraspinatus, middle and lower trapezius* and finally *contralateral quadratus*. In dysfunctional states the most common substitutions are said to involve: shoulder elevation by *levator scapulae and upper trapezius*, as well as early firing by *quadratus lumborum, ipsilateral and contralateral*.

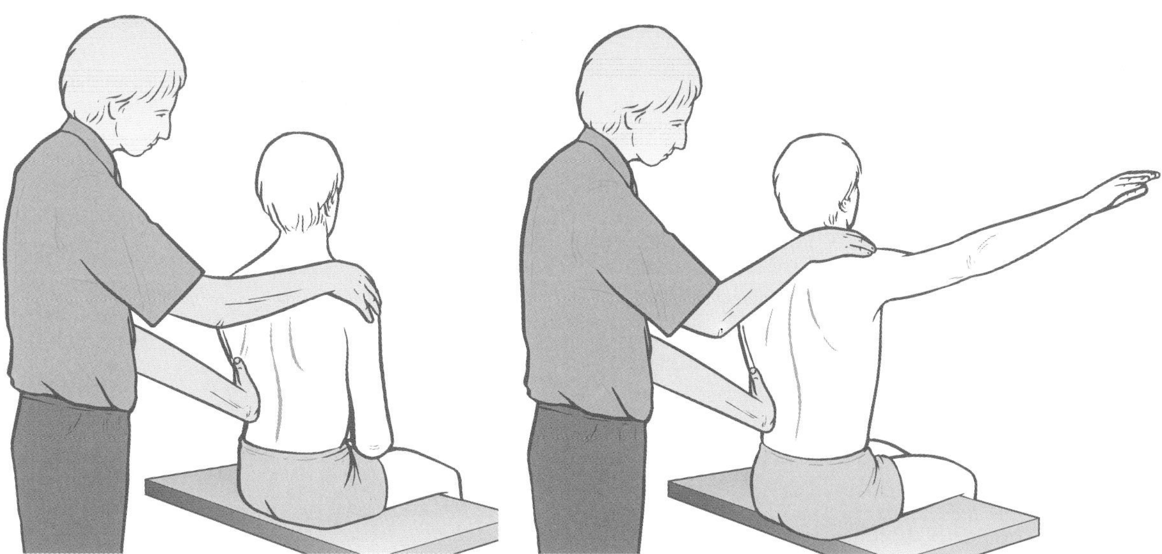

Figure 4.31 Palpation assessment for upper and lower fixators of the shoulder, including upper trapezius (Greenman 1996).

Inappropriate activity of the upper fixators results in shortness, and of the lower fixators in weakness and possible lengthening (see Ch. 2 for discussion of postural/phasic, etc. muscle characteristics).

Test for upper trapezius for shortness (b) The patient is seated and the practitioner stands behind with one hand resting on the shoulder of the side to be tested and stabilising it. The other hand is placed on the ipsilateral side of the head and the head/neck is taken into contralateral sidebending without force while the shoulder is stabilised (see Fig. 4.30).

The same procedure is performed on the other side with the opposite shoulder stabilised. A comparison is made as to which sidebending manoeuvre produced the greater range and whether the neck can easily reach 45° of side-flexion in each direction, which it should. If neither side can achieve this degree of sidebend, then both trapezius muscles may be short. The relative shortness of one, compared with the other, is evaluated.[10]

Test for upper trapezius for shortness (c) The patient is seated and the practitioner stands behind with a hand resting over the muscle on the side to be assessed. The patient is asked to extend the arm at the shoulder joint, bringing the flexed arm/elbow backwards. If the upper trapezius is stressed on that side it will inappropriately activate during this movement. Since it is a postural muscle, shortness in it can then be assumed (see discussion of postural muscle characteristics in Ch. 3).

Test of upper trapezius for shortness (d) The patient is supine with the neck fully (but not forcefully) sidebent contralaterally (away from the side being assessed). The practitioner is standing at the head of the table and uses a cupped hand contact on the ipsilateral shoulder (i.e. on the side being tested) to assess the ease with which it can be depressed (moved caudally) (Fig. 4.32).

[10] If the shoulder towards which the head is being sidebent was stabilised, then assessment would be of the mobility of the cervical structures. By stabilising the side from which the bend is taking place the muscular component is being evaluated.

There should be an easy 'springing' sensation as the practitioner pushes the shoulder towards the feet, with a *soft* end-feel to the movement. If depression of the shoulder is difficult or if there is a *harsh*, sudden end-point, upper trapezius shortness is confirmed.

This same assessment (always with full lateral flexion) should be performed with the head fully rotated away from the side being treated, half turned away from the side being treated, and slightly turned towards the side being treated, in order to respectively assess the relative shortness and functional efficiency of posterior, middle and anterior subdivisions of the upper portion of trapezius.

MET treatment of chronically shortened upper trapezius

MET treatment of upper trapezius, method (a) (Fig. 4.32) In order to treat all the fibres of upper trapezius, MET needs to be applied sequentially. The upper trapezius is subdivided here into *anterior, middle* and *posterior* fibres. The neck should be placed into different positions of rotation, coupled with the sidebending as described in the assessment description above, for precise treatment of the various fibres.

The patient lies supine, arm on the side to be treated lying alongside the trunk, head/neck sidebent away from the side being treated to just short of the restriction barrier, while the practitioner stabilises the shoulder with one hand and cups the ear/mastoid area of the same side of the head with the other:

- With the neck fully sidebent and fully rotated contralaterally, the *posterior* fibres of upper trapezius are involved in the contraction (see below). This will facilitate subsequent stretching of this aspect of the muscle.
- With the neck fully sidebent and half rotated, the *middle* fibres are involved in the contraction.
- With the neck fully sidebent and slightly rotated towards the side being treated the *anterior* fibres of upper trapezius are being treated.

The various contractions and subsequent stretches can be performed with practitioner's

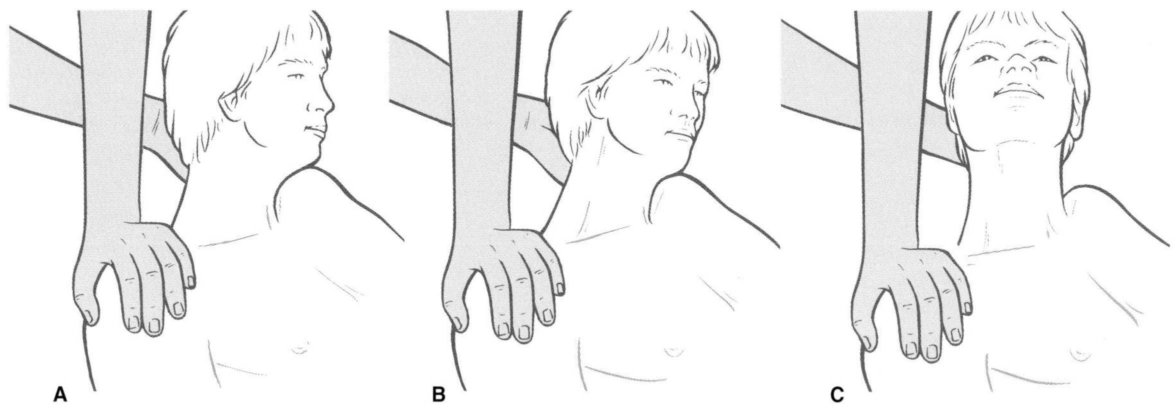

Figure 4.32 MET treatment of right side upper trapezius muscle. **A** Posterior fibres, **B** middle fibres, **C** anterior fibres. Note that stretching in this (or any of the alternative positions which access the middle and posterior fibres) is achieved following the isometric contraction by means of an easing of the shoulder away from the stabilised head, with no force being applied to the neck and head itself.

arms crossed, hands stabilising the mastoid area and shoulder.

The patient introduces a light resisted effort (20% of available strength) to take the stabilised shoulder towards the ear (a shrug movement) and the ear towards the shoulder. The double movement (or effort towards movement) is important in order to introduce a contraction of the muscle from both ends simultaneously. The degree of effort should be mild and no pain should be felt.

The contraction is sustained for 10 seconds (or so) and, upon complete relaxation of effort, the practitioner gently eases the head/neck into an increased degree of sidebending and rotation, where it is stabilised, as the shoulder is stretched caudally.

When stretching is introduced the patient can usefully assist in this phase of the treatment by initiating, on instruction, the stretch of the muscle ('as you breathe out please slide your hand towards your feet'). This reduces the chances of a stretch reflex being initiated. Once the muscle is being stretched, the patient relaxes and the stretch is held for 10–30 seconds.

⚠ **CAUTION:** No stretch should be introduced from the cranial end of the muscle as this could stress the neck. The head is stabilised at its side-flexion and rotation barrier.

Disagreement

There is some disagreement as to the head/neck rotation position as described in the treatment method above, which calls (for posterior and middle fibres) for sidebending and rotation away from the affected side.

Liebenson (1996), suggests that the patient 'lies supine with the head supported in anteflexion and laterally flexed away and rotated towards the side of involvement'.

Lewit (1985b) suggests: 'The patient is supine … the therapist fixes the shoulder from above with one hand, sidebending the head and neck with the other hand so as to take up the slack. He then asks the patient to look towards the side away from which the head is bent, resisting the patient's automatic tendency to move towards the side of the lesion.' (This method is described below.)

The author has used the methods described above with good effect and urges readers to try these approaches as well as those of Liebenson and Lewit, and to evaluate results for themselves.

MET treatment of acutely shortened upper trapezius, method (b) Lewit suggests the use of eye movements to facilitate initiation of PIR before stretching, an ideal method for acute problems in this region.

The patient is supine, while the practitioner fixes the shoulder and the sidebent (away from the treated side) head and neck at the restriction barrier and asks the patient to look, with the eyes only (i.e. not to turn the head), towards the side away from which the neck is bent.

This eye movement is maintained, as is a held breath, while the practitioner resists the slight isometric contraction that these two factors (eye movement and breath) will have created.

On exhalation and complete relaxation, the head/neck is taken to a new barrier and the process repeated. If the shoulder is brought into the equation, this is firmly held as it attempts to lightly push into a shrug.

After this 10 second contraction the muscle will have released somewhat and slack can again be taken out as the head is repositioned before a repetition of the procedure commences.

10. Assessment and treatment of scalenes (see also Box 4.9)

Assessment of shortness in scalenes (14)

Assessment of cervical sidebending (lateral flexion) strength This involves the scalenes and levator scapulae (and to a secondary degree the rectus capitis lateralis and the transversospinalis group).

The practitioner places a stabilising hand on the top of the shoulder to prevent movement and the other on the head above the ear, as the seated patient attempts to flex the head laterally against this resistance.

Both sides are assessed.

Observation assessment (a) There is no easy test for shortness of the scalenes apart from observation, palpation and assessment of trigger point activity/tautness and a functional observation as follows:

- In most people who have marked scalene shortness there is a tendency to overuse these (and other upper fixators of the shoulder and neck) as accessory breathing muscles.
- There may also be a tendency to hyperventilation (and hence for there to possibly be a history of anxiety, phobic behaviour, panic attacks and/or fatigue symptoms).
- These muscles seem to be excessively tense in many people with chronic fatigue symptoms.

Box 4.9 Notes on scalenes

- The scalenes are a controversial muscle since they seem to be both postural and phasic (Lin et al 1994), their status being modified by the type(s) of stress to which they are exposed (see Ch. 3 for discussion of this topic).
- Janda (1988) reports that 'spasm and/or trigger points are commonly present in the scalenes as also are weakness and/or inhibition'.
- The attachment sites of the scalene muscles vary, as does their presence. The scalene posterior is sometimes absent, and sometimes blends with the fibres of medius.
- Scalene medius is noted to frequently attach to the atlas (Gray 1995) and sometimes extend to the 2nd rib (Simons et al 1998).
- The scalene minimus (pleuralis), which attaches to the pleural dome, is present in one-third (Platzer 1992) to three-quarters (Simons et al 1998) of people, on at least one side and, when absent, is replaced by a transverse cupular ligament (Platzer 1992).
- The brachial plexus exits the cervical column between the scalenus anterior and medius. These two muscles, together with the 1st rib, form the scalene hiatus (also called the 'scalene opening' or 'posterior scalene aperture') (Platzer 1992). It is through this opening that the brachial plexus and vascular structures for the upper extremity pass. When scalene fibres are taut, they may entrap the nerves (scalene anticus syndrome) or may elevate the 1st rib against the clavicle and indirectly crowd the vascular, or neurologic, structures (simultaneous compromising of both neural and vascular structures is rare) (Stedman 1998). Any of these conditions may be diagnosed as 'thoracic outlet syndrome', which is 'a collective title for a number of conditions attributed to compromise of blood vessels or nerve fibers (brachial plexus) at any point between the base of the neck and the axilla' (Stedman 1998).

The observation assessment consists of the practitioner placing his relaxed hands over the patient's shoulders so that the fingertips rest on the clavicles, at which time the seated patient is asked to inhale deeply. If the practitioner's hands noticeably rise towards the patient's ears during inhalation then there exists inappropriate use of scalenes, which indicates that they are stressed, which also means that, by definition, they will have become shortened and require stretching treatment.

Observation assessment (b) (Fig. 4.33) Alternatively, during the history taking interview, the patient can be asked to place one hand on the abdomen just above the umbilicus and the other flat against the upper chest.

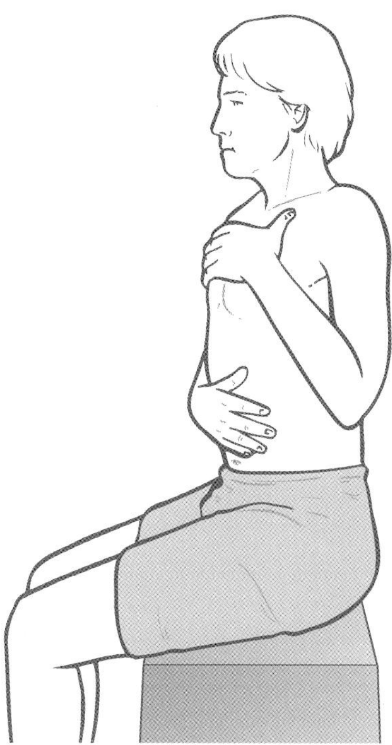

Figure 4.33 Observation assessment of respiratory function. Any tendency for the upper hand to move cephalad, or earlier than the caudad hand, suggests scalene overactivity.

On inhalation, the hands are observed: if the upper hand initiates the breathing process and rises significantly towards the chin, rather than moving forwards, a pattern of upper chest breathing can be assumed, and therefore stress, and therefore shortness of the scalenes (and other accessory breathing muscles, notably sternomastoid).

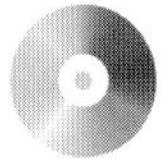

MET treatment of short scalenes (Fig. 4.34A, B, C)

Patient lies supine with a cushion or folded towel under the upper thoracic area so that, unless supported by the practitioner's contralateral hand, the head would fall into extension. The head is rotated contralaterally (away from the side to be treated). There are three positions of rotation required:

1. Full contralateral rotation of the head/neck produces involvement of the more posterior fibres of the scalenes
2. A contralateral 45° rotation of the head/neck involves the middle fibres
3. A position of only slight contralateral rotation involves the more anterior fibres.

The practitioner's free hand is placed on the side of the patient's head to restrain the isometric contraction which will be used to release the scalenes. The patient's head is in one of the above

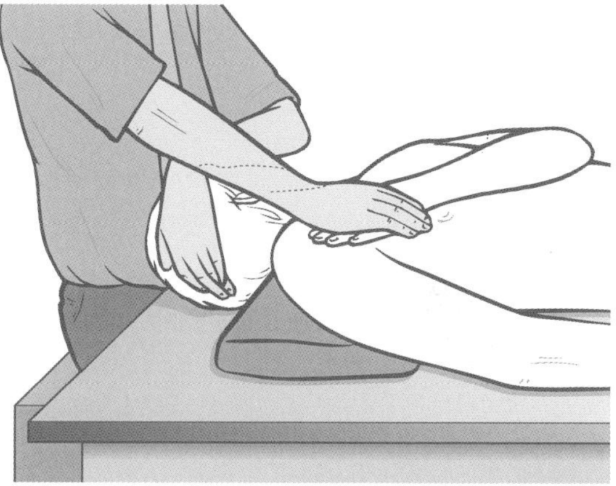

Figure 4.34A MET for scalenus posticus. On stretching, following the isometric contraction, the neck is allowed to move into slight extension while a mild stretch is introduced by the contact hand which rests on the second rib, below the lateral aspect of the clavicle.

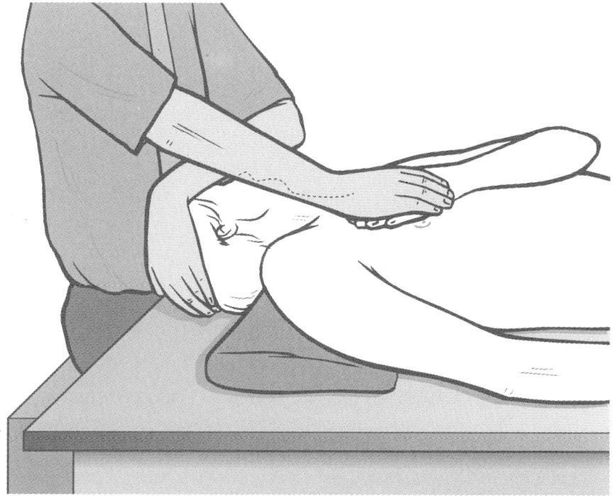

Figure 4.34B MET treatment for the middle fibres of scalenes. The hand placement (thenar or hypothenar eminence of relaxed hand) is on the 2nd rib below the centre of the clavicle.

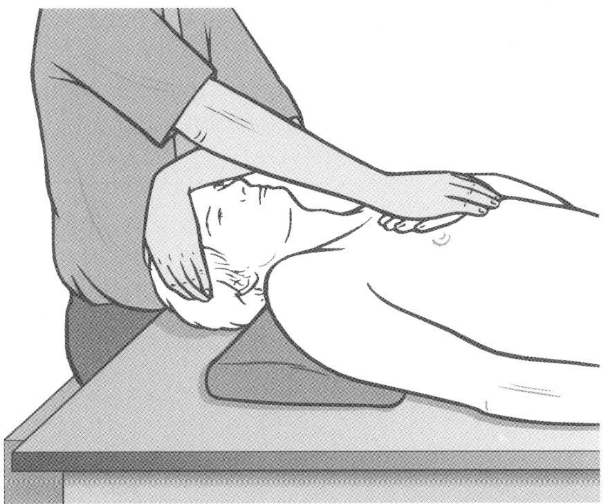

Figure 4.34C MET treatment of the anterior fibres of the scalenes; hand placement is on the sternum.

degrees of rotation, supported by the practitioner's contralateral hand.

The patient is instructed to try to lift the forehead a fraction and to attempt to turn the head towards the affected side, with appropriate breathing cooperation, while resistance is applied by the practitioner's hand to prevent both movements ('breathe in and hold your breath as you "lift and turn", and hold this for 7–10 seconds'). Both the effort and, the counter-pressure should be modest and painless at all times.

After a 7–10 second contraction, the head is placed into extension and one hand remains on it to prevent movement during the scalene stretch.

The patient's contralateral hand is placed (palm down) just inferior to the lateral end of the clavicle on the affected side (for full rotation of the head, posterior scalenes). The practitioner's hand which was acting to produce resistance to the isometric contraction is now placed onto the dorsum of the patient's 'cushion' hand.

As the patient slowly exhales, the practitioner's contact hand, resting on the patient's hand, which is itself resting on the 2nd rib and upper thorax, pushes obliquely away and towards the foot on that same side, following the rib movement into its exhalation position, so stretching the attached musculature and fascia. This stretch is held for at least 20 seconds after each isometric contraction.

The process is then repeated at least once more.

The head is rotated 45° contralaterally and the 'cushion' hand contact, which applies the stretch of the middle scalenes, is placed just inferior to the middle aspect of the clavicle. When the head is in the almost upright facing position for the anterior scalene stretch, the 'cushion' hand contact is on the upper sternum itself.

In all other ways the methodology is as described for the first position above.

NOTE: It is important not to allow heroic degrees of neck extension during any phase of this treatment. There should be some extension, but it should be appropriate to the age and condition of the individual.

A degree of eye movement can assist scalene treatment and may be used as an alternative to the 'lift and turn' muscular effort described above. If the patient makes the eyes look caudally (towards the feet) and towards the affected side during the isometric contraction, she will increase the degree of contraction in the muscles. If during the resting phase, when stretch is being introduced, she looks away from the treated side, with eyes looking towards the top of the head, this will enhance the stretch of the muscle.

This whole procedure should be performed bilaterally several times in each of the three head positions.

Scalene stretches, with all their variable positions, clearly also influence many of the anterior neck structures.

11. Assessment and treatment of sternocleidomastoid (SCM)

(see also Box 4.10)

Assessment for shortness of sternocleidomastoid (15)

Assessment for SCM is as for the scalenes – there is no absolute test for shortness but observation of posture (hyperlordotic neck, chin poked forward) and palpation of the degree of induration, fibrosis and trigger point activity can all alert to probable shortness of SCM. This is an accessory breathing muscle and, like the scalenes, will be shortened

Box 4.10 Notes on sternocleidomastoid

- Sternocleidomastoid (SCM) is a prominent muscle of the anterior neck and is closely associated with the trapezius. SCM often acts as postural compensator for head tilt associated with postural distortions found elsewhere (spinal, pelvic or lower extremity functional or structural inadequacies, for instance) although they seldom cause restriction of neck movement.
- SCM is synergistic with anterior neck muscles for flexion of the head and flexion of the cervical column on the thoracic column, when the cervical column is already flattened by the prevertebral muscles. However, when the head is placed in extension and SCM contracts, it accentuates lordosis of the cervical column, flexes the cervical column on the thoracic column, and adds to extension of the head. In this way, SCM is both synergist and antagonist to the prevertebral muscles (Kapandji 1974).
- SCM trigger points are activated by forward head positioning, 'whiplash' injury, positioning of the head to look upwardly for extended periods of time and structural compensations. The two heads of SCM each have their own patterns of trigger point referral which include (among others) into the ear, top of head, into the temporomandibular joint, over the brow, into the throat, and those which cause proprioceptive disturbances, disequilibrium, nausea and dizziness. Tenderness in SCM may be associated with trigger points in the digastric muscle and digastric trigger points may be satellites of SCM trigger points (Simons et al 1998).
- Simons et al (1998) report:

> When objects of equal weight are held in the hands, the patient with unilateral trigger point [TrP] involvement of the clavicular division [of SCM] may exhibit an abnormal Weight Test. When asked to judge which is heaviest of two objects of the same weight that look alike but may not be the same weight (two vapocoolant dispensers, one of which may have been used) the patient will [give] evidence [of] dysmetria by underestimating the weight of the object held in the hand on the same side as the affected sternocleidomastoid muscle. Inactivation of the responsible sternocleidomastoid TrPs promptly restores weight appreciation by this test. Apparently, the afferent discharges from these TrPs disturb central processing of proprioceptive information from the upper limb muscles as well as vestibular function related to neck muscles.

- Lymph nodes lie superficially along the medial aspect of the SCM and may be palpated, especially when enlarged. These nodes may be indicative of chronic cranial infections stemming from a throat infection, dental abscess, sinusitis or tumour. Likewise, trigger points in SCM may be perpetuated by some of these conditions (Simons et al 1998).
- Lewit (1999) points out that tenderness noted at the medial end of the clavicle and/or at the transverse process of the atlas is often an indication of SCM hypertonicity. This will commonly accompany a forward head position and/or tendency to upper chest breathing, and will almost inevitably be associated with hypertonicity, shortening and trigger point evolution in associated musculature, including scalenes, upper trapezius and levator scapula (see crossed syndrome notes in Ch. 2).

by inappropriate breathing patterns which have become habitual. Observation is an accurate assessment tool.

Since SCM is only just observable when normal, if the clavicular insertion is easily visible, or any part of the muscle is prominent, this can be taken as a clear sign of tightness of the muscle.

If the patient's posture involves the head being held forward of the body, often accompanied by cervical lordosis and dorsal kyphosis (see notes on upper crossed syndrome in Ch. 2), weakness of the deep neck flexors and tightness of SCM is suspected.

Functional SCM test (see Fig. 5.14A, B)

The supine patient is asked to 'very slowly raise your head and touch your chin to your chest'. The practitioner stands to the side with his head at the same level as the patient. At the beginning of the movement of the head, as the patient lifts this from the table, the practitioner would (if SCM were short) note that the chin was lifted first, allowing it to jut forwards, rather than the forehead leading the arc-like progression of the movement. In marked shortness of SCM the chin pokes forward in a jerk as the head is lifted.

If the reading of this sign is unclear then Janda (1988) suggests that a slight resistance pressure be applied to the forehead as the patient makes the 'chin to chest' attempt. If SCM is short this will ensure the jutting of the chin at the outset.

MET treatment of shortened SCM (Fig. 4.35)

The patient is supine with the head supported in a neutral position by one of the practitioner's hands. The shoulders rest on a cushion or folded

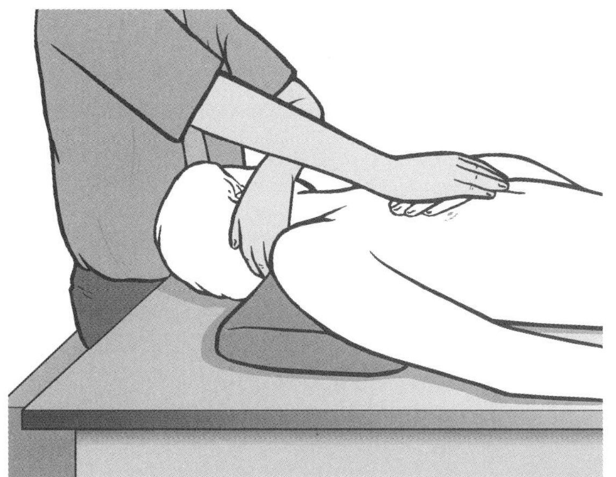

Figure 4.35 MET of sternocleidomastoid on the right.

towel, so that when the head is placed on the table it will be in slight extension. The patient's contralateral hand rests on the upper aspect of the sternum to act as a cushion when pressure is applied during the stretch phase of the operation (as in scalene and pectoral treatment). The patient's head is fully but comfortably rotated, contralaterally.

The patient is asked to lift the fully rotated head a small degree towards the ceiling, and to hold the breath. When the head is raised there is no need for the practitioner to apply resistance as gravity effectively provides this.

After 7–10 seconds of isometric contraction (ideally with breath held), the patient is asked to slowly release the effort (and the breath) and to place the head (still in rotation) on the table, so that a small degree of extension occurs.

The practitioner's hand covers the patient's 'cushion' hand (which rests on the sternum) in order to apply oblique pressure/stretch to the sternum, to ease it away from the head and towards the feet.

The hand not involved in stretching the sternum caudally should gently restrain the tendency the head will have to follow this stretch, but *should not under any circumstances apply pressure to stretch the head/neck while it is in this vulnerable position of rotation and slight extension.*

The degree of extension of the neck should be slight, 10–15° at most.

This stretch, which is applied as the patient exhales, is maintained for not less than 20 seconds to begin the release/stretch of hypertonic and fibrotic structures.

Repeat at least once.

The other side should then be treated in the same manner.

⚠ **CAUTION:** Care is required, especially with middle aged and elderly patients, in applying this useful stretching procedure. Appropriate tests should be carried out to evaluate cerebral circulation problems. The presence of such problems indicates that this particular MET method should be avoided.

12. Assessment and treatment of levator scapulae (Fig. 4.36)

Assessment of levator scapulae (16)

Levator scapula 'springing' test (a) The patient lies supine with the arm of the side to be tested stretched out with the supinated hand and lower arm tucked under the buttocks, to help restrain movement of the shoulder/scapula. The practitioner's contralateral arm is passed across and under the neck to cup the shoulder of the side to be tested, with the forearm supporting the neck.[11] The practitioner's other hand supports the head. The forearm is used to lift the neck into *full pain-free flexion* (aided by the other hand). The head is placed fully towards side-flexion and rotation, *away* from the side being treated.

With the shoulder held caudally and the head/neck in the position described (each at its resistance barrier) stretch is being placed on levator from both ends.

If dysfunction exists and/or levator scapula is short, there will be discomfort reported at the attachment on the upper medial border of the

[11] Lewit (1992) achieves the same control by having the supine patient place their flexed elbow above their head, in contact with the practitioner's thigh or abdomen. This allows pressure through the long axis of the humerus to fix the scapula, while both hands are free to take the head/neck into its desired position.

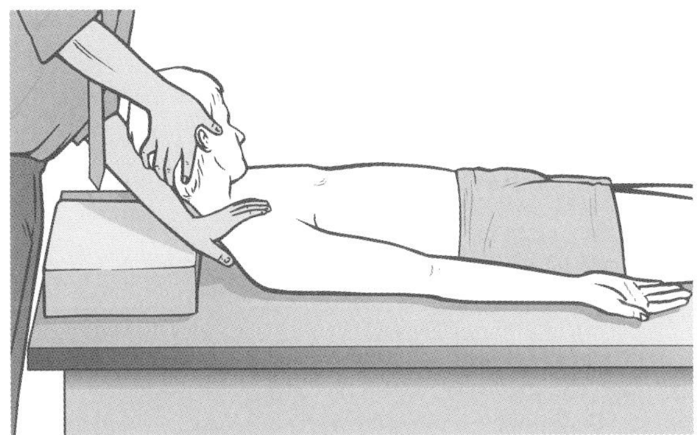

Figure 4.36 MET test (a) and treatment position for levator scapula (right side).

scapula and/or pain reported near the levator attachment on the spinous process of C2.

The hand on the shoulder gently 'springs' it caudally.

If levator is short there will be a *harsh*, wooden feel to this action. If it is normal there will be a soft feel to the springing pressure.

Levator scapula observation test (b) A functional assessment involves applying the evidence we have seen (see Ch. 2) of the imbalances which commonly occur between the upper and lower stabilisers of the scapula. In this process shortness is noted in pectoralis minor, levator scapulae and upper trapezius (as well as SCM), while weakness develops in serratus anterior, rhomboids, middle and lower trapezius – as well as the deep neck flexors.

Observation of the patient from behind will often show a 'hollow' area between the shoulder blades, where interscapular weakness has occurred, as well as an increased (over normal) distance between the medial borders of the scapulae and the thoracic spine, as the scapulae will have 'winged' away from it.

Levator scapula test (c) To see the imbalance described in test (b) in action, Janda (1996) has the patient in the press-up position (see Fig. 5.15). On very slow lowering of the chest towards the floor from a maximum push-up position, the scapula(e) on the side(s) where stabilisation has been compromised will move outwards, laterally and upwards – often into a winged position – rather than towards the spine.

This is diagnostic of weak lower stabilisers, which implicates tight upper stabilisers, including levator scapulae, as inhibiting them.

MET treatment of levator scapula (Fig. 4.36)

Treatment of levator scapulae using MET enhances the lengthening of the extensor muscles attaching to the occiput and upper cervical spine. The position described below is used for treatment, either at the limit of easily reached range of motion, or a little short of this, depending upon the degree of acuteness or chronicity of the dysfunction.

The patient lies supine with the arm of the side to be tested stretched out alongside the trunk with the hand supinated. The practitioner, standing at the head of the table, passes his contralateral arm under the neck to rest on the patient's shoulder on the side to be treated, so that the practitioner's forearm supports the patient's neck. The practitioner's other hand supports and directs the head into subsequent movement (below).

The practitioner's forearm lifts the neck into full flexion (aided by the other hand). The head is turned fully into side-flexion and rotation away from the side being treated.

With the shoulder held caudally by the practitioner's hand, and the head/neck in full flexion, side-flexion and rotation (each at its resistance barrier), stretch is being placed on levator from both ends.

The patient is asked to take the head backwards towards the table, and slightly to the side from which it was turned, against the practitioner's unmoving resistance, while at the same time a slight (20% of available strength) shoulder shrug is also asked for and resisted.

Following the 7–10 second isometric contraction and complete relaxation of all elements of this combined contraction, the neck is taken to further flexion, sidebending and rotation, where it is maintained as the shoulder is depressed caudally with the patient's assistance ('as you breathe out, slide your hand towards your feet'). The stretch is held for 20–30 seconds.

The process is repeated at least once.

⚠ **CAUTION:** Avoid overstretching this sensitive area.

Facilitation of tone in lower shoulder fixators using pulsed MET (Ruddy 1962)

In order to commence rehabilitation and proprioceptive re-education of a weak serratus anterior:

The practitioner places a single digit contact very lightly against the lower medial scapula border, on the side of the treated upper trapezius of the seated or standing patient. The patient is asked to attempt to ease the scapula, at the point of digital contact, towards the spine ('press against my finger with your shoulder blade, towards your spine, just as hard [i.e. very lightly] as I am pressing against your shoulder blade, for less than a second').

Once the patient has learned to establish control over the particular muscular action required to achieve this subtle movement (which can take a significant number of attempts), and can do so for 1 second at a time, repetitively, they are ready to begin the sequence based on Ruddy's methodology (see Ch. 10, p. 75).

The patient is told something such as 'now that you know how to activate the muscles which push your shoulder blade lightly against my finger, I want you to try do this 20 times in 10 seconds, starting and stopping, so that no actual movement takes place, just a contraction and a stopping, repetitively'.

This repetitive contraction will activate the rhomboids, middle and lower trapezii and serratus anterior – all of which are probably inhibited if upper trapezius is hypertonic. The repetitive contractions also produce an automatic reciprocal inhibition of upper trapezius, and levator scapula.

The patient can be taught to place a light finger or thumb contact against their own medial scapula (opposite arm behind back) so that home application of this method can be performed several times daily.

Treatment for eye muscles (Ruddy 1962)

Ruddy's treatment method for the muscles of the eye is outlined in Box 4.11.

Box 4.11 Ruddy's treatment for the muscles of the eye (Ruddy 1962)

Osteopathic eye specialist Dr T. Ruddy described a practical treatment method for application of MET principles to the muscles of the eye:

- The pads of the practitioner's index, middle and ring finger and the thumb are placed together to form four contacts into which the eyeball (eye closed) can rest (middle finger is above the cornea and the thumb pad below it).
- These contacts resist the attempts the patient is asked to make to move the eyes downwards, laterally, medially and upwards – as well as obliquely between these compass points – up and half medial, down and half medial, up and half lateral, down and half lateral, etc.
- The fingers resist and obstruct the intended path of eye motion.
- Each movement should last for a count 'one' and then rest between efforts for a similar count, and in each position there should be 10 repetitions before moving on around the circuit.

Ruddy maintained the method released muscle tension, permitted better circulation, and enhanced drainage. He applied the method as part of treatment of many eye problems.

13. Assessment and treatment of infraspinatus

Assessment of shortness in infraspinatus (17)

Infraspinatus shortness test (a) The patient is asked to reach upwards, backwards and across to touch the upper border of the opposite scapula, so producing external rotation of the humeral head. If this effort is painful infraspinatus shortness should be suspected.

Infraspinatus shortness test (b) (see Fig. 4.37) Visual evidence of shortness is obtained by having the patient supine, upper arm at right angles to the trunk, elbow flexed so that lower arm is parallel with the trunk, pointing caudad with the palm downwards. This brings the arm into internal rotation and places infraspinatus at stretch. The practitioner ensures that the shoulder remains in contact with the table during this assessment by means of light compression.

If infraspinatus is short, the lower arm will not be capable of resting parallel with the floor, obliging it to point somewhat towards the ceiling.

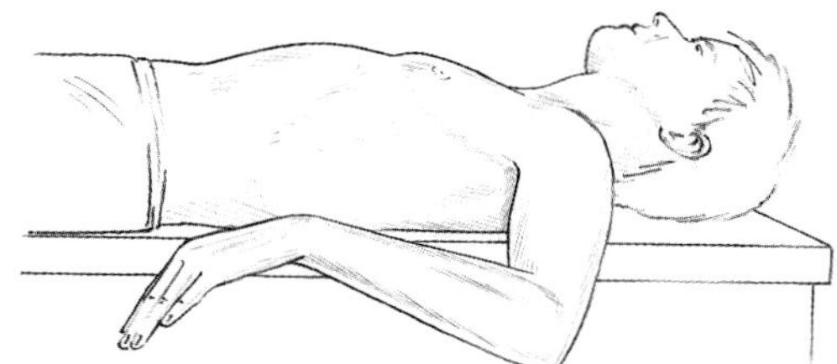

Figure 4.37 Assessment and self-treatment position for infraspinatus. If the upper arm cannot rest parallel to the floor, possible shortness of infraspinatus is indicated.

Assessment for infraspinatus weakness

The patient is seated. The practitioner stands behind. The patient's arms are flexed at the elbows and held to the side, and the practitioner provides isometric resistance to external rotation of the lower arms (externally rotating them and also the humerus at the shoulder). If this effort is painful, an indication of probable infraspinatus shortening exists.

The relative strength is also judged. If weak, the method discussed by Norris (1999) (see Ch. 3) should be used to increase strength (isotonic eccentric contraction performed slowly).

NOTE: In this as in other tests for weakness there may be a better degree of cooperation if the practitioner applies the force, and the patient is asked to resist as much as possible.

Force should always be built slowly and not suddenly.

MET treatment of infraspinatus (Fig. 4.38)

The patient is supine, upper arm at right angles to the trunk, elbow flexed so that lower arm is parallel with the trunk, pointing caudad with the palm downwards. This brings the arm into internal rotation and places infraspinatus at stretch.

The practitioner ensures that the posterior shoulder remains in contact with the table by means of light compression. The patient slowly and gently lifts the dorsum of the wrist towards the ceiling, against resistance from the practitioner, for 7–10 seconds.

After this isometric contraction, on relaxation, the forearm is taken towards the floor (combined patient and practitioner action), so increasing internal rotation at the shoulder and stretching infraspinatus (mainly at its shoulder attachment).

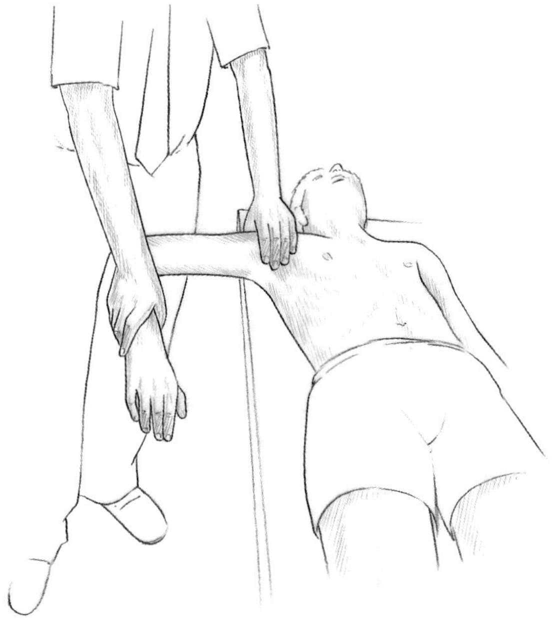

Figure 4.38 MET treatment of infraspinatus. Note that the practitioner's left hand maintains a downward pressure to stabilise the shoulder to the table during this procedure.

Care needs to be taken to prevent the shoulder from rising from the table as rotation is introduced, so giving a false appearance of stretch in the muscle.

And

In order to initiate stretch of infraspinatus at the scapular attachment, the patient is seated with the arm (flexed at the elbow) fully internally rotated and taken into full adduction across the chest. The practitioner holds the upper arm and applies sustained traction from the shoulder in order to prevent subacromial impingement.

The patient is asked to use a light (20% of strength) effort to attempt to externally rotate and abduct the arm, against resistance offered by the practitioner, for 7–10 seconds.

After this isometric contraction, and with the traction from the shoulder maintained, the arm is taken into increased internal rotation and adduction (patient and practitioner acting together) where the stretch is held for at least 20 seconds.

14. Assessment and treatment of subscapularis

Assessment of shortness in subscapularis (18)

Subscapularis shortness test (a) Direct palpation of subscapularis is required to define problems in it, since pain patterns in the shoulder, arm, scapula and chest may all derive from subscapularis or from other sources.

The patient is supine and the practitioner grasps the affected side hand and applies traction while the fingers of the other hand palpate over the edge of latissimus dorsi in order to make contact with the ventral surface of the scapula, where subscapularis can be palpated.

There may be a marked reaction from the patient when this is touched, indicating acute sensitivity.

Subscapularis shortness test (b) (Fig. 4.39) The patient is supine with the arm abducted to 90°, the elbow flexed to 90°, and the forearm in external rotation, palm upwards. The whole arm is resting at the restriction barrier, with gravity as its counterweight.

If subscapularis is short the forearm will be unable to rest easily parallel with the floor but will be somewhat elevated.

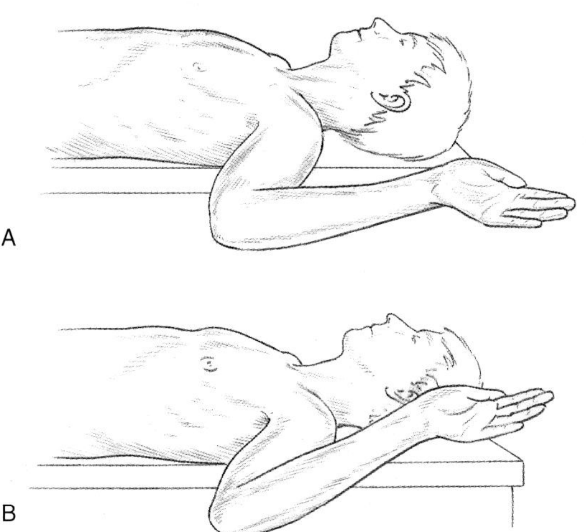

Figure 4.39A, B Assessment and MET self-treatment position for subscapularis. If the upper arm cannot rest parallel to the floor, possible shortness of subscapularis is indicated.

Care is needed to prevent the anterior shoulder becoming elevated in this position (moving towards the ceiling) and so giving a false normal picture.

Assessment of weakness in subscapularis

The patient is prone with humerus abducted to 90° and elbow flexed to 90°. The humerus should be in internal rotation so that the forearm is parallel with the trunk, palm towards ceiling. The practitioner stabilises the scapula with one hand and with the other applies pressure to the patient's wrist and forearm as though taking the humerus towards external rotation, while the patient resists.

The relative strength is judged and the method discussed by Norris (1999) (see Ch. 3) should used to increase strength (isotonic eccentric contraction performed slowly).[12]

MET treatment of subscapularis

The patient is supine with the arm abducted to 90°, the elbow flexed to 90°, and the forearm in external rotation, palm upwards. The whole arm is resting at the restriction barrier, with gravity as its counterweight. (Care is needed to prevent the anterior shoulder becoming elevated in this position (moving towards the ceiling) and so giving a false normal picture.)

The patient raises the forearm slightly, against minimal resistance from the practitioner, for 7–10 seconds and, following relaxation, gravity or slight assistance from the operator takes the arm into greater external rotation, through the barrier, where it is held for not less than 20 seconds.

15. Assessment and treatment of supraspinatus

Assessment for shortness of supraspinatus (19)

Supraspinatus shortness test (a) (see Fig. 4.40) The practitioner stands behind the seated

[12] There could be other reasons for a restricted degree of external rotation, and accurate assessment calls for direct palpation as in (a) above.

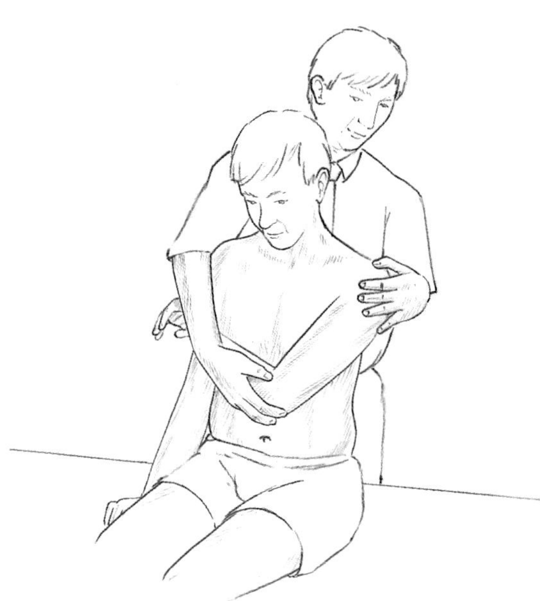

Figure 4.40 Position for test (a) and MET treatment of supraspinatus.

patient, with one hand stabilising the shoulder on the side to be assessed while the other hand reaches in front of the patient to support the flexed elbow and forearm. The patient's upper arm is adducted to its easy barrier and the patient then attempts to abduct the arm.

If pain is noted in the posterior shoulder region during this attempt this is diagnostic of supraspinatus dysfunction and, by implication because it is a postural muscle, of shortness.

Assessment for supraspinatus weakness

The patient sits or stands with arm abducted 15°, elbow extended. The practitioner stabilises the shoulder with one hand while the other hand offers a resistance contact which if forceful would adduct the arm. The patient attempts to resist this, and the degree of effort required to overcome the patient's resistance is graded as weak or strong.

The relative strength is judged and the method discussed by Norris (1999) (see Ch. 3) should be used to increase strength (isotonic eccentric contraction performed slowly).

MET treatment of supraspinatus

The practitioner stands behind the seated patient, with one hand stabilising the shoulder on the side to be treated while the other hand reaches in front of the patient to support the flexed elbow and forearm. The patient's upper arm is adducted to its easy barrier and the patient then attempts to abduct the arm using 20% of strength against practitioner resistance.

After a 10-second isometric contraction, the arm is taken gently towards its new resistance barrier into greater adduction, with the patient's assistance.

Repeat several times, holding each painless stretch for not less than 20 seconds.

16. Assessment and treatment of flexors of the arm

Assessment for shortness in flexors of the arm (20)

Biceps tendon shortness test (a) Long biceps tendon is stressed if pain arises when the semi-flexed arm is raised against resistance.

Biceps tendon shortness test (b) The patient fully flexes the elbow and the practitioner holds it in one hand while holding the patient's hand in the other. The patient is asked to resist as the practitioner attempts to externally rotate the elbow and to straighten the arm. If very unstable, the tendon may momentarily leave its groove and pain will result.

Biceps tendon shortness test (c) The patient sits with extended arm (taking it backwards from the shoulder), half flexes the elbow so that the dorsum of the hand approximates the contralateral buttock. The patient attempts to flex the elbow further against resistance.

If pain is noted, there is stress on the tendon and flexors are probably shortened.

MET treatment for shortness in biceps tendon

Lewit (1992) describes the following method:

The patient sits in front of the practitioner, with the affected arm behind the back, the dorsal aspect of that hand passing beyond the buttock on the opposite side. The practitioner grasps this

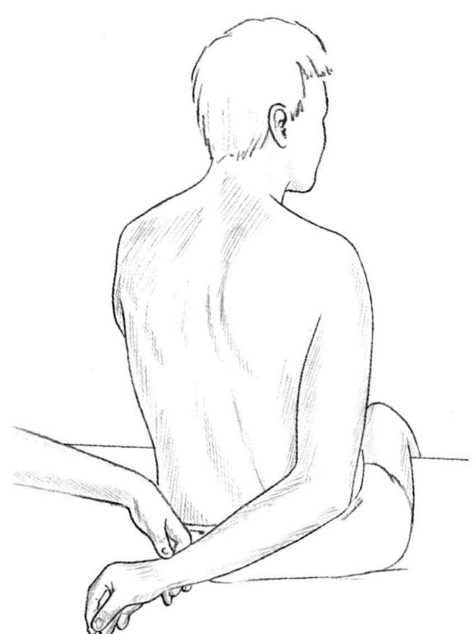

Figure 4.41 Assessment and MET treatment for dysfunction affecting biceps tendon.

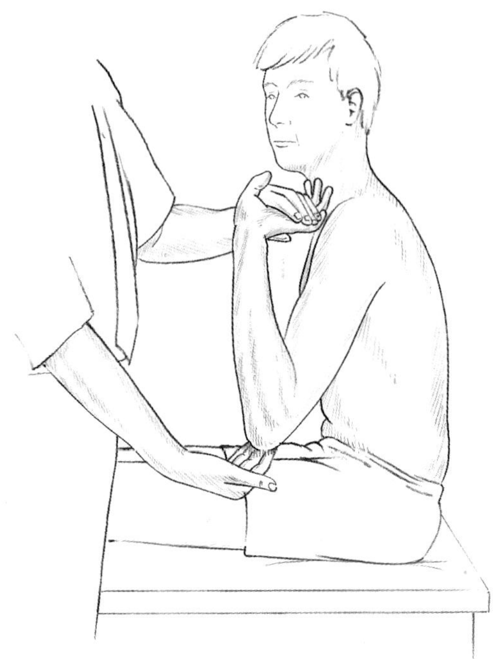

Figure 4.42 Assessment and MET treatment for shortness of the flexors of the forearm.

hand, bringing it into pronation, to take up the slack (see Fig. 4.41).

The patient is instructed to attempt to take the hand back into supination. This is resisted for about 10 seconds by the practitioner, and the relaxation phase is used to take it further into pronation, with simultaneous extension of the elbow.

Three to five repetitions may need to be performed.

Self-treatment is possible, with the patient applying counter-pressure with the other hand.

Flexors of the forearm – assessment for shortness and MET treatment

A painful medial humeral epicondyle usually accompanies tension in the flexors of the forearm.

The patient is seated facing the practitioner, with flexed elbow supported by the practitioner's fingers. The patient's hand is dorsiflexed at the wrist, so that the palm is upwards and fingers face the shoulder (see Fig. 4.42).

The practitioner guides the wrist into greater flexion to an easy barrier, with pronation exaggerated by pressure on the ulnar side of the palm. This is achieved by means of the practitioner's thumb being placed on the dorsum of the patient's hand while the fingers stabilise the palmar aspect, fingertips pressing this towards the floor on the patient's ulnar side of the palm.

The patient attempts to gently supinate the hand against resistance for 7–10 seconds following which, after relaxation, on an exhalation, dorsiflexion is increased to or through (acute/chronic) the new barrier.

Repeat as needed.

This method is easily capable of adaptation to self-treatment by means of the patient applying the counter-pressure.

Biceps brachii – assessment and MET treatment

If extension of the arm is limited, the flexors are probably short. Treatment of biceps brachii involves the affected arm being held in extension at the easy barrier.

The practitioner holds the patient's wrist in order to restrain a light effort to flex the elbow for 7–10 seconds after which, following appropriate rest and breathing cooperation (see notes on breathing, Box 4.2), the arm is extended to or through (acute/chronic) the new resistance barrier.

Repeat several times.

17. Assessment and treatment of paravertebral muscles

Assessment of paravertebral muscles (21) (Fig. 4.43)

Paravertebral muscle shortness test (a) The patient is seated on a treatment table, legs extended, pelvis vertical. Flexion is introduced in order to approximate forehead to knees. An even 'C' curve should be observed and a distance of about 4 in (10 cm) from the knees achieved by the forehead. No knee flexion should occur and the movement should be a spinal one, not involving pelvic tilting (see Fig. 4.43).

Paravertebral muscle shortness test (b) This assessment position is then modified to remove hamstring shortness from the picture by having the patient sit at the end of the table, knees flexed over it. Once again the patient is asked to perform full flexion, without strain, so that forward bending is introduced to bring the forehead towards the knees. The pelvis should be fixed by the placement of the patient's hands on the pelvic crest. If bending of the trunk is greater in this position than in test (a) above, then there is probably shortened hamstring involvement.

During these assessments, areas of shortening in the spinal muscles may be observed as 'flat', or even, in the lumbar area, of a reversed curve. For example, on forward bending a lordosis may be maintained in the lumbar spine, or flexion may be very limited even without such lordosis. There may be evidence of obvious overstretching of the upper back and relative tightness of the lower back.

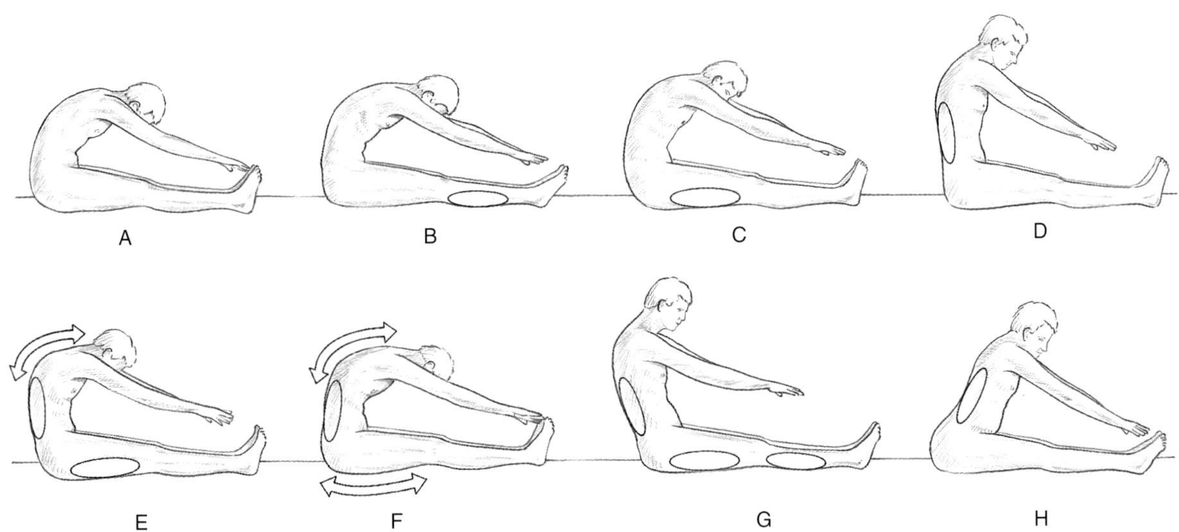

Figure 4.43 Tests for shortness of the erector spinae and associated postural muscles.

A Normal length of erector spinae muscles and posterior thigh muscles.
B Tight gastrocnemius and soleus; the inability to dorsiflex the feet indicates tightness of the plantar – flexor group.
C Tight hamstring muscles, which cause the pelvis to tilt posteriorly.
D Tight low back erector spinae muscles.
E Tight hamstrings; slightly tight low back muscles and overstretched upper back muscles.
F Slightly shortened lower back muscles, stretched upper back muscles and slightly stretched hamstrings.
G Tight low back muscles, hamstrings and gastrocnemius/soleus.
H Very tight low back muscles, with lordosis maintained even in flexion.

All areas of 'flatness' are charted since these represent an inability of those segments to flex, which involves the erector spinae muscles as a primary or a secondary feature.

If the flexion restriction relates to articular factors, the erector group will nevertheless benefit from MET. If they are primary causes of the flexion restriction then MET attention is even more indicated.

Lewit (1999) points out that patients with a long trunk and short thighs may perform the movement without difficulty, even if the erectors are short, whereas if the trunk is short and the thighs long, even if the erectors are supple, flexion will not allow the head to approximate the knees.

In the modified position, with patient's hands on the crest of the pelvis, and the patient 'humping' her spine, Lewit suggests observation of the presence or otherwise of lumbar kyphosis for evidence of shortness in that region. If it fails to appear, erector spinae shortness in the lumbar region is likely. This, together with the presence of flat areas, provides significant evidence of shortness.

Paravertebral muscle shortness test (c) (Fig. 4.44) Once all flat areas are noted and charted, the patient is placed in prone position. The practitioner squats at the side and observes the spinal 'wave' as deep breathing is performed.

There should be a wave of movement starting at the sacrum and finishing at the base of the neck on inhalation. Areas of restriction ('flat areas'), lack of movement, or where motion is not in sequence should be noted and compared with findings from tests (a) and (b) above.

Periodic review of the relative normality of this wave is a useful guide to progress (or lack of it) in normalisation of the functional status of the respiratory and spinal structures.

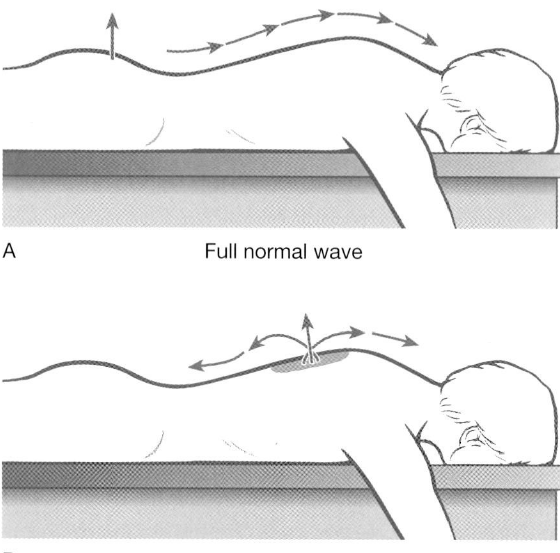

Figure 4.44 Observation of the prone breathing wave indicates areas of paravertebral stiffness or vertebral fixation. Rigid areas tend to move as a block, rather than as a wave.

MET treatment of erector spinae muscle

The patient sits on the treatment table, back towards the practitioner, legs hanging over the side, and hands clasped behind the neck. The practitioner places a knee on the table close to the patient, at the side towards which sidebending and rotation will be introduced.

The practitioner passes a hand in front of the patient's axilla on the side to which the patient is to be rotated, across the front of the patient's neck, to rest on the contralateral shoulder. The patient is drawn into flexion, sidebending and rotation over the practitioner's knee.

The practitioner's free hand monitors the area of tightness (as evidenced by 'flatness' in the flexion test) and ensures that the various forces localise at the point of maximum contraction/tension.

When the patient has been taken to the comfortable limit of flexion, he is asked either to look (eyes only) towards the direction from which rotation has been made while holding the breath for 7–10 seconds, or to do this while also introducing a very slight degree of effort towards rotating back to the upright position, against firm resistance from the practitioner. (See Fig. 6.1B; see also Figs 6.1E, F, 6.2A, B.)

It is useful to have the patient 'breathe into' the tight spinal area which is being palpated and monitored by the practitioner. This will cause an additional increase in isometric contraction of the short muscles. The patient is then asked to release the breath, and completely relax.

The practitioner waits for the patient's second full exhalation and then takes the patient further in all the directions of restriction, towards the new barrier, but not through it.

This whole process is repeated several times, at each level of restriction/flatness.

At the end of each sequence of repetition the patient may be asked to breathe in and to gently attempt to rotate further against resistance, towards the restriction barrier, while holding the breath for 7–10 seconds. This involves contraction of the antagonists. After relaxation, the new barrier is again approached.

Thoracolumbar dysfunction

This important transition region was discussed briefly in the section dealing with quadratus lumborum earlier in this chapter, and deserves special attention due to its particularly vulnerable 'transition' status involving the powerful effect that spasm and tightness of the major stabilising muscles of the region can have on it: notably psoas, the thoracolumbar erector spinae and quadratus lumborum, as well as the influence of rectus abdominis in which weakness is all too common (see lower crossed syndrome notes in Ch. 2).

Screening for lumbodorsal dysfunction involves having the patient straddle the table (so locking the pelvis) in a slightly flexed posture (slight kyphosis). Rotation in either direction enables segmental impairment to be observed at the same time as the spinous processes are monitored.

Restriction of rotation is the most common characteristic of this dysfunction.

MET treatment of thoracolumbar dysfunction

Psoas and/or quadratus lumborum should be treated as described earlier in this chapter.[13]

[13] Not all the muscles involved in thoracolumbar dysfunction pattern described above may need treatment since when one or other is treated appropriately the others tend to normalise. Underlying causes must also always receive attention.

Assessment for shortness in erector spinae muscles of the neck (21)

The patient is supine and the practitioner stands at the head of the table, or to the side, supporting the neck structures in one hand and the occiput in the other, to afford complete support for both. When the head/neck is lifted into flexion the chin should easily be able to be brought into contact with the suprasternal area, *without force*.

If there remains a noticeable gap between the tip of the chin (ignore double chin tissues) and the upper chest wall, then the neck extensors are considered to be short.

MET treatment of short neck extensor muscles (22)

The neck of the supine patient is flexed to its easy barrier of resistance, or short of this (acute/chronic), and the patient is asked to extend the neck ('take the back of your head back to the table, gently') using minimal effort on an inhalation, against resistance.

If the hand positions as described in the test above are not comfortable, then try placing the hands, arms crossed, so that a hand rests on the anterior surface of each shoulder, while the head rests on the crossed forearms.

After the contraction, the neck is flexed further to the new barrier of resistance.

A further aid during the contraction phase is to have the practitioner contact the top of the patient's head with his abdomen, and to use this contact to prevent the patient tilting the head upwards. This allows for an additional isometric contraction which involves the short extensor muscles at the base of the skull ('tip your chin upwards'). The subsequent stretch, as above, will involve these muscles as well.

Repetitions of the stretch to the new barrier should be performed until no further gain is possible, or until the chin easily touches the chest on flexion.

NOTE: No force should be used, or pain produced during this procedure.[14]

[14] If assessment is being made of cervical rotational efficiency/restriction a simple screening device is available. When the head/neck is in full flexion, and rotation is introduced, all rotation below C3 is blocked. Therefore, if rotation is tested in full flexion and there is a limitation to one side, this probably represents a problem in the atlanto-occipital or atlanto-axial joints. When the head is fully extended on the neck, then the atlanto-occipital and C2/3 joints are locked and any rotation restriction relates to problems below that level.

Other MET treatment methods

A variety of MET treatment methods for pelvic and spinal joint restrictions, as well as the shoulder, clavicular and cervical area, will be found in Chapter 6, and these can be used alongside the more general, muscle orientated approaches detailed in this chapter.

REFERENCES

Basmajian J 1974 Muscles alive. Williams and Wilkins, Baltimore

Bergmark A 1989 Stability of the lumbar spine: a study in mechanical engineering. Acta Orthopaedica Scandinavica 230(suppl): 20–24

Bogduk N 1997 Clinical anatomy of the lumbar spine and sacrum, 3rd edn. Churchill Livingstone, Edinburgh

Bogduk N, Pearcy M, Hadfield G 1992 Anatomy and biomechanics of psoas major. Clinical Biomechanics 7: 109–119

Bourdillon J 1982 Spinal manipulation, 3rd edn. Heinemann, London

Cailliet R 1962 Low back pain syndrome. Blackwell, Oxford

Chaitow L 1991 Soft tissue manipulation. Healing Arts Press, Rochester

Dvorak J, Dvorak V 1984 Manual medicine – diagnostics. George Thieme Verlag, New York

Evjenth O 1984 Muscle stretching in manual therapy. Alfta Rehab, Alfta, Sweden

Fryette H 1954 Principles of osteopathic technic. Yearbook of the Academy of Applied Osteopathy, 1954, Indianapolis

Gluck N, Liebenson C 1997 Paradoxical muscle function. Journal of Bodywork and Movement Therapies 1(4): 219–222

Gray 1995 Grays Anatomy, 38th edn. Churchill Livingstone, Edinburgh

Greenman P 1989 Principles of manual medicine, 1st edn. Williams and Wilkins, Baltimore

Greenman P 1996 Principles of manual medicine, 2nd edn. Williams and Wilkins, Baltimore

Janda V 1983 Muscle function testing. Butterworths, London

Janda V 1988 In: Grant R (ed) Physical therapy of the cervical and thoracic spine. Churchill Livingstone, New York

Janda V 1996 Evaluation of muscular imbalance. In: Liebenson C (ed) Rehabilitation of the spine. Williams and Wilkins, Baltimore

Jull G 1994 Active stabilisation of the trunk. Course notes. Edinburgh

Kapandji I 1974 The physiology of the joints, vol 3, 2nd edn. Churchill Livingstone, Edinburgh

Kendall F P, McCreary E K, Provance P G 1993 Muscles, testing and function, 4th edn. Williams and Wilkins, Baltimore

Lehmkuhl L, Smith L 1983 Brunnstrom's clinical kinesiology, 4th edn. F A Davis, Philadelphia

Lewit K 1985a Muscular and articular factors in movement restriction. Manual Medicine 1: 83–85

Lewit K 1985b Manipulative therapy in rehabilitation of the motor system. Butterworths, London

Lewit K 1992 Manipulative therapy in rehabilitation of the locomotor system, 2nd edn. Butterworths, London

Lewit K 1999 Manipulative therapy in rehabilitation of the locomotor system, 3rd edn. Butterworths, London

Liebenson C 1996 Rehabilitation of the spine. Williams and Wilkins, Baltimore

Lin J-P et al 1994 Physiological maturation of muscles in childhood. Lancet (June 4): 1386–1389

McGill S M, Juker D, Kropf P 1996 Quantitative intramuscular myoelectric activity of quadratus lumborum during a wide variety of tasks. Clinical Biomechanics 11: 170–172

Mennell J 1964 Back pain. T and A Churchill, Boston

Mitchell F, Moran P, Pruzzo N 1979 Manual of osteopathic muscle energy technique. Valley Park, Missouri

Moore M et al 1980 Electromyographic investigation manual of muscle stretching techniques. Medicine and Science in Sports and Exercise 12: 322–329

Norris C 1999 Functional load abdominal training (part 1). Journal of Bodywork and Movement Therapies 3(3): 150–158

Norris C 2000 The muscle designation debate. Journal of Bodywork and Movement Therapies 4(4): 225–241

Platzer W 1992 Color atlas/text of human anatomy. Vol. 1: Locomotor System, 4th edn. Thieme, Stuttgart

Retzlaff E 1974 The piriformis muscle syndrome. Journal of the American Osteopathic Association 173: 799–807

Richard R 1978 Lésions ostéopathiques du sacrum. Maloine, Paris

Richardson C, Jull G, Hodges P, Hides J 1999 Therapeutic exercise for spinal segmental stabilisation in low back pain. Churchill Livingstone, Edinburgh

Rolf I 1977 Rolfing – integration of human structures. Harper and Row, New York

Ruddy T 1962 Osteopathic rapid rhythmic resistive technic. Academy of Applied Osteopathy Yearbook, 1962, pp 23–31f

Simons D, Travell J, Simons L 1998 Myofascial pain and dysfunction: the trigger point manual (vol 1), 2nd edn. Williams and Wilkins, Baltimore

Stedman 1998 Stedman's electronic medical dictionary. Version 4.0. Williams and Wilkins, Baltimore

Taylor D, Dalton J, Seaber A, Garrett W 1990 Viscoelastic properties of muscle–tendon units: the biomechanical effects of stretching. American Journal of Sports Medicine 18: 300–309

TePoorten B 1960 The piriformis muscle. Journal of the American Osteopathic Association 69: 150–160

Travell J, Simons D 1992 Myofascial pain and dysfunction: the trigger point manual (vol 2). Williams and Wilkins, Baltimore

van Wingerden J-P 1997 The role of the hamstrings in pelvic and spinal function. In: Vleeming A (ed) Movement, stability and low back pain. Churchill Livingstone, New York

Vleeming A, Mooney A, Dorman T, Snijders C, Stoekart R 1989 Load application to the sacrotuberous ligament: influences on sacroiliac joint mechanics. Clinical Biomechanics 4: 204–209

Williams P 1965 Lumbosacral spine. McGraw Hill, New York

Wolf A 1997 From the archives: osteopathic procedures for the eyes. American Academy of Osteopathy Journal 7(2): 30

CHAPTER CONTENTS

5

Manual resistance techniques in rehabilitation

Craig Liebenson

The goal of rehabilitation is to restore function in the locomotor system. Manual resistance techniques (MRTs) are excellent bridges between passive and active care. The practitioner, or health care provider (HCP), is able to control the direction, magnitude, velocity and time of each force generated by the patient. MRTs can be used to inhibit overactive muscles, to facilitate underactive muscles or to mobilise joints, and are also ideal for self-treatment.

CLINICAL PROGRESSION OF CARE

Once diagnosis of the site of tissue injury or pain generation has been made, treatment matched to the goals of acute care – namely pain relief – can take place. As the patient's acute pain subsides, the recovery phase is entered. During this phase the HCP's assessment attempts to identify the potential sources of biomechanical overload which may have led to tissue injury or pain in the first place. When these sources are identified and linked to the pain generator, then rehabilitation efforts can be utilised to improve function in the relevant kinetic chain.

MRTs can be used during both the acute and recovery phases. Gentle postisometric relaxation (PIR) or hold–relax (HR) methods are ideal during acute care, while facilitation methods such as the diagonal patterns of proprioceptive neuromuscular facilitation (PNF) are more applicable in the recovery phase.

POSTISOMETRIC RELAXATION (PIR) TECHNIQUES

Postisometric relaxation (PIR) is an excellent technique for treating the neuromuscular component of a stiff, shortened or tight muscle (Lewit 1986, Liebenson 1989, 1990, Liebenson & Murphy 1998). In particular, if trigger points are present, PIR is very effective (Lewit & Simons 1984).

First, find the pathological barrier (Fig. 5.1). This occurs the moment resistance starts when taking out the slack. Confirm by feeling a lack of normal resilience or 'spring' at end-feel. Hold tension at the barrier without letting go of the slack and wait for a release of tissue tension. Do not stretch or bounce. If, after a brief latency, no release phenomenon occurs, have the patient gently push away from the barrier against your matched resistance – approximately 10% of their maximum effort – so as to create an isometric contraction. Once the isometric contraction is achieved, have the patient take a deep breath in and 'hold' for 5–8 seconds. Then have the patient 'let go' and again wait to feel the 'release' of the tissue tension. Only after feeling the release should you take up the slack to the new barrier. Repeat this up to three times. At the conclusion perform reciprocal inhibition by contracting antagonist muscles away from the barrier. This can also be performed isometrically in a phasic fashion as resistance is given intermittently over (approximately) a 10-second period.

If no release occurs, the following should be attempted:

1. Utilise respiratory synkinesis (e.g. breathe in during most contractions and exhale during release)
2. Have the patient increase the contraction phase up to 30 seconds
3. Have the patient use more force (i.e. 'as little as possible or as much as necessary')
4. Add visual synkinesis if appropriate (look in the direction of contraction and then the direction of release – see also p. 10)
5. Vary how you 'wind up' the muscle to isolate it. For example, when lengthening the anterior fibres, upper trapezius muscle slack is taken out in flexion of the upper cervical spine, contralateral lateral flexion of the neck, ipsilateral rotation of the neck, and shoulder depression. The order in which the slack is taken out can be altered in order to isolate tension to the part of the muscle where you want it.
6. Treat other related tissue first (joint mobilisation; facilitation of antagonist (reciprocal inhibition)).

According to Lewit (personal communication 1999), muscle is contractile tissue; if a muscle has

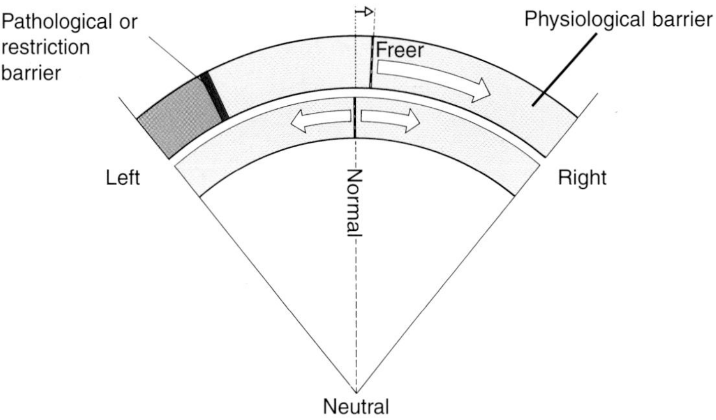

Figure 5.1 The barrier phenomenon.

Box 5.1 Common questions about PIR techniques (answers below)

Questions

1. Should the muscle be lengthened gently or firmly?
2. Is the 'barrier phenomenon' similar in PIR and in thrust techniques?
3. How long does it take to perform PIR on a muscle?
4. If PIR is unsuccessful, what does that suggest?
5. Are these techniques arduous for the HCP to perform?
6. Besides relaxing a muscle, PIR can be used for what other purposes?
7. What are the indications for PIR?

Answers

1. Gently.
2. Yes.
3. Less than a minute.
4. The problem is in the connective tissues.
5. Not typically.
6. To mobilise joints or prepare a muscle for more aggressive stretching techniques.
7. Increased muscle tension, trigger points and joint restriction.

decreased in length, 90% of the time this is due to it being contracted. The treatment in these cases is therefore relaxation. He estimates that in approximately 10% of cases it is due to connective tissue changes, and the treatment is therefore stretching. Do not, however, stretch a muscle containing a trigger point until after it has been inhibited.

PROPRIOCEPTIVE NEUROMUSCULAR FACILITATION

Proprioceptive neuromuscular facilitation (PNF) was originally utilised for neuromuscular re-education in stroke victims (Kabot 1950). Later it was discovered that it was clinically useful in rehabilitating children with cerebral palsy (CP) (Levine et al 1954). This led to its use for a wide range of orthopaedic conditions.

PNF is a philosophy of care which treats the whole body by stimulation of basic movement patterns (Adler et al 1993). These patterns are of neurodevelopmental origin and are incorporated in functional activities such as swimming, running, climbing, throwing, etc. Therefore, in contrast to most isotonic training approaches which are uniplanar, PNF methods resist movement in

Box 5.2 Common clinical applications of manual resistance techniques

A. Trigger point (semi-active)

Indication: palpation of taut band in muscle, with twitch sign and referred pain phenomenon.

Treatment: this is primarily a neuromuscular phenomenon, not a connective tissue problem. Treatment therefore requires a minimum of force. Use postisometric relaxation (PIR). Light ischaemic compression can also be used, especially for trigger points on the surface. The pressure should be just enough to engage a barrier to resistance and, following a latency, should achieve a release phenomenon. Greater force risks facilitating a contraction in the muscle as it 'defends' the barrier.

Experiment: try to find a trigger point in the upper trapezius (using a light pincer grip). Hold the taught band between your fingers. Then roll the taut band through your fingers as you search the length of the muscle for a motor response in the trigger point (i.e. local twitch response (LTR), see Fig. 5.2. Once you have found an LTR try to release the trigger point with PIR and then repalpate.

B. Shortened muscle (passive or semi-active)

Indication: positive length test for decreased range of motion.

Treatment: start with PIR. If PIR is unsuccessful, it is likely that there are connective tissue changes since mere relaxation alone did not result in a release of the muscle to a new resting length. There are two options:

1. Perform myofascial release by folding the muscle perpendicularly against itself and hold until release is 'sensed'. Then take out slack. This avoids the stretch reflex and is ideal for superficial muscles such as the pectoralis major (see Fig. 5.3).

2. If muscle is deep (e.g. iliopsoas), treat with a more forceful technique such as contract–relax antagonist–contract (CRAC) or postfacilitation stretch (PFS). PFS is similar to PIR except that a greater contraction force (25–100% of a patient's maximum) is used, after which a fast stretch is applied (Liebenson 1996). Note: if you are using PFS certain safety rules should be observed. These include the following: stretch over the largest, most stable, least painful joint; joints should be 'loose packed'; avoid uncoupled movements; and do not stretch nerves if they are irritated.

Experiment: test the length of the iliopsoas and adductors and then perform PIR (see Figs 4.9A,B, 4.10A,B).

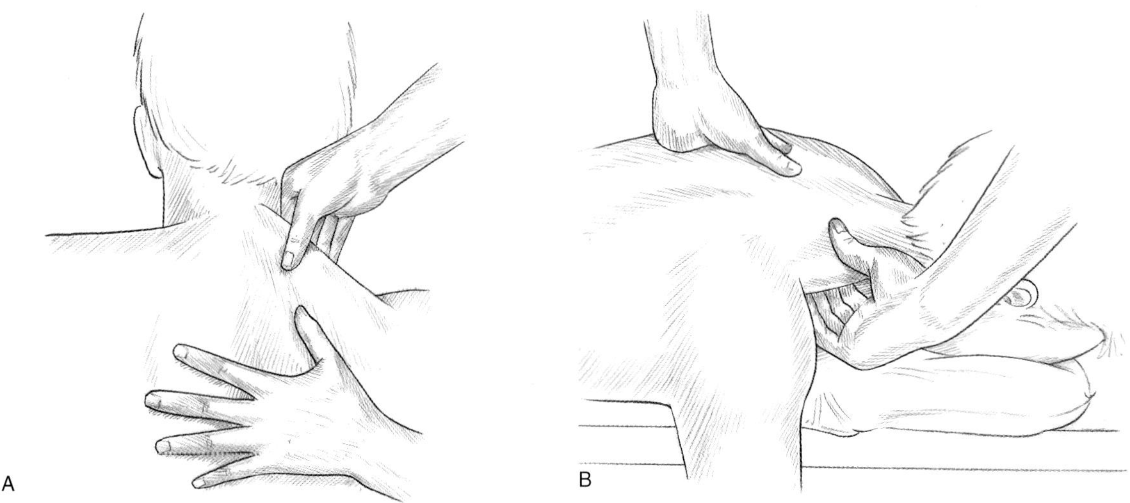

Figure 5.2A, B Palpation of trigger point with local twitch response in upper trapezius.

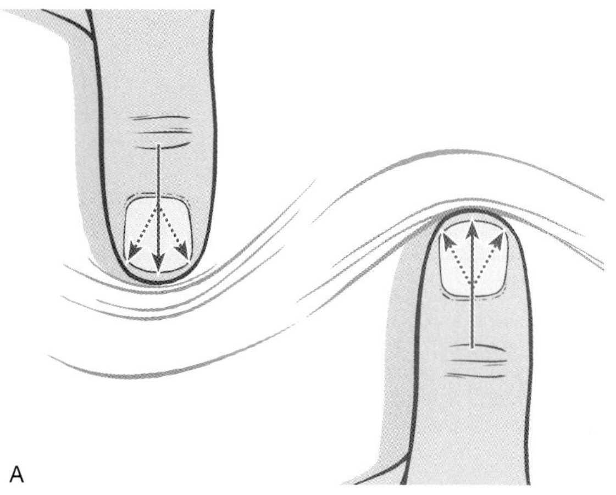

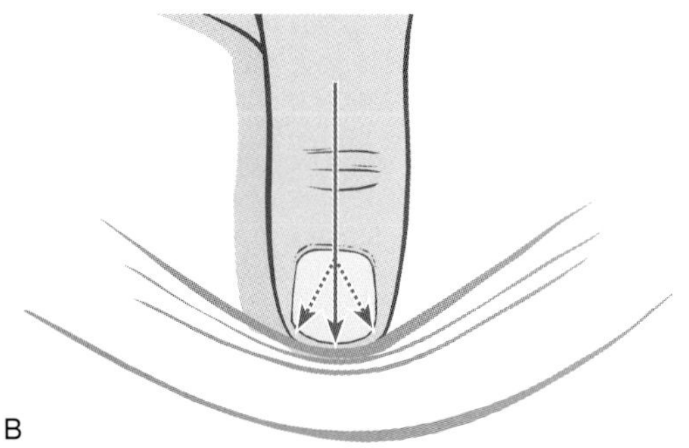

Figure 5.3A, B Myofascial release technique for the pectoralis major muscle.

multiple planes simultaneously. For instance, a diagonal pattern of movement will be resisted at the same time as a flexion/extension and abduction/adduction of an extremity (see Fig. 6.6A, B).

The shoulder girdle is a good example of the clinical utility of PNF principles in rehabilitation of physical performance capacity. Once pain and inflammation begin to subside, PNF patterns can be utilised to restore function in the shoulder (Figs 5.4, 5.5). Such exercises can be combined with muscle balancing approaches, joint mobilisation/manipulation and closed chain stabilisation procedures.

THE NEURODEVELOPMENTAL BASIS FOR MUSCLE IMBALANCE

Janda's model of muscle imbalance drives much of our clinical decision making. Certain muscles active during static postures have a tendency to become overactive or even shorten due to prolonged use of constrained postures (Lewit 1999a). Other muscles active during dynamic activities tend to become inhibited or even weak from disuse. Static postural muscle overactivity is a natural result of modern society's emphasis on constrained postures. Dynamic muscle underactivity is predictable since modern lifestyles are predominantly sedentary.

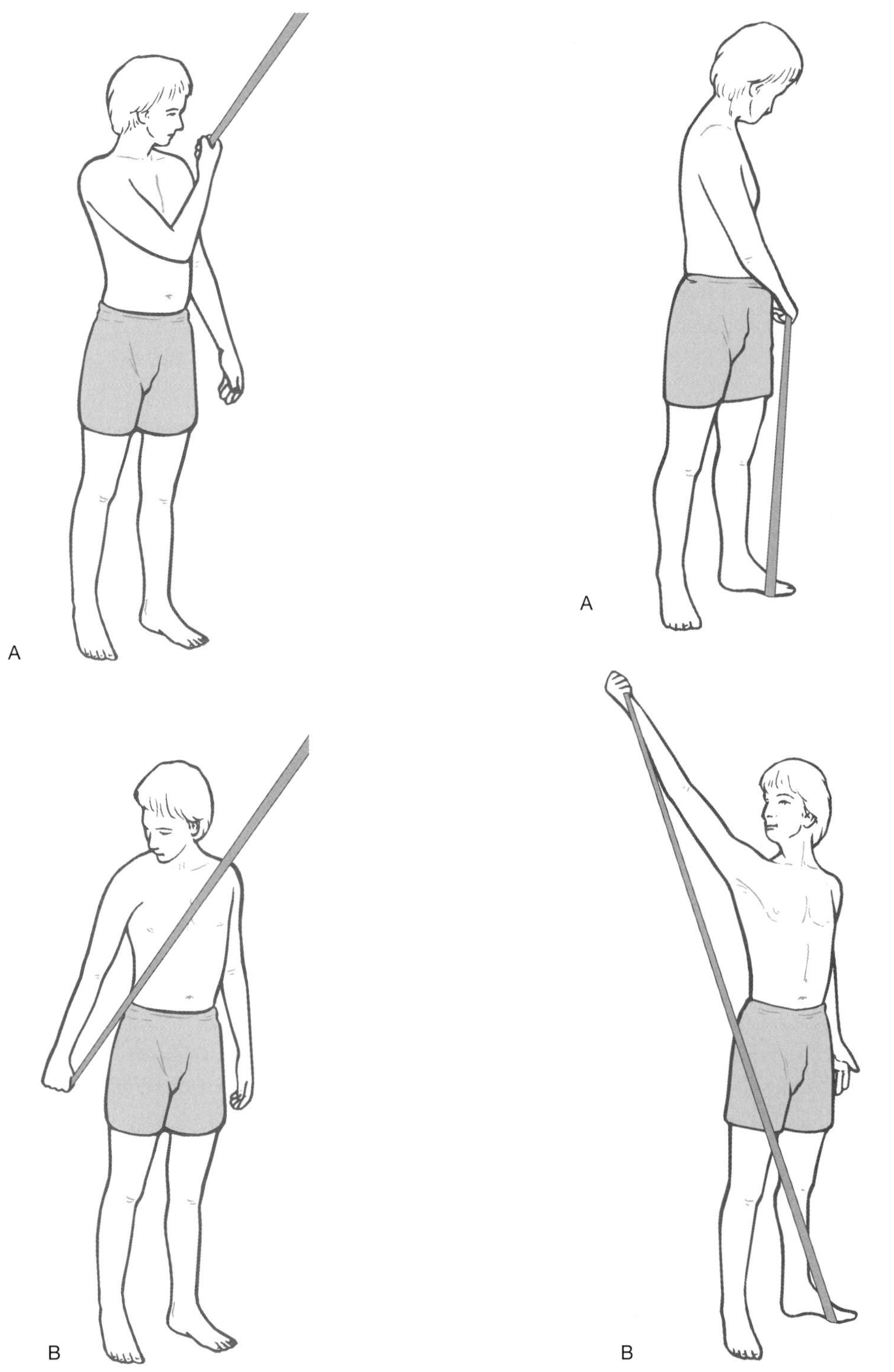

Figure 5.4A,B D1 upper extremity extension technique ('seatbelt').

Figure 5.5A,B D2 upper extremity flexion technique ('drawing a sword').

The static muscle system typically involves superficial muscles such as upper trapezius, sternocleidomastoid, erector spinae and the hamstrings. In contrast, the dynamic muscle system utilises more the deep stabilisers such as transverse abdominus, quadratus lumborum, multifidus and the deep neck flexors. The development of these predictable muscle imbalances is further spurred by the diminished afferent flow of sensory information from the periphery, in particular the sole of the foot, due to sedentarism and a lack of variety of movements. Naturally, movement patterns are altered and fatigueability increased, thus rendering the motor control system less able to adapt to various biomechanical sources of repetitive strain.

The goal of neurodevelopment of the locomotor system is to achieve the upright posture. Brügger and Janda have shown how deleterious sedentarism is (Lewit 1999a). Brügger describes the typical sedentary posture of man via a linkage system. He has shown how approximation of the sternum and symphysis increases both end-range loading, and muscular tension (Lewit 1999a, Liebenson 1999). It is possible, however, to demonstrate that postural correction can immediately improve joint function and muscle tone:

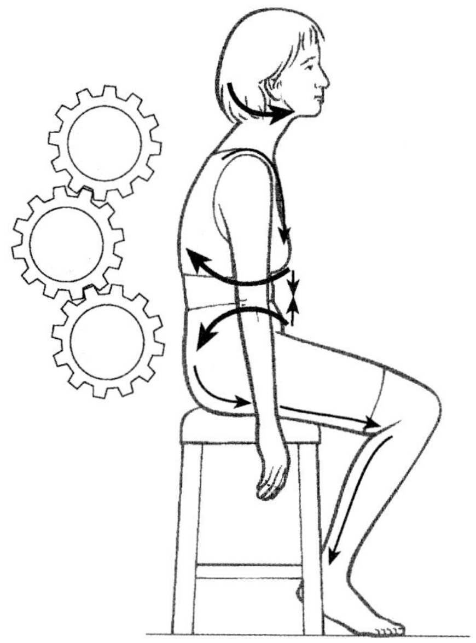

Figure 5.6A Sternosymphyseal syndrome.

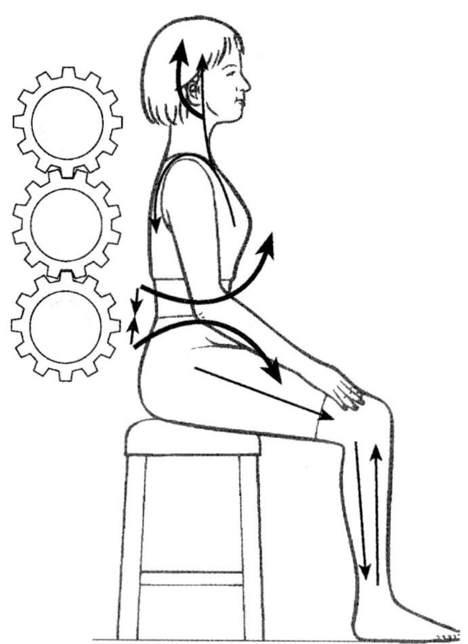

Figure 5.6B Brügger relief position

Experiment in postural correction

(Figs 5.6, 5.7)

- Check upper trapezius tension/trigger points in slump position
- Perform the Brügger relief position recheck
- Check cervical rotation in the slump position; perform the Brügger relief position and recheck
- Check arm abduction in slump; perform the Brügger relief position and recheck.

Brügger's relief position facilitates phasic muscles (muscles which tend to inhibition) and reciprocally inhibits postural muscles (muscles which tend to shortening). His advice is very effective in improving patient compliance with home exercises. It is also an excellent way to increase awareness of postural corrections.

It is worth pointing out that the muscles which Janda has suggested tend to hypertonicity include most of the muscles shortened in the foetal position. These are, in the upper quarter, the finger, hand and wrist flexors, the shoulder internal rotators and adductors, and the shoulder girdle elevators (Kolár 1999). In the lower quarter they are

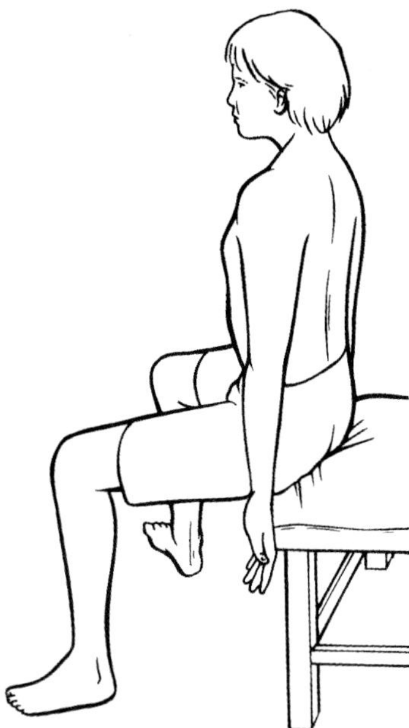

Figure 5.7 Brügger relief position.

the ankle plantar flexors and invertors, the hip flexors, internal rotators and adductors. As the infant's motor control system develops, the antagonists of these muscles become facilitated and the muscles become inhibited. Muscles inhibited in the upper extremity include:

- finger, wrist elbow and shoulder extensors
- forearm supinators
- shoulder external rotators and abductors.

Those in the lower extremity include:

- toe extensors
- ankle dorsiflexors and pronators
- hip abductors and external rotators.

The parallel between the postural muscles which tend to overactivity in adults as a result of sedentarism and the muscles which are used to maintain the foetal position is obvious. Similarly, Janda's phasic muscles are almost identical to the muscles whose activation during neurodevelopment brings about an upright posture. That there is a central neurological programme for these different types of muscles is further reinforced by noting which muscles become spastic in children with CP or which muscles are paralysed in people who have suffered a stroke. It becomes clear that balance between agonist and antagonist muscles is essential for a proper functional motor control system (Kolár 1999, Cholewicki & McGill 1996).

Certain landmark stages exist in the transition from a tonic, reflex motor system (brain stem control) to a balanced postural control system capable of volitional control locomotion (supraspinal control). Each stage of neurodevelopment of posture depends upon a set of specific conditions being met. Specific points of body support, centration of key joints and agonist–antagonist muscular coactivation are all necessary for development of each landmark of neurodevelopment of the postural control system (Kolár 1999).

Kolár (1999) points out that agonist–antagonist coactivation patterns evolve as neurodevelopment progresses to take the infant from a foetal position at birth to a stable upright posture at approximately 3 years of age. In the first month of life the infant's muscles (maintaining the foetal position) are in a state of tonic contraction. At the end of the first month, in response to visual and auditory stimuli from the mother, the child begins to orient its head. This is not a reflex movement, but under higher motor control (Kolár 1999). As posture develops, the tonic contractions, which are reflexly based, begin to relax, thus reducing reciprocal inhibition and facilitating the coactivation patterns necessary for joint centration and load bearing. For instance, at the end of the first month, coactivation of anatagonists at the cervicocranial junction centrates C0–C1:

- Deep neck flexors are facilitated
- Short cervical extensors are no longer tonicly active.

If the tonic contraction of upper cervical extensors does not relax, then joint centration of C0–C1 is not possible, and the infant will not be able to control its head movements for successful orientation.

Coactivation of antagonists occurs proximally at the shoulder and hip by the third month as a prerequisite for weight bearing on all fours (i.e. creeping and crawling):

- Activation of lower scapular fixators, shoulder external rotators, trunk extensors, hip abductors external rotators

- Reduction in tonic activity of scapular elevators, shoulder internal rotators, trunk hip adductors and internal rotators.

Failure of coactivation due to persistent tonic activity results in faulty neurodevelopment of the motor system. This allows a persistence of trunk flexion, eventually promoting both the upper crossed and lower crossed syndromes (see Figs 5.8, 5.9).

Kolár utilises treatments including stimulation of reflex trigger zones at key areas of postural support in the infant such as the symphysis pubis, sternum or occiput to facilitate coactivation patterns (Kolár 1999).

The key role of coactivation of antagonists in producing and maintaining upright posture

Equilibrium is a result of cocontraction of antagonists. This coactivation develops in the first three months of infancy. During the first 3–4 weeks of life the muscles are tonic under reflex control (brain stem). At 4–6 weeks orientation to the mother begins visually with turning of the head. This is the birth of posture and motor control. Postural reactions are supraspinal. The coactivation of antagonists creates maximum congruence of joints, thus promoting equilibrium and joint loading (Kolár 1999).

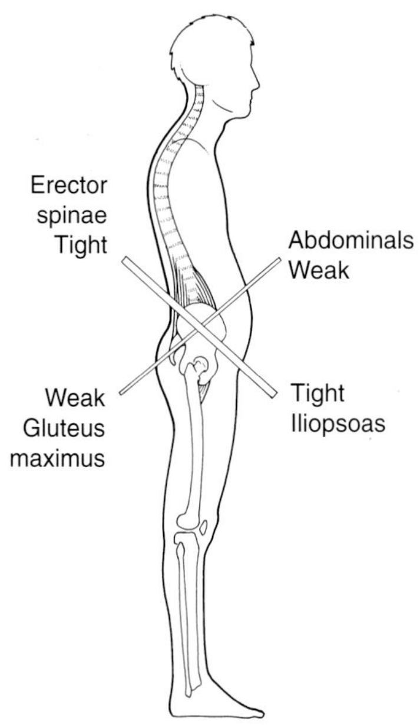

Figure 5.8 Lower crossed syndrome.

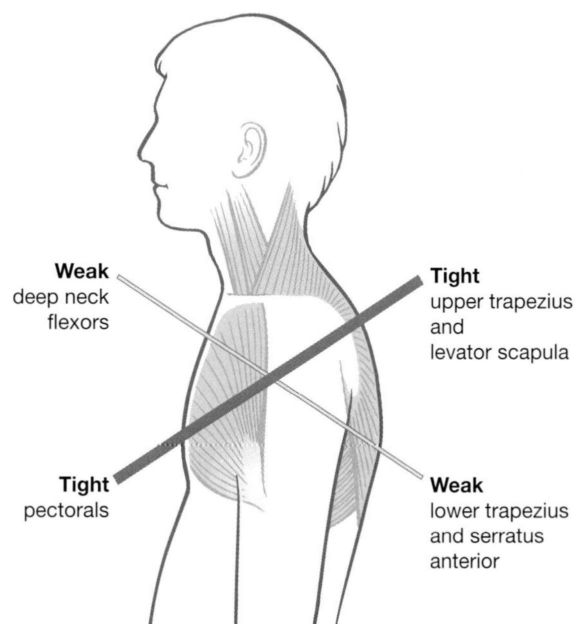

Figure 5.9 Upper crossed syndrome.

During development of upright posture, the upper extremity tonic activity (flexion, internal rotation, adduction and pronation) is joined with phasic activity (extension, external rotation, abduction and supination). In the lower extremity tonic activity (ankle plantar flexion and inversion, hip flexion, internal rotation and adduction) is joined with phasic activity (ankle dorsiflexion and eversion, hip external rotation and abduction). Development from one stage to another requires that balanced muscle contraction of antagonists replaces dominance of tonic muscular activity. This coactivation centrates or aligns joints in maximum congruence. Such coactivation is not reflex (brain stem), but supraspinal, and is the beginning point of postural-motor activity in the human (Kolár 1999).

Sedentarism reduces afferent input – particularly from the sole of the foot – and promotes tension in postural (anti-gravity) muscles while leading to inhibition in dynamic phasic muscles. Janda's muscle imbalances are a predictable result of this with their typical associated faulty movement patterns and repetitive microtrauma to joints. Brügger has developed a systematic approach to improving posture complementing that evolved by Janda (Lewit 1999a).

Certain screening tests have been developed by Janda for identifying agonist, antagonist, synergist relationships during stereotypical movement patterns (Lewit 1999a, Janda 1996, Liebenson & Chapman 1998, Liebenson et al 1998). These kinesiological relationships – called muscle imbalances – alter joint stress by changing movement patterns or the axis of rotation during movement. The screening tests evaluated include hip extension, hip abduction, trunk flexion, scapular fixation during arm abduction, upper cervical flexion, trunk lowering from a push-up and respiration (see Figs 5.10–5.16).

When faulty movement patterns are present they are a key perpetuating factor of myofascial or joint pain (Babyar 1996, Treleaven et al 1994, Watson & Trott 1993, Barton & Hayes 1996,

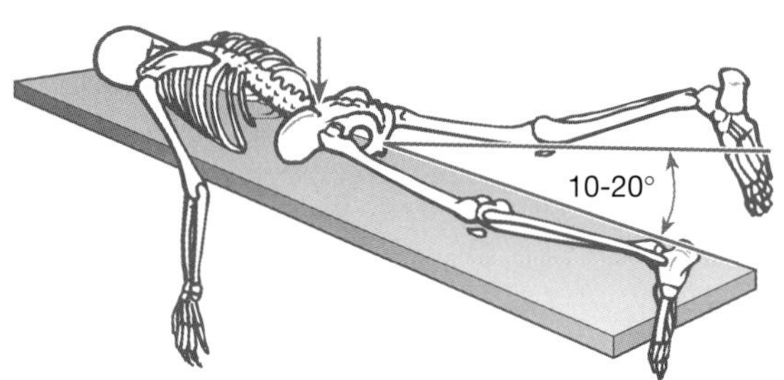

Figure 5.10A Abnormal hip extension movement pattern associated with shortened psoas. Leg raising is initiated with an anterior pelvic tilt.

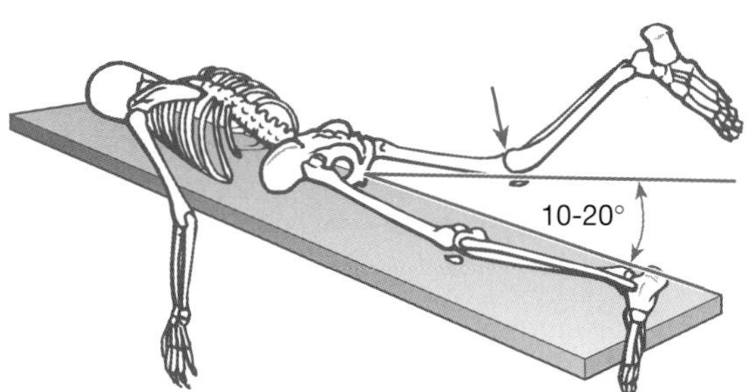

Figure 5.10B Abnormal hip extension movement pattern associated with excessive substitution of the hamstrings. Leg raising is initiated with knee flexion.

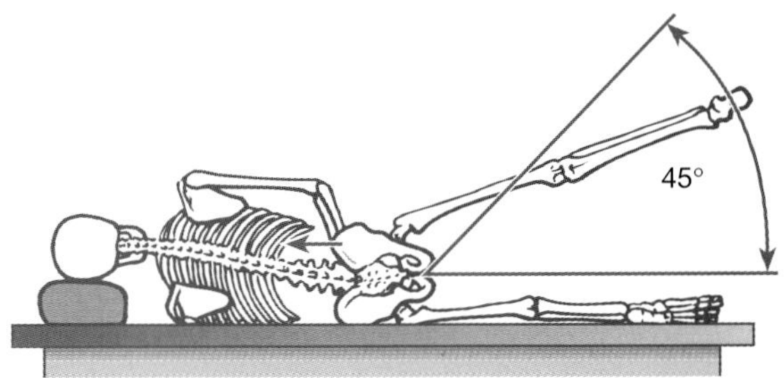

Figure 5.11A Abnormal hip abduction movement pattern associated with excessive substitution of the quadratus lumborum. Leg raising is initiated with a cephalad shift of the pelvis.

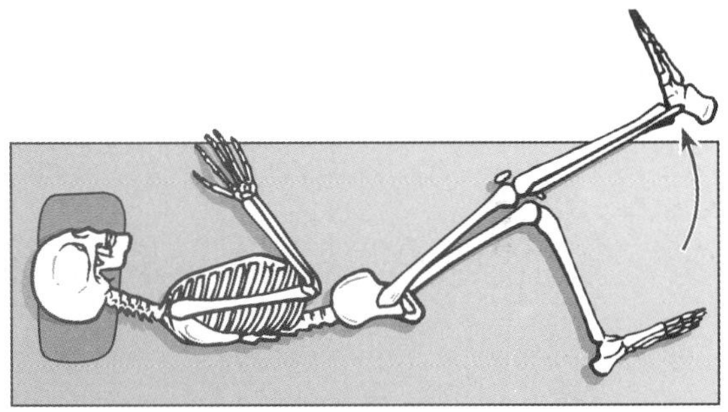

Figure 5.11B Abnormal hip abduction movement pattern associated with excessive substitution of the tensor fascia lata. Leg raising is initiated with flexion of the hip joint.

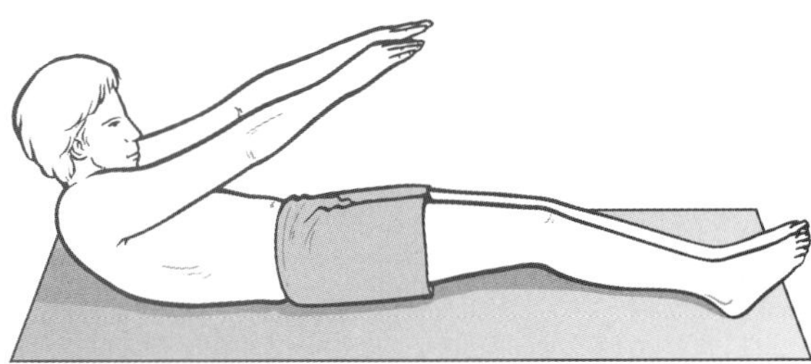

Figure 5.12A Normal trunk flexion movement pattern.

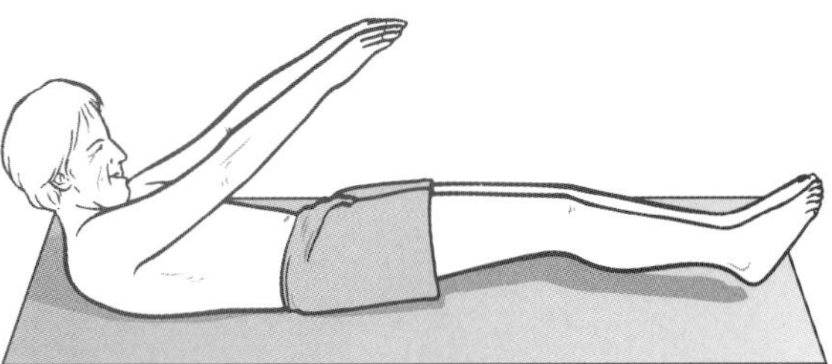

Figure 5.12B Abnormal trunk flexion movement pattern associated with excessive substitution of the psoas. Heels rise up off the table before the shoulder blades are lifted.

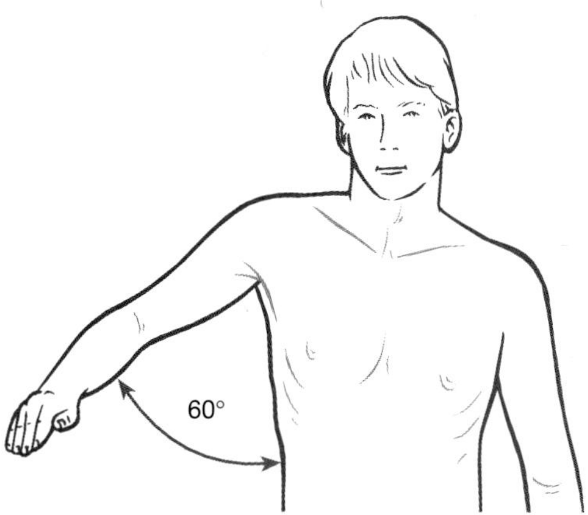

Figure 5.13A Normal scapular fixation during arm abduction movement pattern.

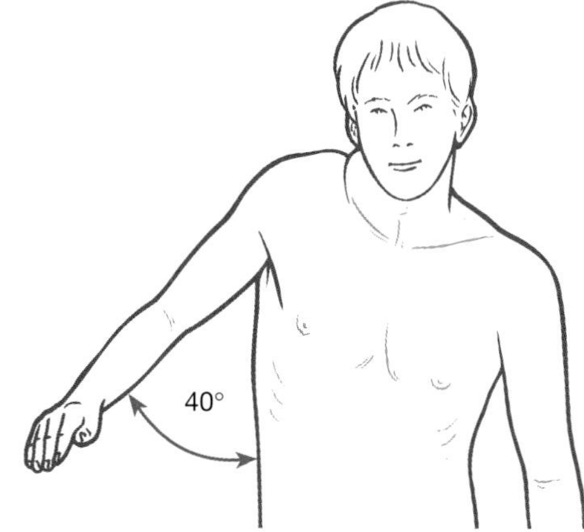

Figure 5.13B Abnormal scapular fixation during arm abduction movement pattern associated with excessive substitution of the upper trapezius and levator scapulae. Scapulae or shoulder girdle elevate before the arm has abducted 45°.

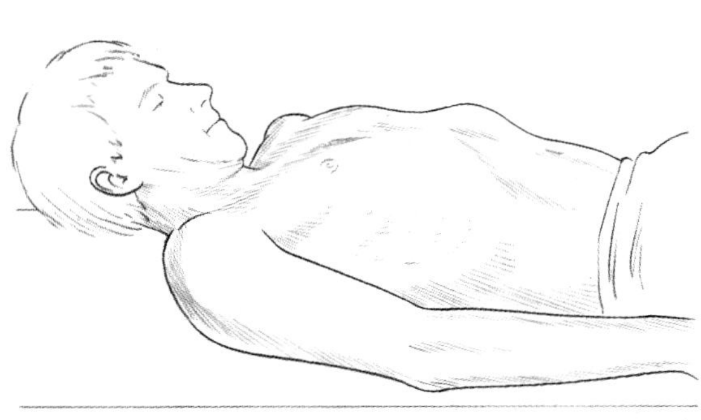

Figure 5.14A Normal upper cervical flexion movement pattern.

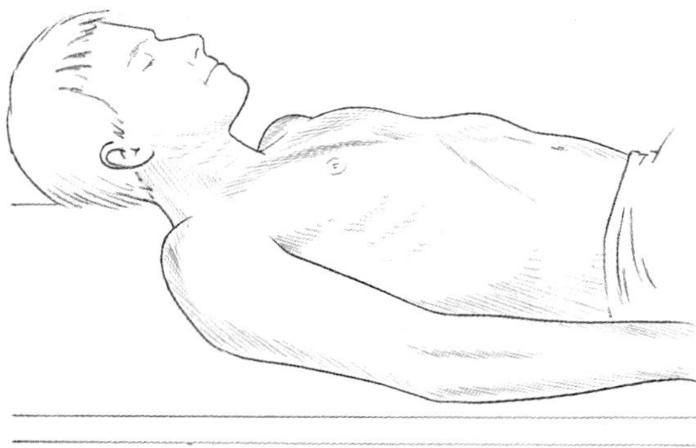

Figure 5.14B Abnormal upper cervical flexion movement pattern associated with excessive substitution of the sternocleidomastoid and/or shortening of the suboccipitals. Head is raised towards the chest with chin poking (i.e. upper cervical extension) occurring.

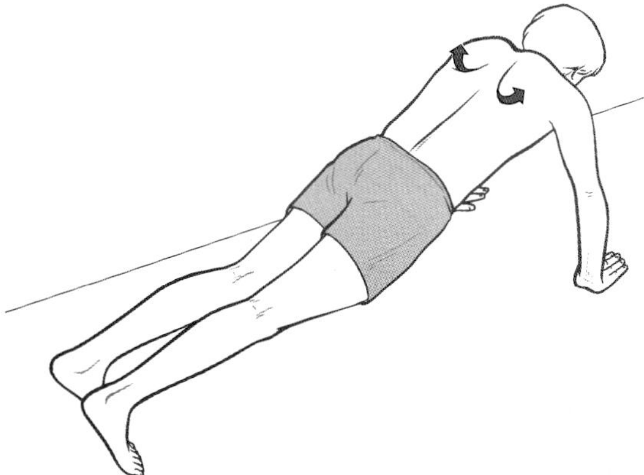

Figure 5.15 Abnormal trunk lowering from a push-up movement pattern associated with inhibition/weakness of the serratus anterior. Winging of the right scapula.

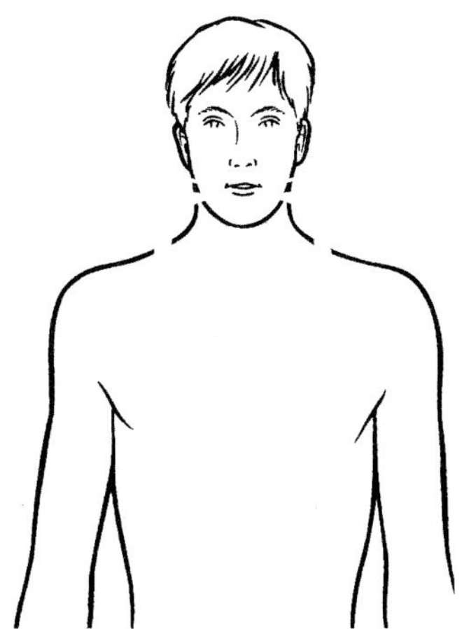

Figure 5.16A Abnormal respiration associated with elevation of the clavicle(s) during relaxed inhalation.

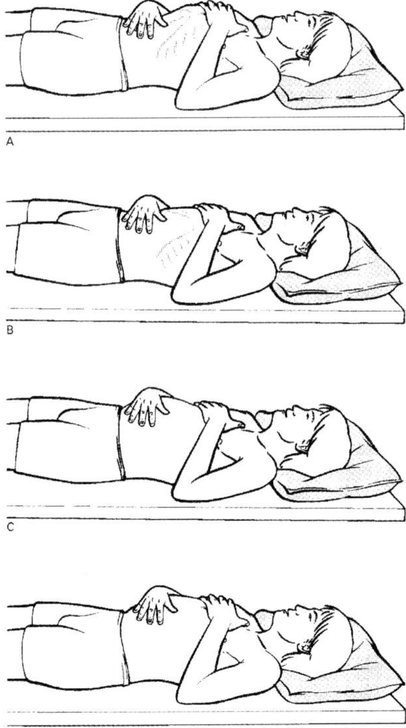

Figure 5.16B The most severe dysfunction occurs when the belly moves inwards during inhalation ('paradoxical breathing').

Edgerton et al 1996). Unless movement patterns are improved during performance of activities of daily life so that joint stability is maintained, then soft tissue or mobilisation/manipulation treatments will fail to achieve a lasting result. In fact, exercises performed without proper form only reinforce such muscle imbalances as 'trick' movement patterns are used due to synergist substitution for inhibited agonists (Edgerton et al 1996, Hodges & Richardson 1996, Paarnianpour et al 1988, Sparto 1997, Grabiner et al 1992, Arendt-Nielson et al 1995, O'Sullivan et al 1997, Hodges & Richardson 1998, 1999).

Experiment in facilitation of an inhibited muscle chain

Eccentric facilitation of a chain of inhibited muscles brings about reciprocal inhibition of the tonic muscle chain. The tonic muscle chain is typically overactivated in individuals with sternosymphyseal syndrome (Lewit 1999a, 1999b). The muscle imbalance is typical in that it involves overactivity in the muscles described by Kolár as tonic and inhibition of those responsible for coactivation during development from a kyphotic to upright posture (Kolár 1999). Such hypertonic muscle chains often involve trigger or tender points in both inhibited and overactive muscle groups (Lewit 1999b). They are expected in chronic pain states as a result of the body's attempt to immobilise the region (Lewit 1999b).

Investigation

To identify a hypertonic muscle chain in the upper extremity look for one-sided predominance of the following dysfunctions:

- Restricted wrist extension mobility
- Palpate trigger points in upper trapezius, pectoralis major
- Palpate tender attachment points in upper ribs 1–3 and the lateral or medial epicondyle.

In the lower extremity look for one-sided predominance of the following dysfunctions:

- Restricted hamstring length
- Palpate trigger points in adductor longus and magnus, pectineus, gluteus medius, gluteus maximus and the longitudinal arch of the foot.

Brügger's facilitation method for inhibited muscle chains in the extremities

Once a predominately one-sided chain has been found in either the upper or the lower extremity, then treatment with a strong (40–80% of maximum effort) contraction of a sequence of movements involving a chain of inhibited muscles can be used to bring about reciprocal inhibition of the chain of hypertonic muscles. An eccentric muscle energy technique is used to maximise reciprocal inhibition of the hypertonic muscle chain. Each of the following movements is resisted individually, one after the other.

Approximately three repetitions of each movement is performed.

The patient contracts against your resistance, then you slowly stretch the muscle while the patient is maintaining resistance, thus achieving an eccentric contraction. The purpose is to facilitate these muscles and reciprocally inhibit the antagonistic muscles.

Indications

- Any time you want to release tension in multiple muscles simultaneously
- When a one-sided chain is present, especially in chronic pain patients.

In the upper quarter eccentricly resist:

- Finger and thumb abduction (Fig. 5.17A, B)
- Wrist and finger extension and thumb abduction (Fig. 5.18A, B)
- Forearm supination (Fig. 5.19A, B)
- Shoulder external rotation (Fig. 5.20A, B)
- Shoulder abduction and external rotation (Fig. 5.21A, B).

In the lower quarter eccentricly resist:

- Toe extension, ankle dorsiflexion and eversion (Fig. 5.22A, B)
- Hip abduction (Fig. 5.23A, B)
- Hip external rotation (Fig. 5.24A, B)

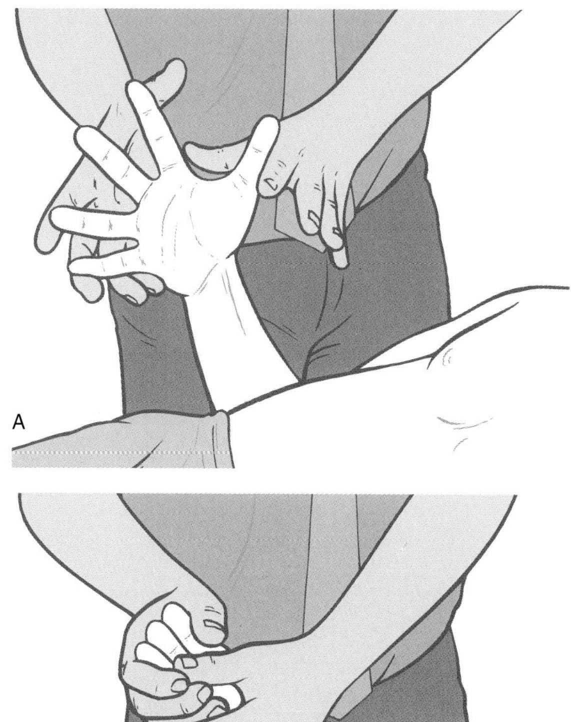

Figure 5.17A,B Eccentric resistance of finger and thumb abduction.

It is notable that the resistance to shoulder abduction and external rotation is almost identical to the final position of the PNF D2 upper extremity flexion – 'drawing a sword' position (see Fig. 5.5).

CONCLUSION

What has been presented here is an exciting new approach to rehabilitation of the motor system. The identification of a nociceptive chain involving agonist/antagonist trigger points enhances our ability to restore muscle balance and improve joint stability. The concept of muscle imbalance

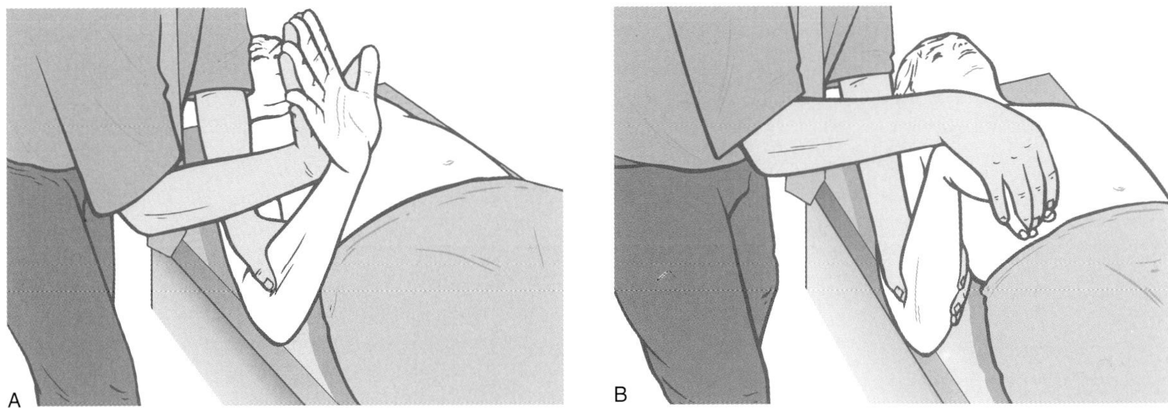

Figure 5.18A,B Eccentric resistance of wrist and finger extension and thumb abduction.

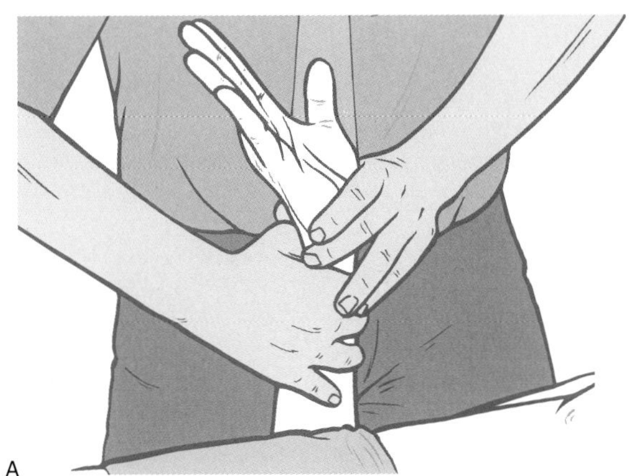

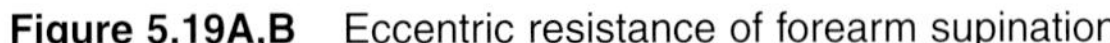

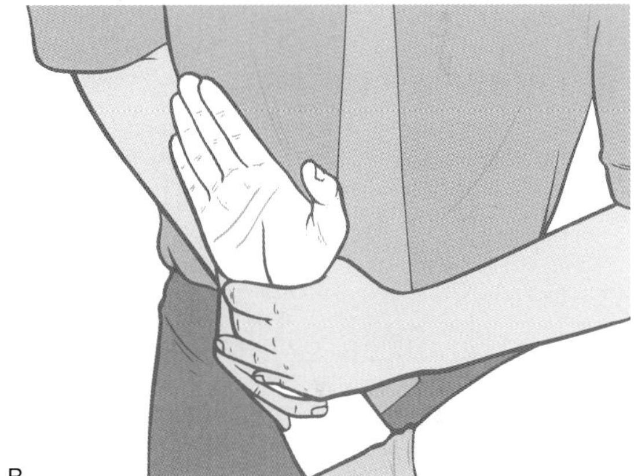

Figure 5.19A,B Eccentric resistance of forearm supination.

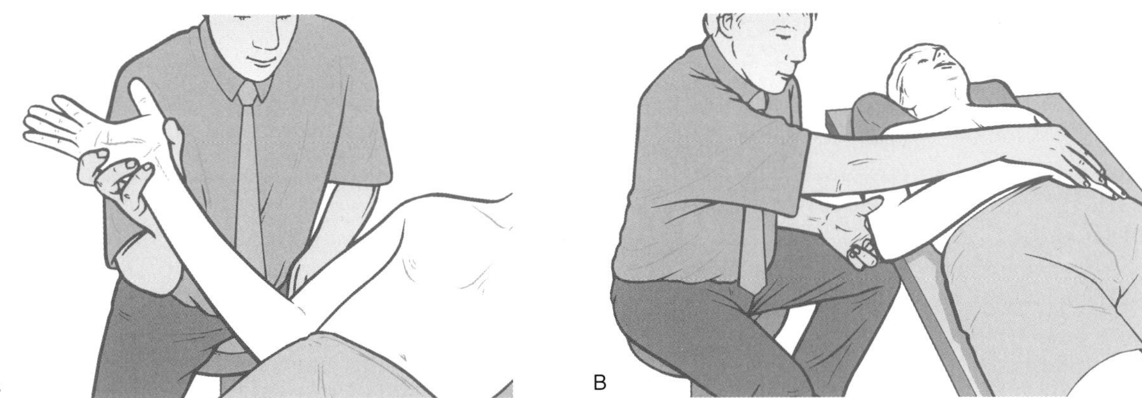

Figure 5.20A,B Eccentric resistance of shoulder external rotation.

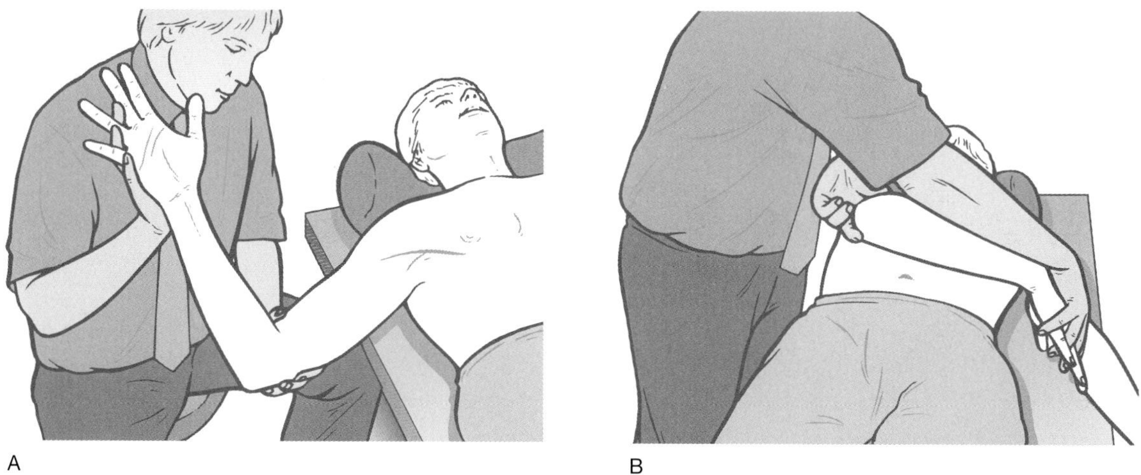

Figure 5.21A,B Eccentric resistance of shoulder abduction and external rotation.

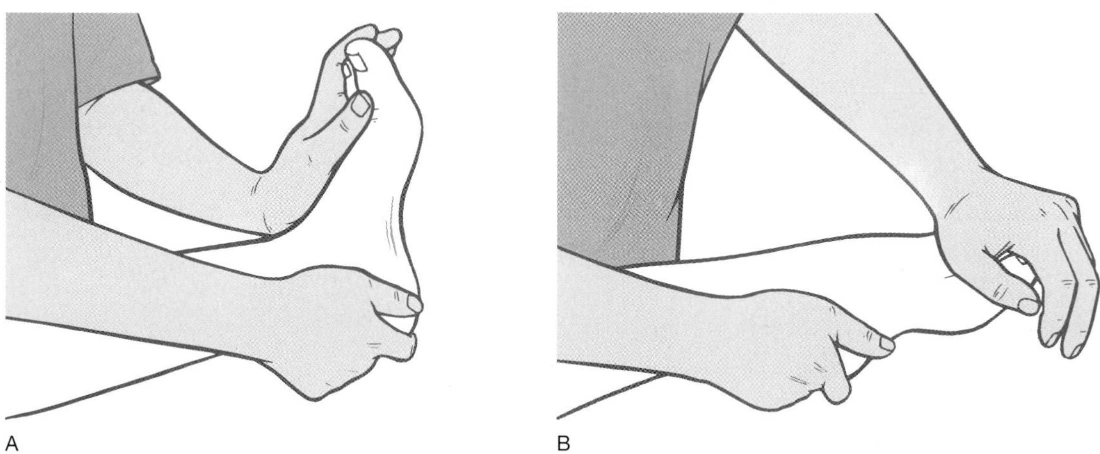

Figure 5.22A,B Eccentric resistance of toe extension, ankle dorsiflexion and eversion.

is reinforced by knowledge of neurodevelopment of the upright posture. Chains form in our patients which are invaluable aids in troubleshooting.

It is not enough simply to identify a muscle imbalance and treat those muscles. The chain which is dysfunctional must also be identified, and treatment of a key link given. Supraspinal control, which begins after 3 weeks of life, is the beginning of voluntary motor control. If chains of agonist–antagonist muscle incoordination hypothetically related to various stages of neurodevelopment of the upright posture are improved, this may be a significant advance in our treatment of motor system problems. Research into agonist–antagonist coactivation, joint congruence, equilibrium, maximisation of joint load handling ability, and neurological programmes in the adult representative of neurodevelopmental stages is eagerly anticipated.

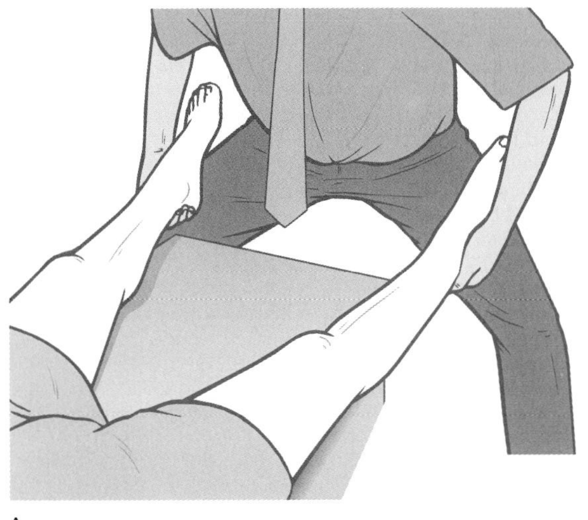
A

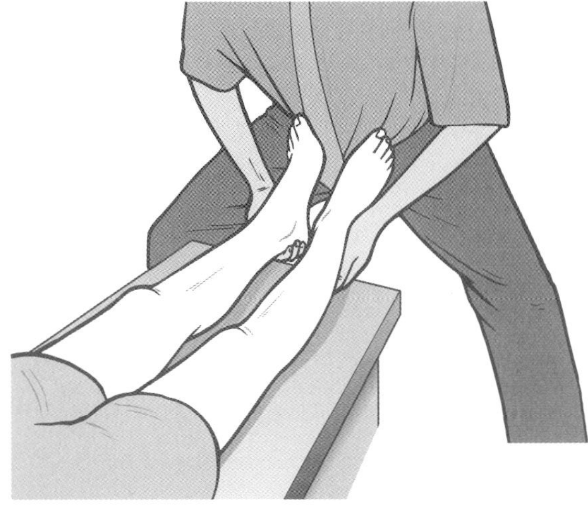
B

Figure 5.23A,B Eccentric resistance of hip abduction.

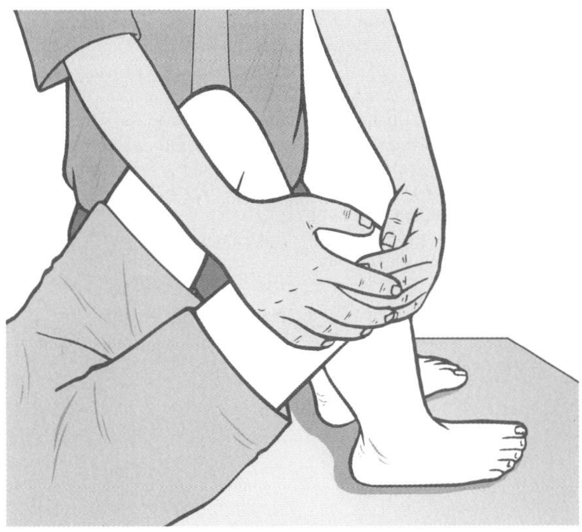
A

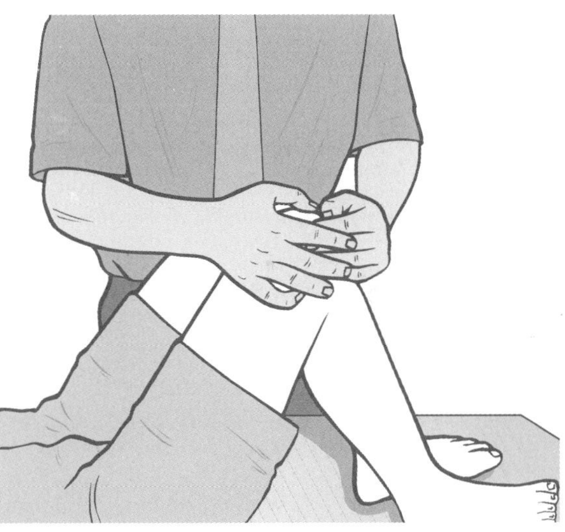
B

Figure 5.24A,B Eccentric resistance of hip external rotation.

REFERENCES

Adler S S, Beckers D, Buck M 1993 PNF in practice – an illustrated guide. Springer-Verlag, Berlin

Arendt-Nielson L, Graven-Nielson T, Svarrer H, Svensson P 1995 The influence of low back pain on muscle activity and coordination during gait. Pain 64: 231–240

Babyar S R 1996 Excessive scapular motion in individuals recovering from painful and stiff shoulders: causes and treatment strategies. Physical Therapy 76: 226–238

Barton P M, Hayes K C 1996 Neck flexor muscle strength, and relaxation times in normal subjects and subjects with unilateral neck pain and headache. Archives of Physical Medicine and Rehabilitation 77: 680–687

Cholewicki J, McGill S M 1996 Mechanical stability of the in vivo lumbar spine: implications for injury and chronic low back pain. Clinical Biomechanics 11(1): 1–15

Edgerton V R, Wolf S L, Levendowski D J, Roy R R 1996 Theoretical basis for patterning EMG amplitudes to assess muscle dysfunction. Medical Science Sports and Exercise 28: 744–751

Grabiner M D, Koh T J, Ghazawi A E 1992 Decoupling of bilateral paraspinal excitation in subjects with low back pain. Spine 17: 1219

Hodges P W, Richardson C A 1996 Inefficient muscular stabilization of the lumbar spine associated with low back pain. Spine 21: 2640–2650

Hodges P W, Richardson C A 1998 Delayed postural contraction of the transverse abdominus associated with movement of the lower limb in people with low back pain. Journal of Spinal Disorders 11: 46–56

Hodges P W, Richardson C A 1999 Altered trunk muscle recruitment in people with low back pain with upper limb movements at different speeds. Archives of Physical Medicine and Rehabilitation 80: 1005–1012

Janda V 1996. Evaluation of muscle imbalances. In: Liebenson C (ed) Rehabilitation of the spine: a practitioner's manual. Williams and Wilkins, Baltimore

Kabot H 1950 Studies on neuromuscular dysfunction XIII: new concepts and techniques of neuromuscular reeducation for paralysis. Permanente Foundation Medical Bulletin 8: 121–143

Kolár P 1999 The sensomotor nature of postural functions, its fundamental role in rehabilitation. Journal of Orthopedic Medicine 21(2): 40–45

Levine M G, Kabat H, Knott M et al 1954 Relaxation of spasticity by physiological techniques. Archives of Physical Medicine and Rehabilitation 35: 214–223

Lewit K, Simons D G 1984 Myofascial pain: relief by post-isometric relaxation. Archives of Physical Medicine and Rehabilitation 65: 452–456

Lewit K 1986 Postisometric relaxation in combination with other methods of muscular facilitation and inhibition. Manual Medicine 2: 101–104

Lewit K 1999a Manipulative therapy in rehabilitation of the motor system, 3rd edn. Butterworths, London

Lewit K 1999b Chain reactions in the locomotor system in the light of coactivation patterns based on developmental neurology. Journal of Orthopedic Medicine 21(2): 52–58

Liebenson C S 1989 Active muscular relaxation techniques, part one. Basic principles and methods. Journal of Manipulative and Physiological Therapeutics 12: 6

Liebenson C S 1990 Active muscular relaxation techniques, part two. Clinical application. Journal of Manipulative and Physiological Therapeutics 13: 1

Liebenson C 1996 Manual resistance techniques. In Liebenson C (ed) Rehabilitation of the spine: a practitioner's manual. Williams and Wilkins, Baltimore

Liebenson C 1999 Advice for the clinician. Journal of Bodywork and Movement Therapies 3: 147–149

Liebenson C, Chapman S 1998 Rehabilitation of the spine: functional evaluation of the lumbar spine. Williams and Wilkins, Baltimore [videotape]

Liebenson C, Murphy D 1998 Rehabilitation of the spine: post-isometric relaxation techniques – low back and lower extremities. Williams and Wilkins, Baltimore [videotape]

Liebenson C, DeFranca C, Lefebvre R 1998 Rehabilitation of the spine: functional evaluation of the cervical spine. Williams and Wilkins, Baltimore [videotape]

O'Sullivan P, Twomey L, Allison G et al 1997 Altered patterns of abdominal muscle activation in patients with chronic low back pain. Australian Journal of Physiotherapy 43: 91–98

Paarnianpour M, Nordin M, Kahanovitz N, Frank V 1998 The triaxial coupling of torque generation of trunk muscles during isometric exertions and the effect of fatiguing isoinertial movements on the motor output and movement patterns. Spine 13: 982–992

Sparto P J, Paarnianpour M, Massa W S, Granata K P, Reinsel T E, Simon S 1997 Neuromuscular trunk performance and spinal loading during a fatiguing isometric trunk extension with varying torque requirements. Spine 10: 145–156

Treleaven J, Jull G, Atkinson L 1994 Cervical musculoskeletal dysfunction in post-concussional headache. Cephalgia 14: 273–279

Watson D H, Trott P H 1993 Cervical headache: an investigation of natural head posture and upper cervical flexor muscle performance. Cephalgia 13: 272–284

CHAPTER CONTENTS

6

MET and the treatment of joints

While Janda (1988) acknowledges that it is not known whether dysfunction of muscles causes joint dysfunction or vice versa, he points to the undoubted fact that each massively influences the other, and that it is possible that a major element in the benefits noted following joint manipulation derives from the effects such methods (high velocity thrust, mobilisation, etc.) have on associated soft tissues.

Steiner (1994) has discussed the influence of muscles in disc and facet syndromes. He describes a possible sequence as follows:

- A strain involving body torsion, rapid stretch, loss of balance, etc., produces a myotatic stretch reflex response in, for example, a part of the erector spinae.
- The muscles contract to protect excessive joint movement, and spasm may result if (for any of a range of reasons, see notes on facilitation in Ch. 2) there is an exaggerated response and they fail to assume normal tone following the strain.
- This limits free movement of the attached vertebrae, approximates them and causes compression and bulging of the intervertebral discs and/or a forcing together of the articular facets.
- Bulging discs might encroach on a nerve root, producing disc syndrome symptoms.
- Articular facets, when forced together, produce pressure on the intra-articular fluid, pushing it against the confining facet capsule which becomes stretched and irritated.
- The sinuvertebral capsular nerves may therefore become irritated, provoking muscular

guarding, initiating a self-perpetuating process of pain–spasm–pain.

Steiner continues: 'From a physiological standpoint, correction or cure of the disc or facet syndromes should be the reversal of the process that produced them, eliminating muscle spasm and restoring normal motion.' He argues that before discectomy or facet rhizotomy is attempted, with the all too frequent 'failed disc syndrome surgery' outcome, attention to the soft tissues and articular separation to reduce the spasm should be tried, in order to allow the bulging disc to recede and/or the facets to resume normal motion.

Clearly, osseous manipulation often has a place in achieving this objective, but the evidence of clinical experience indicates that a soft tissue approach which either relies largely on MET or at least incorporates MET as a major part of its methodology is frequently likely to produce excellent results in at least some such cases, and research evidence of this is available (see Ch. 7).

MET APPLICATION

Preparing joints for manipulation using MET

What if high velocity thrust or mobilisation methods of joint manipulation are the appropriate method of choice in treatment of a restricted joint? How can MET fit into the picture?

Muscle energy methods are versatile, and while they certainly have applications which are aimed at normalising soft tissue structures such as shortened or tense muscles, with no direct implications as to the joints associated with these, they can also be used to help to normalise joint mobility via their influence on the associated soft tissues, which may be the major obstacle to the restoration of free movement.

As we have seen in previous chapters, MET may be employed to relax tight, tense musculature, or even spasm, and can also help to reduce the fibrotic changes in chronic soft tissue problems and tone weakened structures which may be present in the antagonists of shortened soft tissues. MET may therefore be employed in a pre-manipulative mode. In this instance, the conventional manipulative procedure is prepared for as it would normally be, whether this involves leverage or a thrust technique. The practitioner could then – having adopted an appropriate position, made suitable manual contacts and prepared the tissues for the high velocity or mobilisation adjustment by engaging the restriction barrier – take out available slack (manipulative effort) and then ask the patient to 'push back' from this position against solid resistance.

The practitioner will have engaged the barrier in this preparation for manipulation, and will have taken out the slack that was available in the soft tissues of the joint(s), in order to achieve this position.

When the patient is asked to firmly but painlessly resist or 'push back', against the practitioner's contact hands, this produces a patient-indirect (practitioner pushing towards the resistance barrier while the patient pushes away from it) isometric contraction, which would have the effect of contracting the presumably shortened muscles associated with the restricted joint.

After holding this effort for several seconds (ideally with a held breath), both practitioner and patient would simultaneously release their efforts, in a slow, deliberate manner.

This can be repeated several times, with the additional slack being taken out after appropriate relaxation by the patient.

Having engaged and re-engaged the barrier a number of times, the practitioner would decide when adequate release of restraining tissues had taken place and would then make the high velocity or mobilisation adjustment as normal.

Laurie Hartman (1985) states that: 'If the patient is in the absolute optimum position for a particular thrust technique during one of these repetitions (of MET), the joint in question will be felt to release. Even if this has not occurred, when retesting the movement range there is often a considerable increase in range and quality of play.' He suggests that the practitioner use the temporary rebound reflex relaxation in the muscles, which will have followed the isometric contraction, to perform the technique. This will allow successful completion of the adjustment with minimal force. This refractory period of relaxation lasts for quite a few seconds and is valuable in all cases, but especially where the patient is tense or resistant to a manipulative effort.

Joint mobilisation using MET

The emphasis of MET on soft tissues should not be taken to indicate that intra-articular causes of dysfunction are not acknowledged. Indeed, Lewit (1985) addressed this controversy in an elegant study which demonstrated that some typical restriction patterns remain intact even when the patient is observed under narcosis with myorelaxants. He tries to direct attention to a balanced view when he states, 'The naive conception that movement restriction in passive mobility is necessarily due to articular lesion has to be abandoned. We know that taut muscles alone can limit passive movement and that articular lesions are regularly associated with increased muscular tension.'

He then goes on to point to the other alternatives, including the fact that many joint restrictions are not the result of soft tissue changes, using as examples those joints not under the control of muscular influences: tibiofibular, sacroiliac, acromioclavicular. He also points to the many instances where joint play is more restricted than normal joint movement. Since joint play is a feature of joint mobility which is not subject to muscular control, the conclusion has to be made that there are indeed joint problems which have the soft tissues as a secondary factor in any general dysfunctional pattern of pain and/or restricted range of motion (blockage).

He continues: 'This is not to belittle the role of the musculature in movement restriction, but it is important to re-establish the role of articulation, and even more to distinguish clinically between movement restriction caused by taut muscles and that due to blocked joints, or very often, to both.' Fortunately MET is capable of offering assistance in normalisation of both forms of dysfunction.

Basic criteria for treating joint restriction with MET (Fig. 6.1A–F)

In treating joint restriction with MET, Sandra Yates (1991) suggests the following simple criteria be maintained:

1. The joint should be positioned at its physiological barrier (specific in three planes if spinal segments are being considered: flexion–extension, sidebending, rotation).
2. The patient should be asked to statically contract muscles towards their freedom of motion (i.e. away from the barrier(s) of restriction) as the practitioner resists totally any movement of the part. The contraction, Yates suggests, is held for about 3 seconds (many MET experts suggest longer – up to 10 seconds).
3. The patient is asked to relax for 2 seconds or so between the contraction efforts, at which time

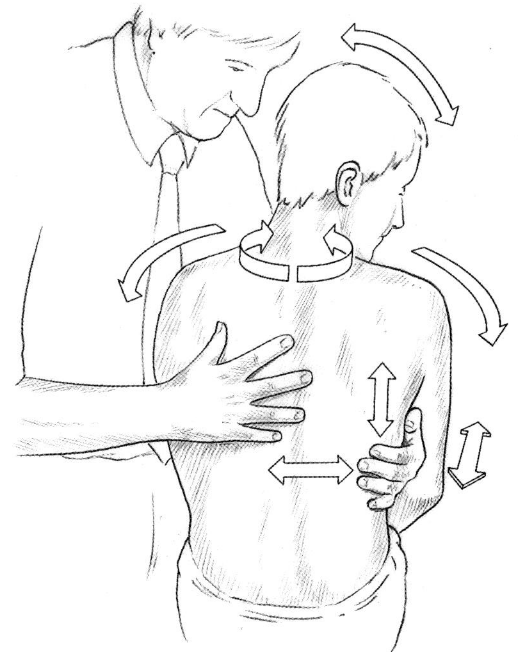

Figure 6.1A General assessment for restriction in thoracic spine, showing the possible directions of movement – flexion, extension, sidebending and rotation right and left, translation forwards, backwards, laterally in both directions, compression and distraction. MET treatment can be applied from any of the restriction barriers (or any combination of barriers) elicited in this way, with the area stabilised at the point of restriction.

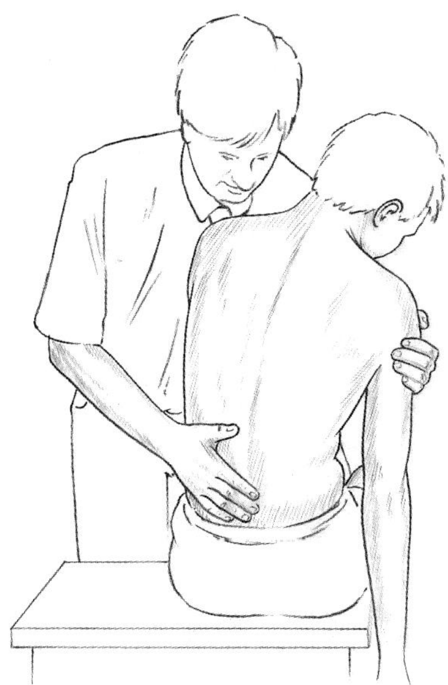

Figure 6.1B Assessment and possible MET treatment position for restriction in sidebending and rotation to the right, involving the lumbar spine.

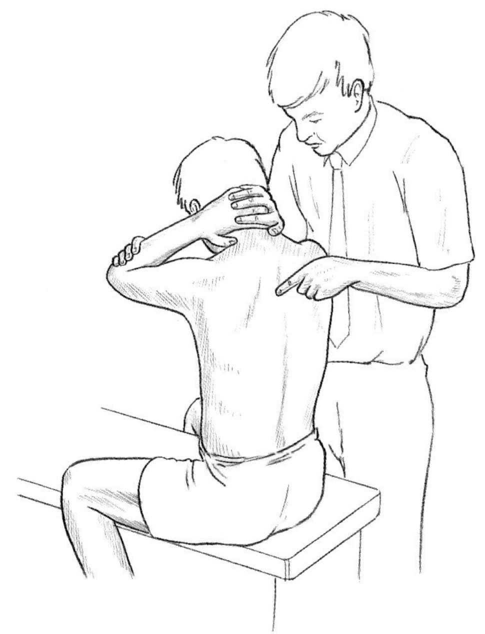

Figure 6.1D Assessment and possible MET treatment position for extension restriction (inability to adequately flex) in the upper thoracic area. MET treatment should commence from the perceived restriction barrier.

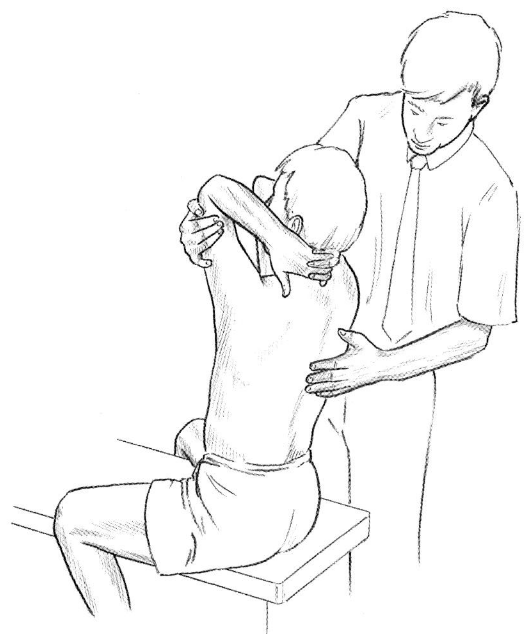

Figure 6.1C Assessment and possible MET treatment position for flexion restriction (inability to adequately extend) in the mid-thoracic area. MET treatment should commence from the perceived restriction barrier.

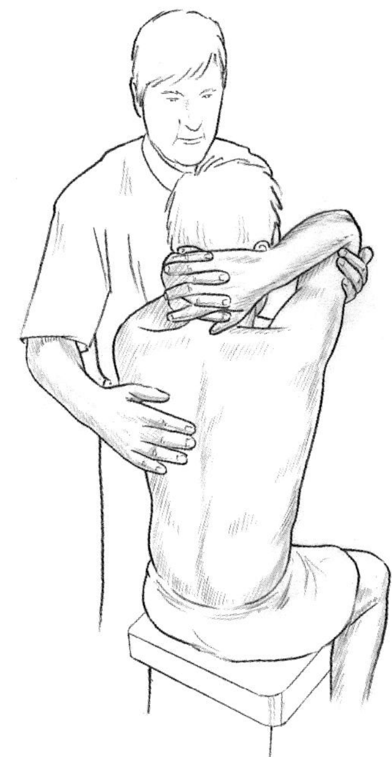

Figure 6.1E Assessment and possible MET treatment position for sidebending restriction (inability to adequately sidebend left) in the mid-thoracic area. MET treatment should commence from the perceived restriction barrier.

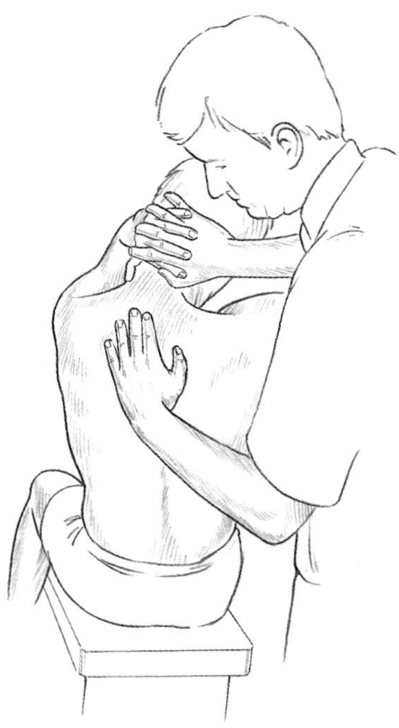

Figure 6.1F Assessment and possible MET treatment position for rotation restriction (inability to adequately rotate right) in the upper thoracic area. MET treatment should commence from the perceived restriction barrier.

the practitioner re-engages the joint at its new motion barrier(s).

This process is repeated until free movement is achieved or until no further gain is apparent following a contraction.

Precise focus of forces – example of lumbar dysfunction

Stiles (1984a), like most other practitioners using muscle energy methods, stresses the importance of accurate and precise structural diagnosis if MET is to be used effectively in treatment of joint dysfunction. By careful motion palpation, determination is made as to restricted joints or areas, and which of their motions is limited. Precise, detailed localisation is required if there is to be accuracy in determining the direction in which the patient is to apply their forces so that the specific restricted barrier can be engaged. If MET applications are poorly focused, it is possible to actually create hypermobility in neighbouring segments, instead of normalising the restricted segment, by inappropriately introducing stretch into already adequately mobile tissues above or below the restricted area.

For example, if a particular restriction is present in lumbar vertebrae – say limitation in gapping of the L4–L5 left side facets on flexion – should a general MET mobilisation attempt not localised to this segment be used, which involved the joints above and/or below the restricted segment, hypermobility of these joints could result, leading, on retesting for general mobility, to an incorrect assumption that the restriction had been cleared.

In order to localise the effort at this segment, the patient would require to be positioned so as to precisely engage the barrier in that joint. For example:

One of the practitioner's hands could palpate the facets of L4–L5, while the seated patient was guided into a flexed and sidebent position which brought the affected segment to its barrier of motion (see Fig. 6.1B). At that point an instruction for the patient to attempt to return to an upright position would involve the muscles (agonists) which are restraining the joint from movement to its normal barrier. At the same time the practitioner's force would be restraining any movement.

This isometric contraction should ideally be maintained for 3–5 seconds (Stiles's timing) with no more than perhaps 20% of the patient's strength being employed in the effort (and synchronised to breathing, see Box 4.2).

After this, when all efforts have ceased, the barrier would normally be found to have retreated, so that greater flexion and sidebending could be achieved, without effort, before re-engaging the barrier.

Repetition would continue several times, until the maximum degree of motion had been obtained.

Alternatively: precisely the opposite method could also be employed, in which, having engaged the barrier, the patient attempted to move through it, while being restrained. This would bring into play reciprocal inhibition of the contracted muscles which are restraining normal range of motion. Were this an acute problem, using the antagonists instead of these dysfunctional muscles would reduce the likelihood of pain being produced.

Goodridge (1981) cautions that 'Monitoring of force is more important than intensity of force. Localisation depends on the practitioner's palpatory proprioceptive perception of movement (or resistance to movement) at or about the specific articulation.' He continues: 'Monitoring and confining forces to the muscle group, or level of somatic dysfunction involved, are important in achieving desirable changes. Poor results are most often due to improperly localised forces, usually too strong.'

Precise localisation of restrictions and identification of muscular contractions and fibrotic changes depend on careful palpation, a set of skills which require constant refinement and maintenance by virtue of use. Identification of the particulars of each restriction is critical, and this can only be achieved via the development of the skills required to assess joint mechanics combined with a sound anatomical grasp. Assessment, via motion palpation, is called for. If forces are misdirected, then results will not only be poor but may also exacerbate the problem. In joint problems, localisation of the point of restriction is the major determining factor of the success (or otherwise) of MET (as in all manipulation).

Harakal's cooperative isometric technique

(Harakal 1975) (Fig. 6.2A–D)

When there is a specific or general restriction in a spinal articulation (for example):

- The area should be placed in neutral (patient seated usually).
- The permitted range of motion should be determined by noting the patient's resistance to further motion.
- The patient should be rested for some seconds at a point just short of the resistance barrier, termed the 'point of balanced tension', in order to 'permit anatomic and physiologic response' to occur.
- The patient is asked to reverse the movement towards the barrier by 'turning back towards where we started', thus contracting any agonists which may be influencing the restriction. (The degree of patient participation at this stage can be at various levels, ranging from 'just think about turning' to 'turn as hard as you would like', or by giving specific instructions.)
- Following a holding of this effort for a few seconds and then relaxing completely, the patient is taken further in the direction of the previous barrier, to a new point of restriction determined by their resistance to further motion as well as tissue response (feel for 'bind').

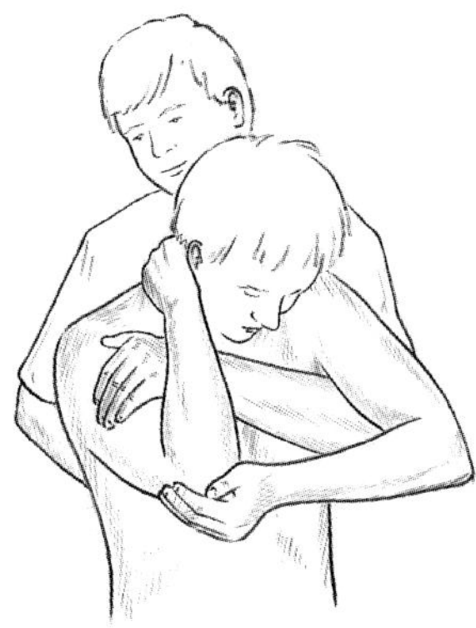

Figure 6.2A Harakal's approach requires the dysfunctional area (mid-thoracic in this example, in which segments cannot easily sidebend right and rotate left) to be taken to a position just short of the assessed restriction barrier. This is termed a point of 'balanced tension' where, after resting for a matter of seconds, an isometric contraction is introduced as the patient attempts to return towards neutral (sitting upright) against the practitioner's resistance.

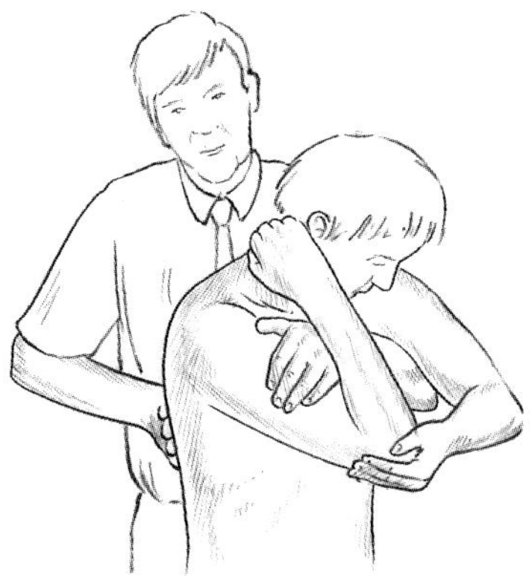

Figure 6.2B Following this effort, the restriction barrier should have eased and the patient can be guided through it towards a new point of balanced tension, just short of the new barrier, and the procedure is repeated.

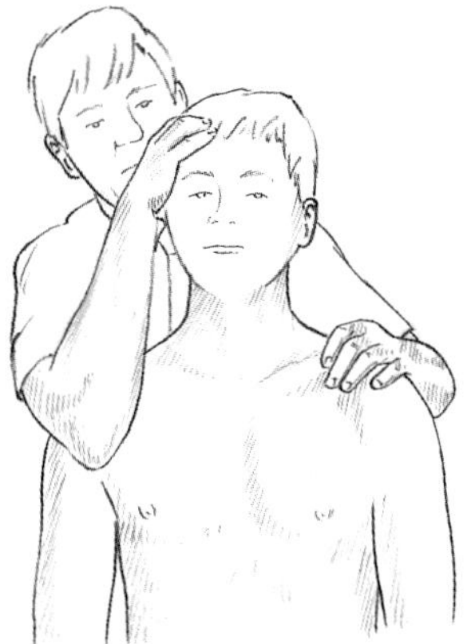

Figure 6.2C In this example the patient, who cannot easily sidebend and rotate the neck towards the left, is held just short of the present barrier in order to introduce an isometric contraction by turning the head to the right against resistance.

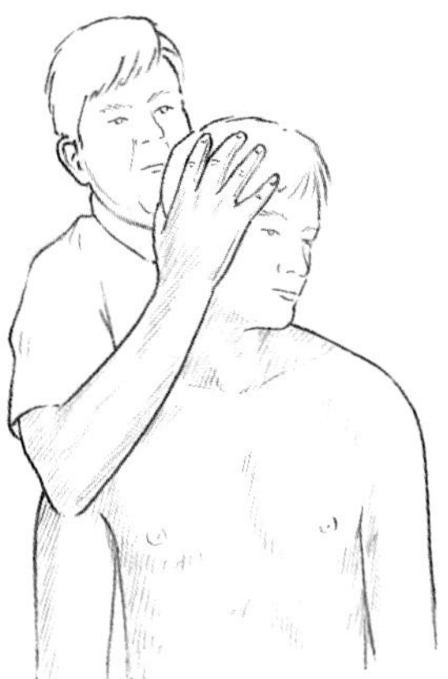

Figure 6.2D Following the contraction described in Figure 6.2C, it is possible for the practitioner to ease the neck into a greater degree of sidebending and rotation towards the left.

- The procedure is repeated until no further gain is being achieved.

It would also, of course, be appropriate to use the opposite direction of rotation, for example asking the patient to 'turn further towards the direction you are moving', so utilising the antagonists to the muscles which may be restricting free movement.

More on MET and the low back

Grieve (1984) describes a low back approach, using MET, which provides insights which can be adapted for use in other spinal regions. The example he gives is of a spine which is capable of full flexion, but in which palpable left sidebending and left rotation fixation exists (i.e. it is locked in left sidebending rotation, and therefore cannot freely sidebend and rotate to the right) in the lumbar spine.

Grieve's low back approach (see Fig. 6.3)

In Grieve's example, the patient sits on a stool, feet apart and flat on the floor. The patient's left arm hangs between his knees, taking him into slight flexion and right rotation/sidebending. The practitioner stands at the patient's left side, with his left leg straddling the patient's left leg.

The practitioner reaches across and holds the patient's right shoulder, while the right hand palpates the vertebral interspace between the spinous processes immediately below the vertebra which is restricted in its ability to rotate to the right. The patient is asked to slump forwards in this twisted posture until the segment under inspection is most prominent, posteriorly.

At this point the practitioner presses his left pectoral area against the patient's left shoulder and, with the patient still flexed, the spine is sidebent by the practitioner, without resistance, so that the patient's right hand approximates the floor. The practitioner then rotates the patient to the right until maximum tension (bind) is felt to build at the segment being palpated. This is the barrier.

At this time the first MET procedure is brought into play. The patient is asked to attempt to reach the floor with his right hand, and this is resisted by the practitioner.

This may last for 5–10 seconds, after which the patient relaxes (exhaling). The practitioner increases the sidebending and rotation to the right, before increasing the degree of flexion. No force is used, simply removal of whatever additional degree of slack has been produced by the isometric effort.

This is the new barrier, and the procedure of attempting to increase these directions of spinal movement (sidebending and rotation to the right and flexion) is repeated, against resistance, a further three or four times.

These movements all involve reciprocal inhibition of the shortened muscle fibres, which are holding the restricted area in left sidebending and left rotation. The antagonists are being contracted isometrically to induce relaxation of the tense (agonist) structures.

After the repetitions, the patient (who is still flexed and rotated, and sidebent to the right) attempts to push against the practitioner's chest with the left shoulder (i.e. attempts to rotate left and sidebend left, as well as to extend).

This effort is maintained for a few (5–10) seconds before relaxation, re-engagement of the barrier, and repetition.

This contraction involves those structures which have shortened and so the isometric contraction produces postisometric relaxation in them.

After each such contraction the slack is again taken out by taking the patient further into right sidebending, rotation and flexion.

The practitioner's position alters after the isometric efforts to the left and right, so that he now stands behind the patient with a hand on each shoulder. Grieve then suggests that the patient be asked to perform a series of stretching movements to the floor, first with the left hand and then with the right hand, against resistance, before being brought into an upright position by the practitioner, against slight resistance of the patient. The condition is then reassessed.

Notice that Grieve uses both reciprocal inhibition and postisometric relaxation in this manoeuvre. He states: 'Whether autogenic (PIR) or reciprocal inhibition is used is totally dependent on which technique effects the best neurophysiological change in the joint environment.' In practice, however, it may not be clear which to choose; the author's experience is that PIR incorporating use of the agonists – those structures thought to be most restricted and negatively influencing joint movement – produces the most satisfying results. Reciprocal inhibition methods are, nevertheless, valuable – for example, in situations in which PIR is painful, or where agonist and antagonist both require therapeutic attention (e.g. following trauma such as whiplash in which all soft tissues will have been stressed).

In short, PIR works best in chronic settings and RI in acute settings, but both can usefully be used in either type of condition if the guideline is adhered to that no pain should be produced, and if no attempt is made to force or 'stretch' joint structures.

Unlike the approach adopted in treating muscles as such, joint applications of MET require that the barrier is all that is approached, with no attempt at pushing through it.

Additional choices

Goodridge (1981) describes two additional MET procedures (the same pattern of dysfunction is assumed):

> If the left transverse process of L5 is more posterior, when the patient is flexed, one postulates that the left caudad facet did not move anteriorly and superiorly along the left cephalad facet of S1, as did the right caudad facet. There would therefore seem to be restrictions in movements in the directions of flexion, lateral flexion (side-bending) to the right, and rotation to the right. It is conceptualised that the restricted motion involves hypertonicity (or shortening) of some muscle fibres. Therefore, the practitioner devises a muscle energy procedure to decrease the tone of (or to lengthen) the affected shortened or hypertonic fibres.

First (Fig. 6.3) the position described by Grieve (see above) is adopted. The patient is seated, left hand hanging between thighs, with the practitioner at his left, the patient's right hand lateral to his right hip and pointing to the floor. The practitioner's right hand monitors either L5 spinous or transverse process. The patient's left shoulder is contacted against the practitioner's left axillary fold, and upper chest. The practitioner's left hand is holding the patient's right shoulder.

The patient slouches to flex the lumbar spine, so that the apex of the posterior convexity is located at the L5–S1 articulation. The practitioner induces first right sidebending and then right rotation (patient's right hand approaches the floor) and localises movement at L5 when a sense of bind and restriction is noted there by the palpating hand.

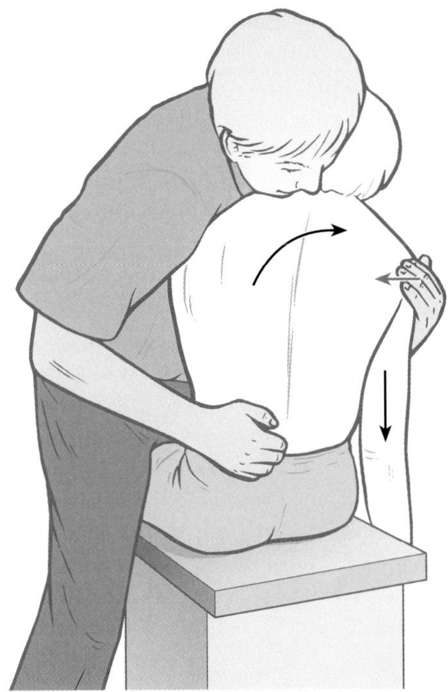

Figure 6.3 Localisation of forces before using MET to release low back restriction.

The patient is then asked to attempt to move in one or more directions, singly or in combination with each other. These would involve left sidebending, rotation left and/or extension, all against practitioner's counterforces.

The patient is, in all of these efforts, contracting muscles on the left side of the spine, but is not changing the distance between the origin and insertion in muscles on either side of the spine. This achieves postisometric relaxation, and subsequent contractions would be initiated after appropriate taking up of slack and engagement of the new barrier.

Additionally, as in the Grieve example above, having attained the position of flexion, right sidebending and right rotation, localised at the joint in question, the patient is asked to move both shoulders in a translation to the left, against resistance from the practitioner's chest and left anterior axillary fold. Neither of the shoulders should rise or fall as this is done, during the translation effort.

While the patient is attempting to move in this manner, the practitioner palpates the degree of increased right sidebending which it induces, at L5–S1. As the patient eases off from this contraction, as described, the practitioner should be able to increase right rotation and sidebending until once again resistance is noted.

The objective of this alternative method is the same as in Grieve's example, but the movement involves, according to Goodridge, a concentric-isotonic procedure, because it allows right lateral flexion of the thoracolumbar spine during the effort.

As this demonstrates, some MET methods are very simple, while others involve conceptualisation of multiple movements and the localisation of forces to achieve their ends. The principles remain the same, however, and can be applied to any muscle or joint dysfunction since the degree of effort, duration of effort and muscles utilised provide so many variables which can be tailored to meet most needs.

Questions and answers

What if pain is produced when using MET in joint mobilisation?

- Evjenth & Hamberg (1984) have a practical solution to the problem of pain being produced when an isometric contraction is employed. They suggest that the degree of effort be markedly reduced and the duration of the contraction increased from 10 seconds to 30 seconds. If this fails to allow a painless contraction, then use of the antagonist muscle(s) for the isometric contraction is another alternative.

Following the contraction, if a joint is being moved to a new resistance barrier and this produces pain, what variations are possible?

- If, following an isometric contraction and movement towards the direction of restriction, there is pain, or if the patient fears pain, Evjenth suggests, 'then the therapist may be more passive and let the patient actively move the joint'.
- Pain experienced may often be lessened considerably if the therapist applies gentle traction while the patient actively moves the joint.

- Sometimes pain may be further reduced if, in addition to applying gentle traction, the therapist simultaneously either aids the patient's movement at the joint, or provides gentle resistance while the patient moves the joint.

Cervical application of MET

Edward Stiles (1984b) has described some of the most interesting applications of MET in treatment of joint restrictions. Some of his thoughts on cervical assessment and treatment are explained below:

General procedure using MET for cervical restriction

Prior to any testing, Stiles suggests a general manoeuvre in which the patient is sitting upright. The practitioner stands behind and holds the head in the midline, with both hands stabilising it, and possibly employing his chest to prevent neck extension.

The patient is told to try (gently) to flex, extend, rotate and sidebend the neck, in all directions, alternately. (No particular sequence is necessary as long as all directions are engaged five or six times.) Each muscle group should undergo slight contraction against unyielding force. This relaxes the tissues in a general manner. Traumatised muscles will relax without much pain via this method.

Upper cervical dysfunction assessment and MET treatment

To test for dysfunction in the upper cervical region, the patient lies supine. The practitioner flexes the head on the neck slightly with one hand while the other cradles the neck. (Flexion of this small degree stabilises the cervical area below C2 so that evaluation of atlantoaxial rotation may be carried out. The region C1 and C2 is usually responsible for half the gross rotation of the neck.)

With the neck flexed (effectively 'locking' everything below C2), it is then passively rotated to both left and right.

If the range is greater on one side, then this is indicative of a probable restrictive barrier, which may be amenable to MET. If rotation towards the left is normally about 85°, but in this instance it is restricted, then palpation of muscle tissues at the level of the facets of C2 (just below the level of joint dysfunction) should indicate contraction or tension locally on the right.

This may or may not be tender, but the likelihood is that it will be so if there is dysfunction. (Pain is often more noticeable at the level of any hypermobile joint rather than where the actual restriction is noted. This may be ascertained by palpation and motion palpation, feeling the tissues as the joint is moved.)

If dysfunction is suspected at the atlantoaxial joint, then C2 is stabilised, in order to isolate C1 for treatment. A fingertip is placed on the left transverse process of C2 so that it cannot turn left when the patient's head is turned left. The second finger of the practitioner's left hand (which is cradling the neck in flexion) is rested as a barrier to prevent left rotation of C2, and the head is then taken gently into left rotation. C1 and the head move, and C2 remains fixed. The barrier is engaged when C2 starts to move (i.e. 'bind' is noted by the palpating finger).

The slack is removed, and at that point the patient is asked to try to turn the head gently to the right, away from the barrier. The practitioner's right hand should be resting on the right side of the patient's head, to prevent this right rotation. The patient's light rotation force is exerted against the practitioner's hand and this is maintained for a few (5–7) seconds.

Both patient and practitioner release their efforts simultaneously, and the practitioner then attempts to take the head further to the left, without force, to engage the new barrier.

This is repeated two or three times.

The monitoring and stabilising pressure on C2 should be minimal, since the patient's effort is not a strong one (this must be stressed to the patient). The patient is using the muscles which are in spasm or contracted (preventing rotation left) and, according to Stiles, 'the exertion builds up tension in the contracted muscles; the Golgi receptor system starts reporting the increased tension in relation to surrounding muscles, and spasm is reflexively inhibited.'

This is a practitioner-direct approach, involving postisometric relaxation.

Stiles' comments regarding whiplash injury and MET

In such conditions X-ray pictures are often normal, as are neurological examinations. Pain, often of major proportions, is nevertheless present. Careful examination should show some segments which are not capable of achieving a full range of movement. These would normally correlate with palpable tissue change and sensitivity. More often than not there is a restriction in which a vertebra is caught in flexion (forward bending). Less commonly, extension fixations may be noted. Each vertebra should be tested to note its ability to flex, extend, sidebend and rotate. MET is applied to whatever specific restrictions are found, as in the example described above.

Wherever a restriction is noted in any particular direction, MET should be used. For example:

- If C3–C4 facets close properly as the neck is sidebent to the left, a characteristic physiological 'springing' will be noted as the barrier is reached.
- If on the right, however, there is dysfunction as the neck is sidebent to that side, the facets will not be felt to close, and a pathological barrier will be noted, which is characterised by a lack of 'give', or increased resistance.

This restriction may be expressed in two ways:

1. The positional diagnosis would be that the segment is flexed and sidebent to the left (and therefore, because of the nature of spinal mechanics, rotated left).

2, The functional diagnosis would be that the joint will not extend, sidebend, or rotate to the right.

The patient should be in the same position as was used in diagnosis (supine, neck slightly flexed). The practitioner's right middle fingers would be placed over the right pillars of C3–C4 and the neck taken to the maximum position of sidebending rotation to the right, engaging the barrier. The left hand is placed over the patient's left parietal and temporal areas. With this hand offering counterforce, the patient is invited to sidebend and rotate to the left, for a few seconds.

This employs the muscles which are presumed to be shortened, and which are therefore preventing the joint from easily sidebending and rotating to the right.

Postisometric relaxation of these muscles will follow the 5–7 second mild contraction, after which the neck should be taken to its new barrier, and the same procedure repeated two or three times.

An alternative would be for the patient to engage the barrier while the practitioner resisted, so incorporating reciprocal inhibition. A further alternative would be to have the patient use Ruddy's pulsating contractions (described in Ch. 3).

Greenman's exercise in cervical palpation and MET application

The following exercise sequence is based on the work of Philip Greenman (1996), and is suggested as an excellent way of becoming familiar with both the mechanics of the neck joints and safe and effective MET applications to whatever is found to be restricted.

In performing this exercise it is important to be aware that normal physiology dictates that sidebending and rotation in the cervical area (C3–C7) is usually 'type 2' (see Box 6.1), which means that segments which are sidebending will automatically rotate towards the same side (i.e. a sidebend to the right means that rotation will take place to the right). Most cervical restrictions are compensations and will involve several segments, all of which will adopt this type 2 pattern. Exceptions occur if a segment is traumatically induced into a different format of dysfunction, in which case there could be sidebending to one side and rotation to the other – termed 'type 1', which it is claimed is the physiological pattern for the rest of the spine, unless the region is in flexion or extension, when type 2 coupling could

Box 6.1 Spinal coupling concepts

Fryette (1954) described spinal biomechanics and defined basic 'laws' as follows (summarised by Mitchell (1995)):

- Law 1 – sidebending with the spine in neutral results in rotation to the contralateral side (i.e. rotation into the convexity). This is known as 'type 1' coupling.
- Law 2 – sidebending with the spine in hyperextension or hyperflexion results in rotation to the ipsilateral side (i.e. into the concavity). This is known as 'type 2' coupling.
- Law 3 – when motion is introduced to a joint in one plane its mobility in other planes is reduced.

In the past MET has been taught with this model utilised to predict probable directions of motion. Gibbons & Tehan (1998) have extensively examined current research and maintain that:

'1. Coupled motion occurs in all regions of the spine
2. coupled motion occurs independently of muscular activity but muscular activity might influence the direction and the magnitude of coupled movement
3. coupling of sidebending and rotation in the lumbar spine is variable in degree and direction
4. there are many variables that can influence the degree and direction of coupled movement and include pain, vertebral level, posture and facet tropism
5. there does not appear to be any simple and consistent relationship between conjunct rotation and intervertebral motion segment level in the lumbar spine.'

However, they state that the evidence of research and the literature is that 'in the cervical spine, below C2, Fryette's laws do seem to be applicable'. The use of these biomechanical laws therefore allows application of Greenman's cervical spine method, as described in this chapter, to be used with confidence.

occur (Ward 1997, Greenman 1996). The concepts of spinal coupling taking place in a predictable manner have been challenged (Gibbons & Tehan 1998). This is discussed in Box 6.1.

Exercise in cervical palpation (Fig. 6.4A, B)

To easily palpate for sidebending and rotation, a side-to-side *translation* ('shunt') movement is used, with the neck in slight flexion or slight extension. When the neck is absolutely neutral (no flexion or extension – an unusual state in the neck), true translation side-to-side is possible. As a segment is translated to one side it is therefore automatically sidebending and, because of the anatomical and physiological rules governing it, it will be rotating to the same side.

In order to evaluate cervical function using this knowledge, Greenman suggests that the practitioner places the fingers as follows, on each side of the spine (see Fig. 6.4A):

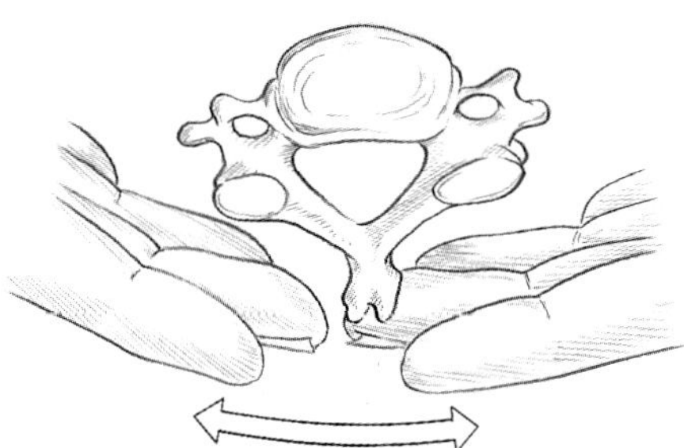

Figure 6.4A The finger pads rest as close to the articular pillars as possible, in order to be able to palpate and guide vertebral motion in a translatory manner.

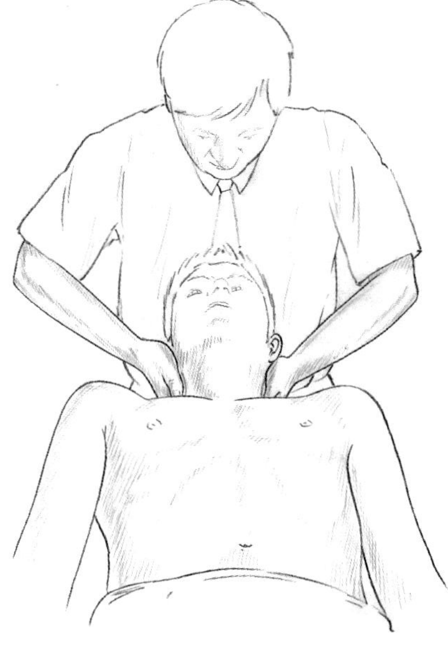

Figure 6.4B With the neck/head in a neutral position, the practitioner sequentially guides individual segments into translation in both directions in order to sense indications of restriction and tissue modification. If a restriction is sensed, its increase or decrease is evaluated by retesting with the segment held in greater flexion and then extension. MET would be applied from the position of greatest unforced bind/restriction, using muscles which would either take the area through (antagonists to shortened muscles) or away from (shortened muscles themselves – the agonists) the barrier.

- The index finger pads rest on the articular pillars of C6, just above the transverse processes of C7, which can be palpated just anterior to the upper trapezius.
- The middle finger pads will be on C6 and the ring fingers on C5, with the little finger pads on C3.

Then:

1. With these contacts (practitioner seated at the head of the supine patient) it is possible to examine for sensitivity, fibrosis, hypertonicity, as well as being able to apply lateral translation to cervical segments with the head in flexion or extension. In order to do this effectively, it is necessary to stabilise the superior segment to the one about to be examined. The heel of the hand controls movement of the head.
2. With the head/neck in relative neutral (no flexion and no extension), translation to the right and then left is introduced (any segment) to assess freedom of movement (sidebending and rotation) in each direction.

Say C5 is being stabilised with the finger pads, as translation to the left is introduced, the ability of C5 to freely sidebend and rotate on C6 is being evaluated with the neck in neutral. If the joint (and/or associated soft tissues) is normal, this translation will cause a gapping of the left facet and a 'closing' of the right facet as left translation is performed, and vice versa. There will be a soft end-feel to the movement, without harsh or sudden braking. If, however, translation of the segment towards the right from the left produces a sense of resistance/bind, then the segment is restricted in its ability to sidebend left and (by implication) to rotate left:

3. If such a restriction is noted, the translation should be repeated, but this time with the head in extension instead of neutral. This is achieved by lifting the contact fingers on C5 (in this example) slightly towards the ceiling before reassessing the side-to-side translation.
4. The head and neck are then taken into flexion, and left-to-right translation is again assessed.

The objective is to ascertain which position creates the greatest degree of bind as the barrier is engaged – is it more restricted in neutral, extension, flexion?

If this restriction is greater with the head extended, the diagnosis is of a joint locked in flexion, sidebent right and rotated right (meaning that there is difficulty in the joint extending and of sidebending and rotating to the left).

If this (C5 on C6 translation left to right) restriction is greater with the head flexed, then the joint is locked in extension and sidebent right and rotated right (meaning there is difficulty in the joint flexing, sidebending and rotating to the left).

MET treatment of the cervical area

Using MET, and using the same example (C5 on C6 as above, translation right is restricted with the greatest degree of restriction noted in extension) the procedure would be as follows:

One hand palpates both of the articular pillars of the inferior segment of the pair which is dysfunctional. (In this instance, this hand will stabilise the C6 articular pillars, holding the inferior vertebra so that the superior segment can be moved on it.) The other hand will introduce movement to, and control the head and neck above the restricted vertebra.

The articular pillars of C6 are held and are lifted towards the ceiling, introducing extension, while the other hand introduces sidebending and rotation to the left until the restriction barrier is reached.

A slight isometric contraction is introduced using sidebending, rotation or flexion (or all of these). The patient is asked to try to lightly turn his head to the right and to sidebend it that way while straightening the neck, or any one of these movements, which should be firmly restrained.

After 5–7 seconds the patient relaxes, and extension, sidebending and rotation left are increased to the new resistance barrier, with no force at all. Repeat three or four times.

NOTE: Eye movement can be used instead of muscular effort in cases where effort results in pain. Looking upwards will encourage isometric contraction of the extensors and vice versa, and looking towards a direction encourages contraction of the muscles on that side.

EXAMPLES OF MET IN JOINT TREATMENT

As we have seen, joints are treatable via MET, and some additional examples are given below. It is, however, not possible to provide a comprehensive body-wide, joint-by-joint description of MET application in joint restriction, especially in a text focusing its attention on soft tissue dysfunction. Nevertheless, sufficient information is provided in this chapter to allow the interested therapist/practitioner to pursue this approach further, providing insights into possible technique applications involving spinal joints quite specifically, as well as generally, and also, more surprisingly perhaps, in dealing with joints which have no obvious muscular control, the iliosacral and acromioclavicular joints, both of which respond dramatically well to MET.

As a learning exercise in practical clinical application of MET to a dysfunctional joint, the well known osteopathic Spencer shoulder sequence has been modified (below). This sequence is based on a clinically useful and practical approach, first described nearly a century ago and still taught in most osteopathic schools in its updated form utilising MET or positional release methods.

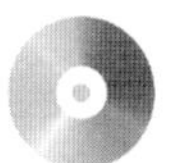

Spencer shoulder sequence modified to incorporate MET

(Spencer 1976, Patriquin 1992; Fig. 6.5A–F)

Assessment and MET treatment of shoulder extension restriction (Fig. 6.5A)

The practitioner's cephalad hand cups the shoulder of the side-lying patient, firmly compressing the scapula and clavicle to the thorax, while the patient's flexed elbow is held by the practitioner's caudad hand, as the arm is taken into extension towards the optimal 90° of extension.

Try to sense any restriction in range of motion, ceasing movement at the first indication of resistance to movement.

At that barrier the patient is instructed to push the elbow towards the feet or anteriorly, or to push further towards the direction of extension – utilising no more than 20% of their strength, building up force slowly.

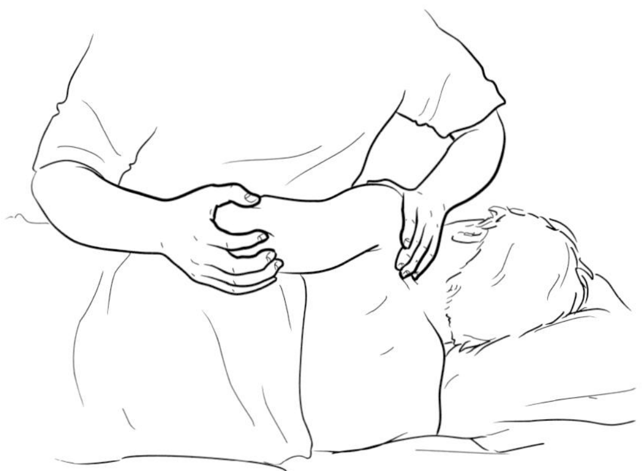

Figure 6.5A Shoulder extension.

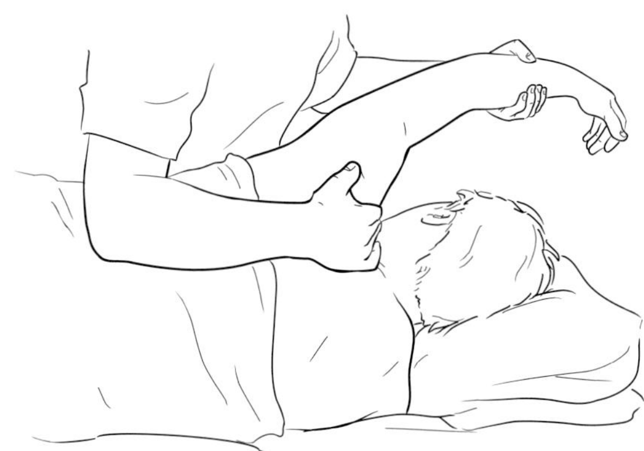

Figure 6.5B Shoulder flexion.

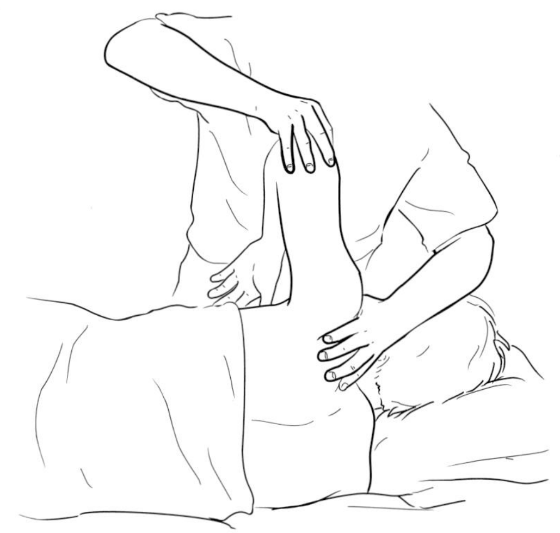

Figure 6.5C Circumduction with compression.

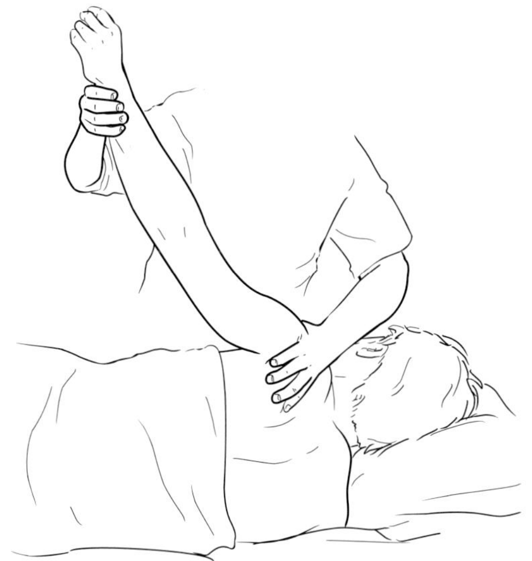

Figure 6.5D Circumduction with traction.

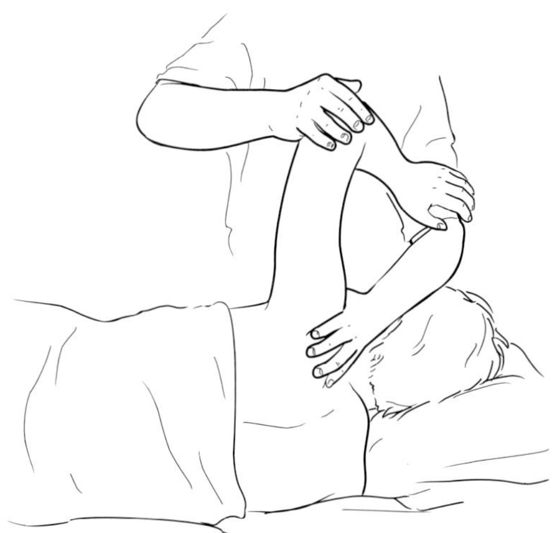

Figure 6.5E Adduction with external rotation of shoulder.

This effort is firmly resisted by the practitioner, and after 7–10 seconds the patient is instructed to slowly cease the effort.

After complete relaxation, and on an exhalation, the practitioner moves the elbow to take the shoulder further into extension, to the next restriction barrier, and the MET procedure is repeated. A degree of active patient participation in the movement towards the new barrier is usually helpful.

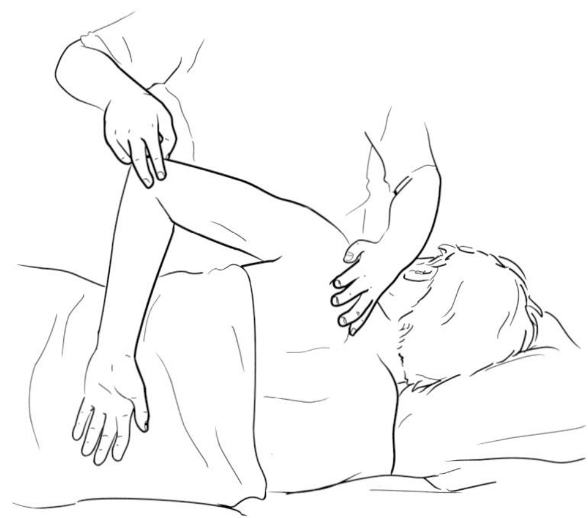

Figure 6.5F Internal rotation of the shoulder.

Assessment and MET treatment of shoulder flexion restriction (Fig. 6.5B)

The patient has the same starting position as in the test above. The practitioner stands at chest level, half-facing cephalad. The practitioner's non-table-side hand grasps the patient's forearm while the table-side hand holds the clavicle and scapula firmly to the chest wall.

The practitioner slowly introduces shoulder flexion in the horizontal plane, as range of motion to 180° is assessed, by which time the elbow will be in extension. At the position of very first indication of restriction in movement, the patient is instructed to pull the elbow towards the feet or posteriorly, or to push further towards the direction of flexion – utilising no more than 20% of their strength, building up force slowly.

This effort is firmly resisted, and after 7–10 seconds the patient is instructed to slowly cease the effort simultaneously with the practitioner.

After complete relaxation, and on an exhalation, the practitioner moves the arm to take the shoulder further into flexion, to the next restriction barrier, where the MET procedure is repeated. A degree of active patient participation in the movement towards the new barrier is usually helpful.

Articulation and assessment of circumduction with compression (Fig. 6.5C)

The patient is side-lying with flexed elbow. The practitioner's cephalad hand cups the patient's shoulder, firmly compressing scapula and clavicle to the thorax. The practitioner's caudad hand grasps the patient's elbow and takes the shoulder through a slow clockwise circumduction, while adding compression through the long axis of the humerus.

This is repeated several times in order to assess range, freedom and comfort of the circumduction motion, as the humeral head moves on the surface of the glenoid fossa.

The same procedure is then performed anticlockwise.

If any restriction is noted, Ruddy's pulsed MET may be usefully introduced, in which the patient attempts to execute a series of minute contractions, towards the restriction barrier, 20 times in a period of 10 seconds, before articulation is continued.

Articulation and assessment of circumduction with traction (Fig. 6.5D)

The patient is side-lying with arm straight. The practitioner's cephalad hand cups the patient's shoulder, compressing scapula and clavicle to the thorax, while the caudad hand grasps the patient's wrist and introduces slight traction, before taking the arm through slow clockwise circumduction. This articulates the joint while assessing range of motion in circumduction, as well as the status of the joint capsule.

The same process is repeated anticlockwise.

If any restriction is noted, Ruddy's pulsed MET (as described above) can usefully be introduced before articulation is continued.

Assessment and MET treatment of shoulder abduction restriction (Fig. 6.5E)

The patient is side-lying. The practitioner cups the patient's shoulder and compresses the scapula and clavicle to the thorax with the cephalad hand, while cupping flexed elbow with the caudad hand. The patient's hand is supported on the practitioner's cephalad forearm/wrist to stabilise the arm.

The elbow is abducted towards the patient's head as range of motion is assessed. A degree of internal rotation is involved in this abduction. Pain-free easy abduction should be close to 180°.

Note any restriction in range of motion. At the position of the very first indication of resistance to movement, the patient is instructed to pull the elbow towards the waist, or to push further towards the direction of abduction – utilising no more than 20% of their strength, building up force slowly.

This effort is firmly resisted, and after 7–10 seconds the patient is instructed to slowly cease the effort simultaneously with the practitioner.

After complete relaxation, and on an exhalation, the practitioner moves the elbow to take the shoulder further into abduction, to the next restriction barrier, where the MET procedure is repeated if necessary (i.e. if there is still restriction). A degree of active patient participation in the movement towards the new barrier is usually helpful.

Assessment and MET treatment of shoulder adduction restriction

The patient is side-lying. The practitioner cups the patient's shoulder and compresses the scapula and clavicle to the thorax with the cephalad hand, while cupping the elbow with the caudad hand. The patient's hand is supported on the practitioner's cephalad forearm/wrist to stabilise the arm.

The elbow is taken in an arc forward of the chest so that it moves both cephalad and medially as the shoulder adducts and externally rotates. The action is performed slowly, and any signs of resistance are noted.

At the position of the very first indication of resistance to movement, the patient is instructed to pull the elbow towards the ceiling, or to push further towards the direction of adduction – utilising no more than 20% of their strength, building up force slowly.

This effort is firmly resisted, and after 7–10 seconds the patient is instructed to slowly cease the effort.

After complete relaxation, and on an exhalation, the elbow is moved to take the shoulder further into adduction, to the next restriction barrier, where the MET procedure is repeated if restriction remains. A degree of active patient participation in the movement towards the new barrier is usually helpful.

Assessment and MET treatment of internal rotation restriction (Fig. 6.5F)

The patient is side-lying. The patient's flexed arm is placed behind his back to evaluate whether the dorsum of the hand can be painlessly placed against the dorsal surface of the ipsilateral lumbar area (see Fig. 6.5F). This arm position is maintained throughout the procedure.

The practitioner stands facing the side-lying patient and cups the patient's shoulder and compresses the scapula and clavicle to the thorax with his cephalad hand while cupping the flexed elbow with the caudad hand.

The practitioner slowly brings the patient's elbow (ventrally) towards his body, and notes any sign of restriction as this movement, which increases internal rotation, is performed.

At the position of first indication of resistance to this movement, the patient is instructed to pull his elbow away from the practitioner, either posteriorly, or medially, or both simultaneously – utilising no more than 20% of his strength, building up force slowly.

This effort is firmly resisted, and after 7–10 seconds the patient is instructed to slowly cease the effort simultaneously with the practitioner.

After complete relaxation, and on an exhalation, the elbow is moved to take the shoulder further into abduction and internal rotation, to the next restriction barrier, where the MET procedure is repeated.

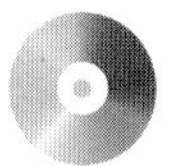

Modified PNF 'spiral stretch' techniques (Fig. 6.6A, B)

Proprioceptive neuromuscular facilitation (PNF) methods have been incorporated into useful assessment and treatment sequences (McAtee & Charland 1999). These ideas have been modified to take account of MET principles (Chaitow 1996)

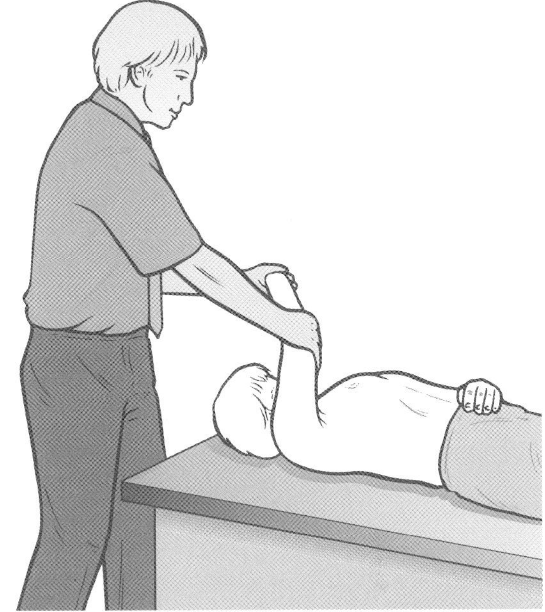

Figure 6.6A Spiral MET starts with shoulder in flexion, adduction and external rotation. Following compound isometric contraction all these directions are taken to new barriers.

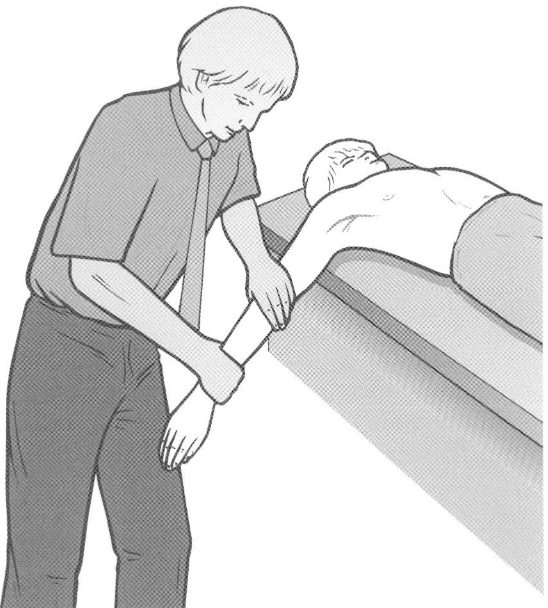

Figure 6.6B Spiral MET2 starts with shoulder in extension, abduction and internal rotation. Following compound isometric contraction all these directions are taken to new barriers.

Spiral MET method 1. Shoulder 'spiral' stretch into extension to increase the range of motion in flexion, adduction and external rotation The patient lies supine and ensures that her shoulders remain in contact with the table throughout the procedure. The head is turned left. The patient flexes, adducts and externally rotates the (right) arm fully, maintaining the elbow in extension (palm facing the ceiling). The practitioner stands at the head of the table and supports the patient's arm at proximal forearm and elbow.

The patient is asked to begin the process of returning the arm to her side, in stages, against resistance. The amount of force used by the patient should not exceed 25% of their strength potential.

The first instruction is to pronate and internally rotate the arm ('turn your arm so that your palm faces the other way'), followed by abduction and then extension ('bring your arm back outwards and to your side').

All these efforts are combined by the patient into a sustained effort which is resisted by the practitioner so that a 'compound' isometric contraction occurs involving infraspinatus, middle trapezius, rhomboids, teres minor, posterior deltoid and pronator teres.

On complete relaxation the practitioner, with the patient's assistance, takes the arm further into flexion, adduction and external rotation, stretching these muscles to a new barrier.

The same procedure is repeated two or three times.

Spiral MET method 2. Shoulder 'spiral' stretch into flexion to increase the range of motion in extension, abduction and internal rotation The patient lies supine and ensures that her shoulders remain in contact with the table throughout the procedure. She extends, abducts and internally rotates the (right) arm fully, maintaining the elbow in extension (wrist pronated). The practitioner stands at the head of the table and supports the patient's arm at proximal forearm and elbow.

The patient is asked to begin the process of returning the arm to her side, in stages, against resistance. The amount of force used by the patient should not exceed 25% of their strength potential.

The first instruction is to supinate and externally rotate the arm, ('turn your arm outwards so that your palm faces the other way'), followed by adduction and then flexion ('bring your arm back towards the table and then up to your side').

All these efforts are combined by the patient into a sustained effort which is resisted by the practitioner, so that a 'compound' isometric contraction occurs involving the clavicular head of pectoralis major, anterior deltoid, coracobrachialis, biceps brachii, infraspinatus and supinator.

On complete relaxation the practitioner, with the patient's assistance, takes the arm further into extension, abduction and internal rotation, stretching these muscles to a new barrier.

The same procedure is repeated two or three times.

MET treatment of acromioclavicular and sternoclavicular dysfunction

Whereas spinal/neck and most other joints are seen to be moved by and to be under the postural influence of muscles, and therefore to an extent to be capable of having their function modified by muscle energy techniques, articulations such as those of the sternoclavicular, acromioclavicular and iliosacral joints seem far less amenable to such influences. Hopefully, some of the methods detailed below will modify this impression, since MET is widely used in the osteopathic profession to help normalise the functional integrity of these joints.

Acromioclavicular (AC) dysfunction (Fig. 6.7A, B)

Stiles (1984b) suggests beginning evaluation of AC dysfunction at the scapulae, the mechanics of which closely relate to AC function.

The patient sits erect and the spines of both scapulae are palpated by the practitioner, standing behind. The hands are moved medially, until the medial borders of the scapulae are identified, at the level of the spine.

Using the palpating fingers as landmarks, the levels are checked to see whether they are the same. Inequality suggests AC dysfunction.

The side of dysfunction remains to be assessed, and each side is tested separately (see Fig. 6.7A). To test the right side AC joint, the practitioner is

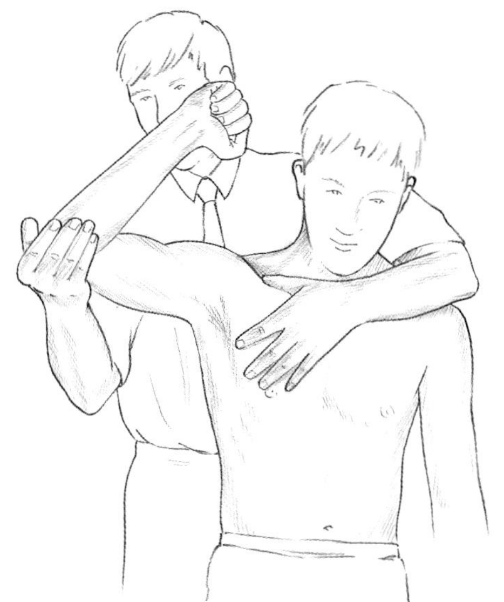

Figure 6.7A MET treatment of right side acromioclavicular restriction. Patient attempts to return the elbow to the side against resistance.

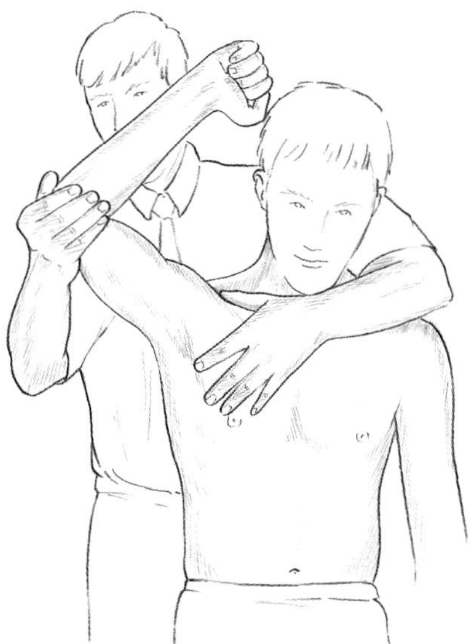

Figure 6.7B Following the isometric contraction, the arm is elevated further while firm downward pressure is maintained on the lateral aspect of the clavicle.

behind the patient, with the left hand palpating over the joint. The right hand holds the patient's right elbow. The arm is lifted in a direction, 45° from the sagittal and frontal planes. As the arm approaches 90° elevation, the AC joint should be carefully palpated for hinge movement, between the acromion and the clavicle.

In normal movement, with no restriction, the palpating hand should move slightly caudad, as the arm is abducted beyond 90°. If the AC is restricted, the palpating hand/digit will move cephalad and little or no action will be noted at the joint itself as the arm goes beyond 90° elevation.

Muscle energy technique is employed with the arm held at the restriction barrier, as for testing above.

If the scapula on the side of dysfunction had been shown to be more proximal than that on the normal side, then the humerus is placed in external rotation, which takes the scapula caudad against the barrier, before the isometric contraction commences.

If, however, the scapula on the side of the AC dysfunction was more distal than the scapula on the normal side, then the arm is internally rotated, taking the scapula cephalad against the barrier before the isometric contraction commences.

The left hand (we assume this to be a right-sided problem in this example) stabilises the distal end of the clavicle, with caudad pressure being applied by the left thumb which rests on the proximal surface of the scapula. The first finger of the left hand lies on the distal aspect of the clavicle.

The combination of the rotation of the arm as appropriate (externally if the scapula on that side was high and internally if it was low) as well as the caudad pressure exerted by the left hand on the clavicle and the scapula, provides an unyielding counterforce.

The arm will have been raised until the first sign of inappropriate movement at the AC joint was noted (as a sense of 'bind'). This is the barrier, and at this point the various stabilising holds (internal or external arm rotation, etc.) are introduced.

An unyielding counter-pressure is applied at the point of the patient's elbow by the right hand, and the patient is asked to try to take that elbow towards the floor with less than full strength.

After 7–10 seconds the patient and practitioner relax, and the arm is once more taken towards the barrier.

Again, greater internal or external rotation is introduced to take the scapula higher or lower, as appropriate, as firm but not forceful pressure is sustained on the clavicle and scapula in a caudad direction.

The mild isometric contraction is again called for, and the procedure repeated several times. (It is worth recalling that respiratory accompaniment to the efforts described is helpful, with inhalation accompanying effort, and exhalation accompanying relaxation and the engagement of the new barrier.)

The procedure is repeated until no further improvement is noted in terms of range of motion or until it is sensed that the clavicle has resumed normal function.

Assessment and MET treatment of restricted abduction in the sternoclavicular joint

As the clavicle abducts it rotates posteriorly. To test for this motion, the patient lies supine, or is seated, with arms at side (Fig. 6.8A). The practitioner places his index fingers on the superior surface of the medial end of the clavicle.

The patient is asked to shrug the shoulders as the practitioner palpates for the expected caudal movement of the medial clavicle. If it fails to do so, there is a restriction preventing normal abduction.

MET treatment of restricted abduction in the sternoclavicular joint (Fig 6.8B)

The practitioner stands behind the seated patient with his thenar eminence on the superior margin of the medial end of the clavicle to be treated. The other hand grasps the patient's flexed elbow and holds this at 90°, with the upper arm externally rotated and abducted.

The patient is asked to adduct the upper arm for 5–7 seconds against resistance, using about 20% of available strength.

Following the effort and complete relaxation, the arm is abducted further, and externally rotated further, until a new barrier is sensed, with the practitioner all the while maintaining firm caudad pressure on the medial end of the clavicle.

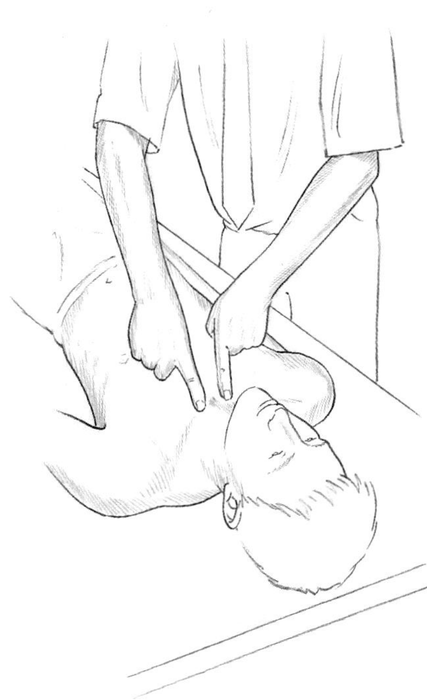

Figure 6.8A Assessment ('shrug test') for restriction in clavicular mobility.

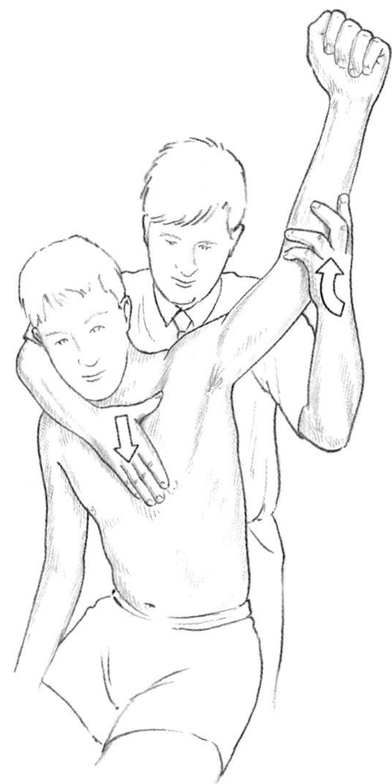

Figure 6.8B MET treatment of restricted sternoclavicular joint. Following an isometric contraction, the arm is elevated and extended while firm downward pressure is maintained on the medial aspect of the clavicle with the thenar eminence.

The process is repeated until free movement of the medial clavicle is achieved.

Assessment and MET treatment of restricted horizontal flexion of the upper arm (sternoclavicular restriction)

The patient lies supine and the practitioner stands to one side with the index fingers resting on the anteromedial aspect of each clavicle.

The patient is asked to extend his arms forwards in front of his face in a 'prayer' position, palms together, pointing to the ceiling (Fig. 6.9A). On the patient pushing the hands forwards towards the ceiling, the clavicular heads should drop towards the floor and not rise up to follow the hands. If one or both fail to drop, there is a restriction.

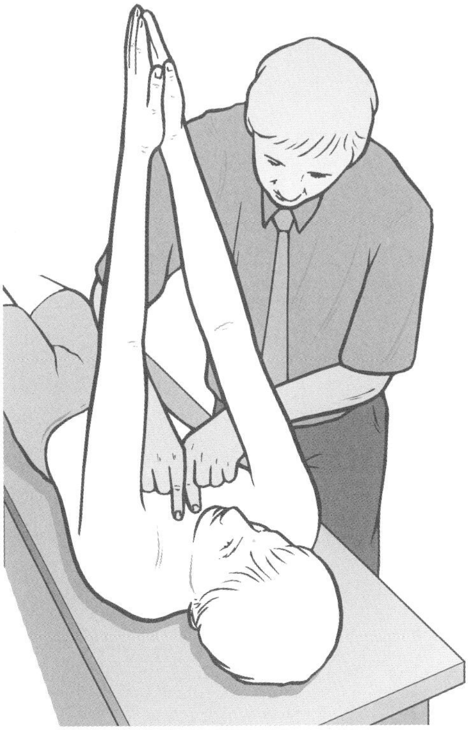

Figure 6.9A Assessment ('prayer test') for restricted horizontal flexion of the sternoclavicular joint.

MET treatment of restricted horizontal flexion of the upper arm (sternoclavicular restriction)

The patient is supine and the practitioner stands on the contralateral side facing the patient at shoulder level. The practitioner places the thenar eminence of his cephalad hand over the medial end of the dysfunctional clavicle, holding it towards the floor. His caudad hand lies under the shoulder on that side to embrace the dorsal aspect of the lateral scapula (Fig. 6.9B).

The patient is asked to stretch out the arm on the side to be treated so that the hand can rest behind the practitioner's neck or shoulder.

The practitioner leans back to take out all the slack from the extended arm and shoulder while at the same time lifting the scapula on that side slightly from the table. At this time the patient is asked to pull the practitioner towards himself, against firm resistance, for 7–10 seconds.

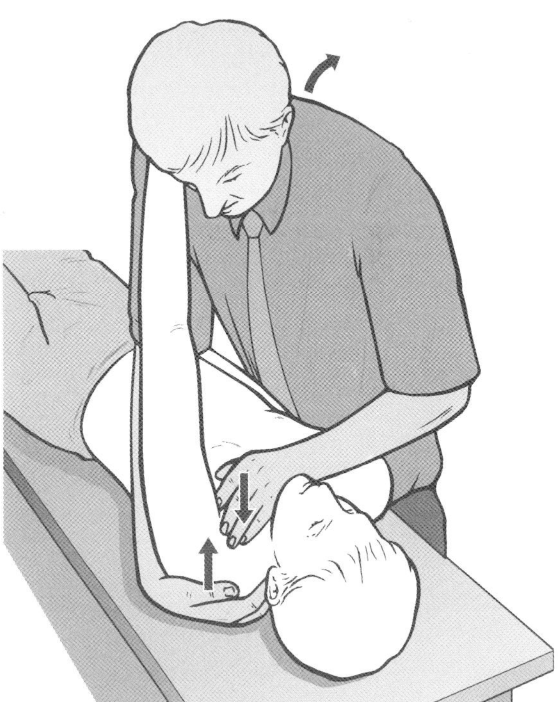

Figure 6.9B MET treatment of horizontal flexion restriction. After isometric contraction (patient attempts to pull practitioner towards himself) the practitioner simultaneously lifts the shoulder while maintaining firm downwards pressure (to the floor) with the hypothenar eminence on the medial aspect of the clavicle.

Following complete release of all the patient's efforts, the downwards (to the floor) thenar eminence pressure is maintained (painlessly) and more slack is taken out (practitioner keeps in place all elements of the procedure throughout, only the patient releases effort between contractions).

The process is repeated once or twice more or until the 'prayer' test proves negative.

NOTE: No pain should be noted during this procedure.

MET for rib dysfunction (Goodridge & Kuchera 1997, Greenman 1996)

In order to use MET successfully to normalise rib dysfunction the nature of the problem requires identification. In this section of the chapter only a limited number of rib problems are considered, in order to illustrate MET usefulness. Study is recommended of Greenman (1996) and Ward (1997) for a wider range of MET choices.

Restrictions in the ability of a given rib to move fully (as compared with its pair) during inhalation indicates a depressed status, while an inability to move fully (as compared with its pair) into exhalation indicates an elevated status.

As a rule, unless there has been direct trauma, rib restrictions of this sort are compensatory, and involve groups of ribs. Osteopathic clinical experience suggests that if a group of depressed ribs is located, the 'key' rib is likely to be the most superior of these, which, if successfully released, will 'unlock' the remaining ribs in that group. Similarly, if a group of elevated ribs is located, the key rib is likely to be the most inferior of these; if successfully released, it will unlock the remaining ribs in that group.

If palpation commences at the most cephalad aspect of the thorax, the 2nd rib is the most easily palpatated. The ribs are sequentially assessed, and if a depressed rib is noted this is clearly the most cephalad and is the one to be treated (see below). Similarly, if an elevated rib is identified, the ribs continue to be evaluated until a normal pair is located and the dysfunctional rib cephalad to these is treated.

MET methods described below are one way of releasing such restrictions. However, there are also extremely useful positional release methods for treating such problems, based on Jones's strain/counterstrain methods (Jones 1981).

As in all forms of somatic dysfunction, causes should be sought and addressed, in addition to mobilisation of restrictions, using MET or other methods, as described in this text.

Rib palpation test: rib 1 (Fig. 6.10) The patient is seated and the practitioner stands behind. The practitioner places his hands so that the fingers can draw posteriorly the upper trapezius fibres lying superior to the 1st rib. The tips of the practitioner's middle and index (or middle and ring) fingers can then most easily be placed on the superior surface of the posterior shaft of the 1st rib.

Symmetry is evaluated as the patient breathes lightly.

The commonest dysfunction is for one of the pair of 1st ribs to be 'locked' in an elevated position ('inhalation restriction'). The superior aspect of this rib will palpate as tender and attached scalene structures are likely to be short and tight (Greenman 1996).

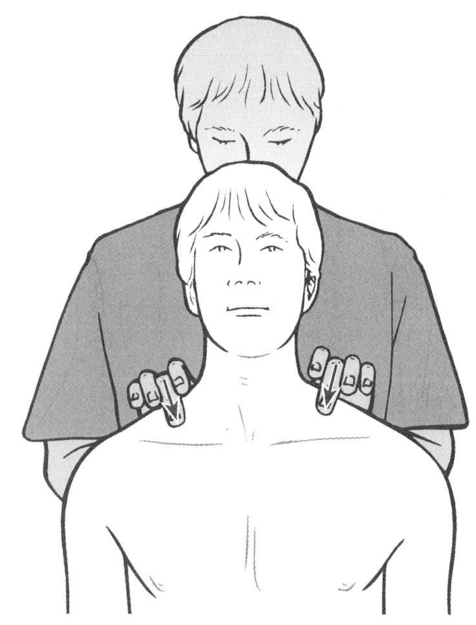

Figure 6.10 Palpation of 1st rib anterior to upper trapezius fibres.

Or
The patient is seated and the practitioner stands behind. The practitioner places his hands so that the fingers can draw posteriorly the upper trapezius fibres lying superior to the 1st rib. The tips of the practitioner's middle and index (or middle and ring) fingers can then most easily be placed on the superior surface of the posterior shaft of the 1st rib.

The patient exhales and shrugs his shoulders and the palpated 1st ribs behave asymmetrically (one moves superiorly more than the other); or: the patient inhales fully and the palpated 1st ribs behave asymmetrically (one moves more than the other).

The commonest restriction of the 1st rib is into elevation and the likeliest soft tissue involvement is of anterior and medial scalenes (Goodridge & Kuchera 1997).

Rib palpation test: ribs 2–10 (Fig. 6.11) The patient is supine. The practitioner stands at waist level facing the patient's head, with a single finger contact on the superior aspect of one pair of ribs. The practitioner's dominant eye determines the side of the table from which he is approaching the observation of rib function (right eye dominant calls for standing on the patient's right side).

The fingers are observed as the patient inhales and exhales fully (eye focus is on an area between the palpating fingers so that peripheral vision assesses symmetry of movement). If, on inhalation, one of a pair of ribs fails to rise as far as its pair, it is described as a depressed rib, unable to move fully to its end of range on inhalation ('exhalation restriction'). If, on exhalation, one of a pair of ribs fails to fall as far as its pair, it is described as an elevated rib, unable to move fully to its end of range on exhalation ('inhalation restriction').

Rib palpation test: ribs 11 and 12 (Fig. 6.12) Assessment of 11th and 12th ribs is usually performed with the patient prone and palpation performed with a hand contact on the posterior shafts to evaluate full inhalation and exhalation motions.

The 11th and 12th ribs usually operate as a pair so that if any sense of reduction in posterior motion is noted on one side or the other, on inhalation, the pair is regarded as depressed,

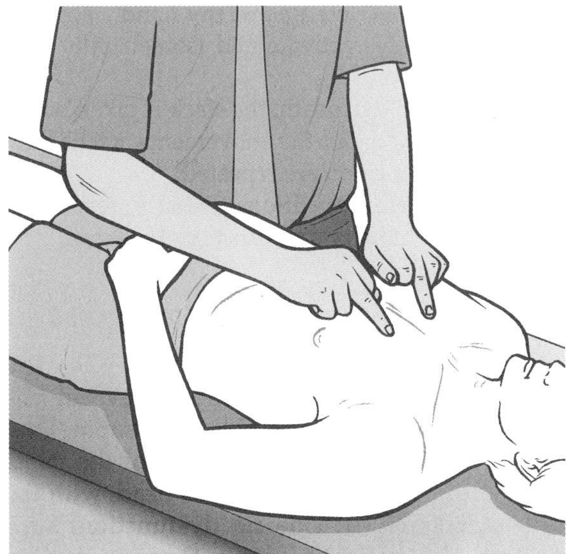

Figure 6.11 Palpation of ribs 2–10.

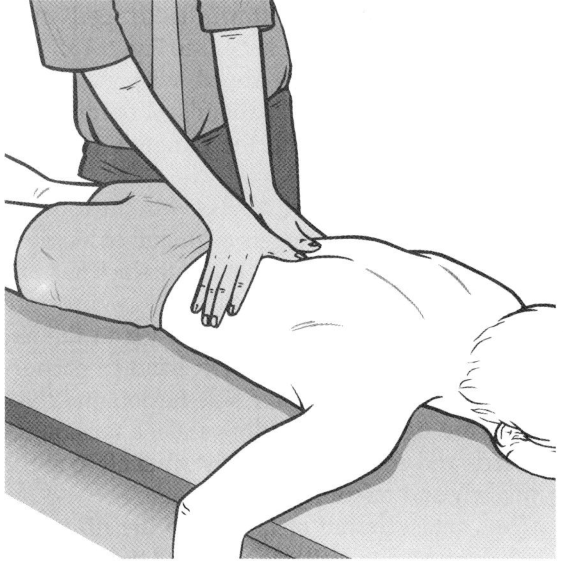

Figure 6.12 Palpation of ribs 11 and 12.

unable to fully inhale ('exhalation restriction'). If any sense of reduction in anterior motion is noted on one side or the other, on exhalation, the pair is regarded as elevated, unable to fully exhale ('inhalation restriction').

General principles of MET for rib dysfunction

Before using MET on rib restrictions identified in tests such as those summarised above, appropriate attention should be given to the attaching musculature, for example the scalenes for the upper ribs, and pectorals, latissimus, quadratus lumborum and others for the lower ribs (see Ch. 4).

Additionally, before specific attention is given to rib restrictions, evaluation and appropriate treatment should be given to any thoracic spine dysfunction which may be influencing the function of associated ribs. Attention should also be given to postural and breathing habits which may be contributing to thoracic spine and/or rib dysfunction, and appropriate re-education and exercise protocols prescribed.

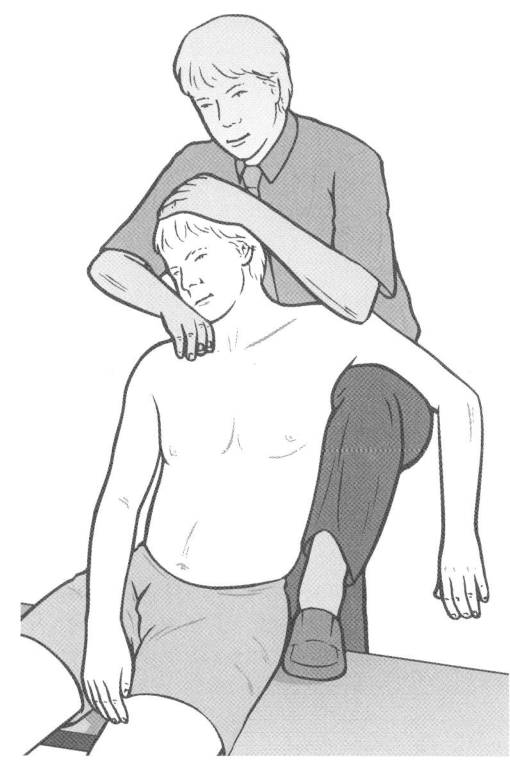

Figure 6.13 Position for MET treatment of restricted (elevated) 1st rib on the right.

MET treatment for restricted 1st rib (Fig. 6.13)

The patient is seated. To treat a right elevated 1st rib, the practitioner's left foot is placed on table and the patient's left arm is 'draped' over the practitioner's flexed knee (see Fig. 6.13). The practitioner's left arm is flexed, with the elbow placed anterior to the patient's shoulder and the left hand supporting the patient's (side of) head.

The practitioner makes contact with the tubercle of the 1st rib with the fingers or thumb of his right hand, taking out available soft tissue slack as force is applied in an inferior direction.

The practitioner eases his flexed leg to the left and simultaneously uses his left hand to encourage the patient's neck into a side-flexion and rotation to the right, so unloading scalene tension on that side and encouraging the 1st rib shaft to move anteriorly and inferiorly.

The contact thumb or fingers on the rib tubercle/shaft take out available slack and the patient is asked to 'inhale and hold your breath for a few seconds and at the same time gently press your head towards the left against my hand'. This 5–7 second effort will activate and isometrically contract the scalenes.

On releasing the breath, the slack is taken out of the soft tissues as all the movements which preceded the contraction are repeated.

Two or three repetitions usually results in greater rib symmetry and functional balance.

MET treatment for restricted 2nd to 10th ribs

Method for elevated ribs (Fig. 6.14) The most inferior of a group of elevated ribs is identified. The patient is supine and the practitioner stands at the head of the table, slightly to the left of the patient's head, with the right hand (for left side rib dysfunction) supporting the patient's upper thoracic region, forearm supporting neck and head. The left

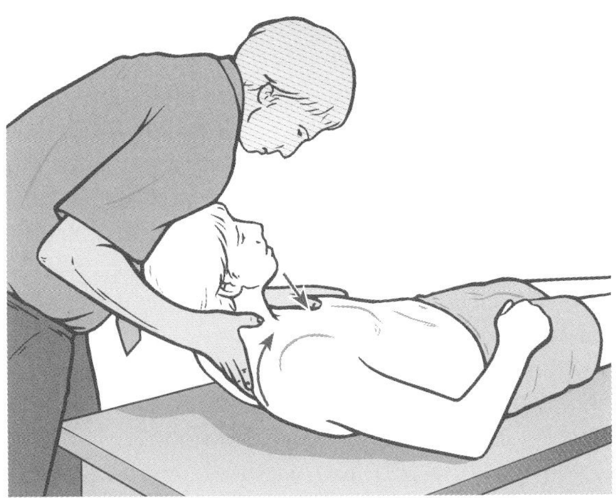

Figure 6.14 MET treatment of elevated rib.

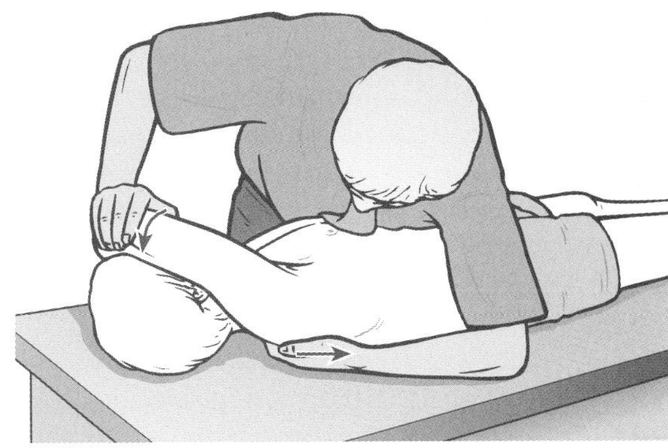

Figure 6.15 MET treatment of depressed 2nd rib.

hand is placed so that the thenar eminence rests on the superior aspect of the costochondral junction of the designated rib, close to the mid-clavicular line (for upper ribs; for ribs 7–10 the contact would be more lateral, closer to the mid-axillary line), directing the rib caudally.

The upper thoracic and cervical spine is eased into flexion, as well as side-flexion towards the treated side, until motion is sensed at the site of the rib stabilisation. If introduction of side-flexion is difficult, the patient should be asked to ease the left hand (in this example) towards the feet until motion is noted at the palpated rib.

The patient should then be asked to 'inhale fully and hold your breath' (isometric contraction of intercostals as well as scalenes) and to attempt to return the back and head to the table, against the practitioner's resistance.

On release and full exhalation, the slack is removed from the local tissues (thenar eminence holding the rib towards its caudad position) as increased flexion and side-flexion is introduced.

This sequence is repeated once or twice only and usually results in release of the group of 'elevated' ribs.

Method for depressed ribs (Fig. 6.15) Various muscles are used for different depressed rib restrictions (see method below), based on their attachments. Goodridge & Kuchera (1997) list (and recommend patient positioning to treat) these as:

1. *Rib 1: anterior and middle scalenes.* The patient's arm is flexed, forearm resting on forehead, head rotated away from the side to be treated (towards the left in this example); the patient is instructed to attempt to flex the neck and head further, against resistance for 5–7 seconds.
2. *Rib 2: posterior scalene.* The patient's arm is flexed, forearm resting on forehead, head rotated away from the side to be treated (towards the left in this example); the patient is instructed to attempt to move the elbow and head anteriorly against resistance for 5–7 seconds (see Fig. 6.15).
3. *Ribs 3–5: pectoralis minor.* The patient's head is in neutral, the arm flexed and placed alongside of the head; the patient is asked to bring the elbow towards the sternum against resistance for 5–7 seconds.
4. *Ribs 6–9: serratus anterior.* The patient's head is in neutral, the elbow flexed, the dorsum of the hand resting on the forehead. The patient is asked to bring the hand anteriorly against resistance for 5–7 seconds.
5. *Ribs 10–12: latissimus dorsi.* The patient is prone, the arm, elbow flexed, lies in abduction between 90° and 130°, depending on localisation of forces to rib being treated; the patient is asked to abduct the arm against resistance (Fig. 6.16).

Method The most superior of an identified group of depressed ribs is treated. The patient is supine and the practitioner stands on the contralateral side, and places his table-side arm across the patient's trunk, inserting the hand beneath the patient's torso so that he can engage, with fingertips, the superior aspect of the costal angle of the designated rib (the most superior of the group).

The patient's head or arm is placed in the most suitable position so that an isometric contraction will engage the muscle(s) most likely to influence the key rib (see the list and suggestions above). The patient is asked to move the head or arm as appropriate (see list above), against practitioner resistance, while holding the breath (this is an isometric contraction of the intercostals), for 5–7 seconds.

On complete relaxation the fingers draw the rib inferiorly to take out available slack and the process is repeated at least once more before reassessment of rib movement is carried out.

MET treatment for restricted (depressed) 11–12th ribs (Fig. 6.16)

The patient is prone, and the practitioner stands on the ipsilateral side, facing the patient.

For left side depressed 11th rib, the patient places his left arm above his head and the practitioner holds that elbow with his cephalad hand. The practitioner locates the depressed 11th rib and draws it superiorly to its barrier, with his finger pads.

The patient is asked to breathe in and hold the breath, while simultaneously attempting to bring the elevated and abducted left elbow sideways, back towards the side, against resistance.

After 5–7 seconds, and complete relaxation by the patient, the rib is drawn superiorly towards its new barrier via the finger contact.

A repetition of the procedure should then be carried out and the rib reassessed for motion.

MET treatment for restricted (elevated) 11–12th ribs (Fig. 6.17)

The patient is prone, arms at his side, and the practitioner stands on the contralateral side to the dysfunctional ribs.

For right side 11th and 12th elevated ribs, the practitioner places the thenar and hypothenar eminences of his cephalad hand on the medial aspects of the shafts of both the 11th and 12th ribs (these two ribs usually act in concert in the way they become dysfunctional). The practitioner's caudad hand grasps the patient's right ASIS.

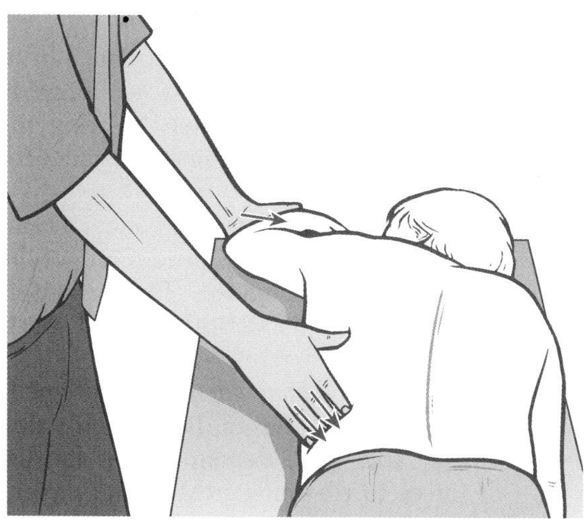

Figure 6.16 MET treatment of depressed 11th and/or 12th ribs.

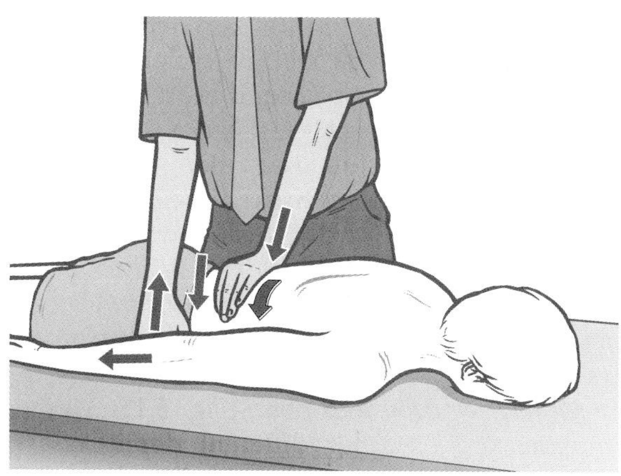

Figure 6.17 MET treatment of elevated 11th and/or 12th ribs.

The patient is asked to exhale fully, and hold this out, and to reach towards the right foot with the right hand, so introducing sidebending to the right, taking the elevated ribs towards their normal position. At the end of the exhalation the patient is asked to bring the ASIS firmly into the practitioner's hand ('push your pelvis towards the table').

After 5–7 seconds and complete relaxation, the practitioner takes out all slack with his contact hand and the process is repeated, before retesting.

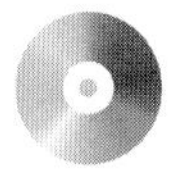

General thoracic cage release using MET (Fig. 6.18)

The patient is supine and the practitioner stands at waist level facing cephalad and places his hands over the middle and lower thoracic structures, fingers along the rib shafts.

Treating the structure being palpated as a cylinder, the hands test the preference this cylinder has to rotate around its central axis, one way and then the other:

- 'Does the lower thorax rotate with more difficulty to the right or to the left?'

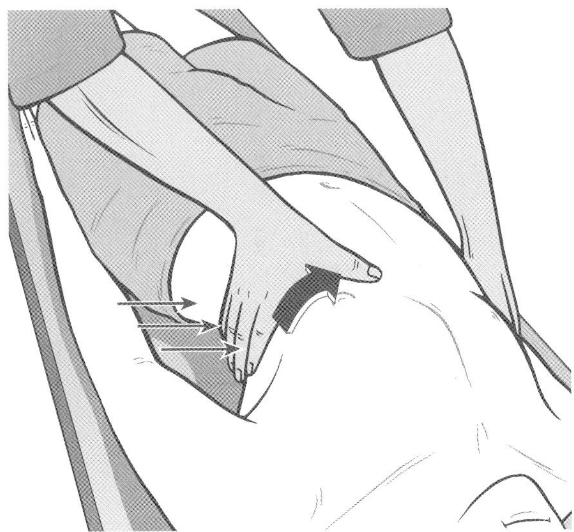

Figure 6.18 General MET for release of lower thorax and diaphragm.

Once the direction of greatest rotational restriction has been established, the sidebending one way or the other is evaluated:

- 'Does the lower thorax side-flex with more difficulty to the right or to the left?'

Once these two pieces of information have been established, the combined positions of restriction, so indicated, are introduced.

By sidebending and rotating *towards the tighter* directions, the combined directions of restriction are engaged, at which time the patient is asked to inhale and hold the breath, and to 'bear down' slightly (Valsalva manoeuvre). These efforts introduce isometric contractions of the diaphragm and intercostal muscles.

On release and complete exhalation and relaxation the diaphragm should be found to function more normally, accompanied by a relaxation of associated soft tissues and a more symmetrical rotation and side-flexion potential of the previously restricted tissues.

Assessment and MET treatment of pelvic and iliosacral restrictions

In order to apply certain useful MET applications to pelvic dysfunction involving the iliosacral joint it is necessary to carry out a few basic assessments.

⚠ **CAUTION:** The evidence derived from the standing flexion test as described below is invalid if there is concurrent shortness in the hamstrings, since this will effectively give either:

- A false positive sign on the contralateral side with unilateral hamstring shortness due to the restraining influence on the side of hamstring shortness, creating a compensating iliac movement on the other side during flexion, or
- False negative signs if there is bilateral hamstring shortness (i.e. there may be iliosacral motion which is masked by the restriction placed on the ilia via hamstring shortness).

The hamstring tests as described in Chapter 4 should therefore be carried out first, and if this proves positive these structures should be normalised as far as is possible, prior to the assessment methods described here being utilised.

Test (a): pelvic balance (Fig. 6.19A) The practitioner stands or squats behind the standing patient and places the medial side of his hands on the lateral pelvis below the crests, pushing inwards and upwards until the index fingers lie superior to the crest:

- If these are judged to be level then no anatomical leg length discrepancy exists.
- If an inequality of height of pelvic crests is observed, the heights of the greater trochanters should also be assessed, by direct palpation.
- If both the pelvic crest height and the height of the greater trochanter on the same side appear to be greater than the opposite side, an anatomical leg length difference is likely (Greenman 1996).
- If pelvic crest height OR trochanter height are greater on one side than the other, pelvic imbalance is a possible explanation, commonly involving postural muscle shortening and imbalance, or actual osseous asymmetry.

Test (b): iliosacral The PSIS positions are assessed just below the pelvic dimples:

- Are they symmetrical?
- Is one superior or anterior to the other?

Anteriority may involve shortness of the external rotators on that side (iliopsoas, quadratus femoris, piriformis) or internal rotators on the other side (gluteus medius, hamstrings).

Inferiority may indicate hamstring shortness or pelvic/pubic dysfunction.

Test (c): standing flexion (iliosacral) (Fig. 6.19A) With the patient still standing and any inequality of leg length having been compensated for by insertion of a pad under the foot on the short side, the practitioner's thumbs are placed firmly (a light contact is useless) on the inferior slope of the PSIS.

The patient is asked to go into full flexion while thumb contact is maintained (see Fig. 6.19A). The patient's knees should remain extended during this bend.

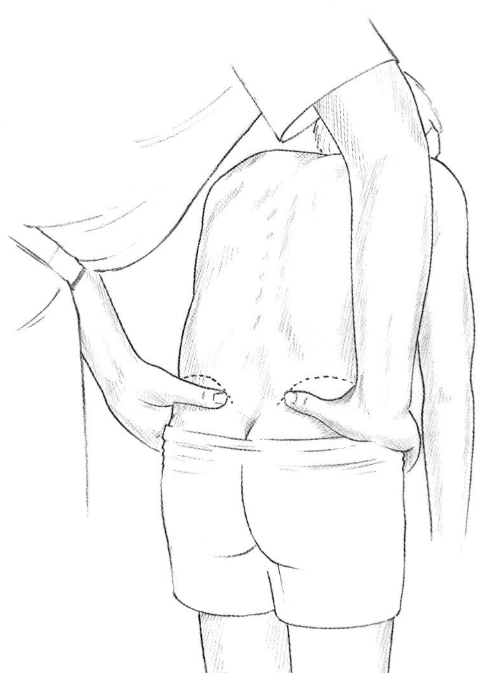

Figure 6.19A Standing flexion test for iliosacral restriction. The dysfunctional side is that on which the thumb moves during flexion.

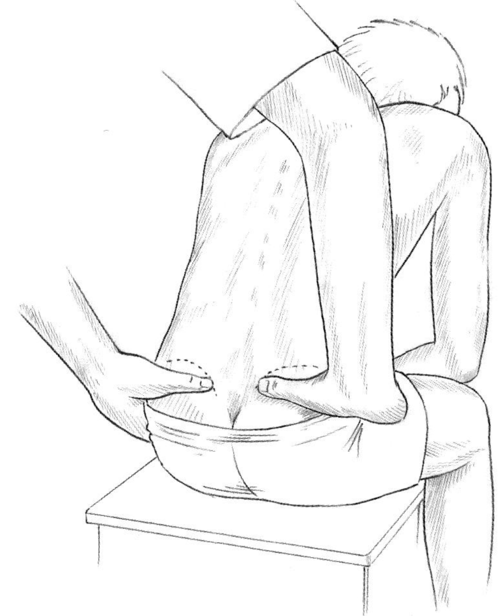

Figure 6.19B Seated flexion test for sacroiliac restriction. The dysfunctional side is that on which the thumb moves during flexion.

The practitioner observes, especially near the end of the excursion of the bend, whether one or other thumb seems to start to travel with the PSIS.

Interpretation. If one thumb moves superiorly during flexion it indicates that the ilium is fixed to the sacrum on that side (or that the contralateral hamstrings are short, or that the ipsilateral quadratus lumborum is short: therefore these muscles should have been assessed prior to the standing flexion test).

Test (d): standing spinal rotation Before performing the seated flexion test, the practitioner moves to the front of the fully flexed patient and looks down the spine for evidence of greater 'fullness' on one side or the other of the lumbar spine, indicating muscular mounding, possibly in association with spinal rotoscoliosis (or due to excessive tension in quadratus lumborum or hypertrophy of the erector spinae).

Test (e): seated flexion (sacroiliac) The seated flexion test involves exactly the same hand placement as in the standing flexion test (test (c) above) and observation of the thumb movement, if any, during full flexion, while the patient is seated on the table, legs over the side, knees in flexion (see Fig. 6.19B).

Interpretation. In this instance, since the ischial tuberosities are being 'sat upon', the ilia cannot easily move, and if one thumb travels forward during flexion it means that the sacrum is stuck to the ilium on that side, dragging the ilium with it in flexion.

Test (f): seated spinal rotation With the seated patient still fully flexed, move to the front and look down the spine for fullness in the paravertebral muscles, in the lumbar area.

- If greater fullness exists in a paraspinal area of the lumbar spine with the patient standing as opposed to seated, then this is evidence of a compensatory process, involving the postural muscles of the lower limbs and pelvic area, as a prime cause.
- If, however, fullness in the lumbar paraspinal region is the same when seated, or greater when seated, this indicates some primary spinal dysfunction and not a compensation for postural muscle imbalances.

Test (g): confirmation of iliosacral restriction test The patient stands, practitioner is behind, kneeling, with thumbs placed so that on the side being assessed the contact is on the PSIS, while the other hand palpates the median sacral crest directly parallel to the PSIS.

The patient is asked to slowly and fully flex the ipsilateral hip to waist level.

A normal response is for the thumb on the PSIS to move caudally in relation to the thumb on the sacral base as the hip and knee are flexed. If on the flexing of the hip there is a movement of the PSIS and the median sacral crest 'as a unit', together with a compensating adaptation in the lumbar spine, this indicates *iliosacral* restriction on the side being palpated.

If this combined (PSIS and sacral thumb contact) movement occurred when the contralateral hip was being flexed, it would indicate a *sacroiliac* restriction on the side being palpated.

What type of iliosacral dysfunction exists?

Once an iliosacral restriction has been identified, it is necessary to define precisely what type of restriction it is. In this text only anterior rotation, posterior rotation, inflare and outflare will be considered. This part of the evaluation process depends upon observation of landmarks.

Test (h) The patient lies supine and straight while the practitioner locates the inferior slopes of the two ASISs with thumbs, and views these contacts from directly above the pelvis with the dominant eye over the centre line (bird's eye view – see Fig. 6.20A):

- Which thumb is nearer the head and which nearer the feet?
- Is one side superior or is the other inferior?

In other words, has one ilium rotated posteriorly or the other anteriorly? This is determined by referring back to the standing flexion test (test (c) above).

The side of dysfunction – as determined by the standing flexion test 'travelling thumb' (test (c) above) and/or the standing hip flexion test (test (g) above) – defines which observed anterior landmark is taken into consideration (Fig. 6.20Bi–iv).

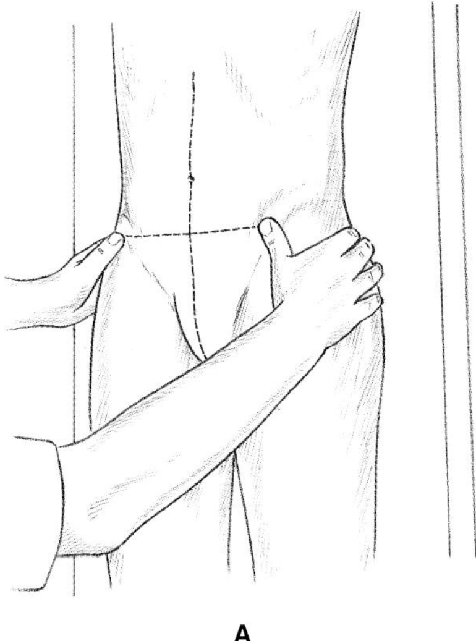

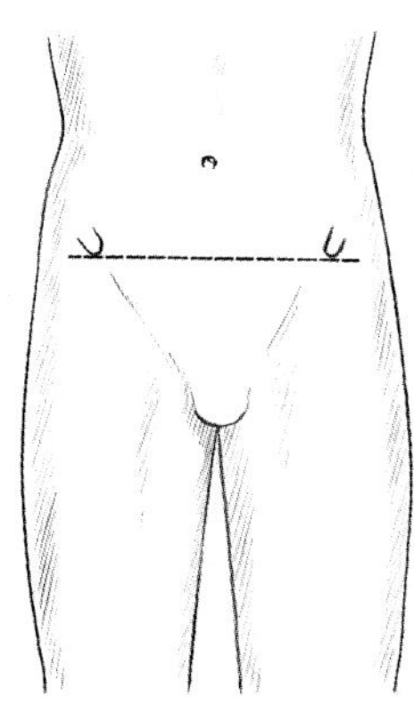

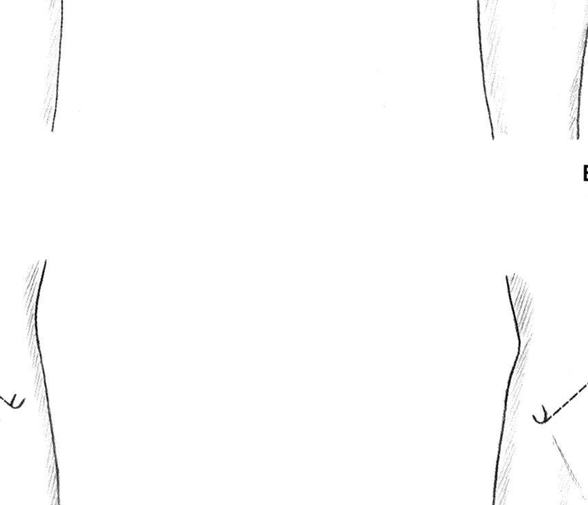

Figure 6.20 (**A**) Practitioner adopts a position providing a bird's-eye view of ASIS prominences on which rest the thumbs. (**Bi**) The ASISs are level and there is no rotational dysfunction involving the iliosacral joints. (**Bii**) The right ASIS is higher than the left ASIS. If a thumb 'travelled' on the right side during the standing flexion test this would represent a posterior right iliosacral rotation dysfunction. If a thumb 'travelled' on the left side during the test this would represent an anterior left iliosacral rotation dysfunction. (**Biii**) The ASISs are equidistant from the umbilicus and the midline, and there is no iliosacral flare dysfunction. (**Biv**) The ASIS on the right is closer to the umbilicus/midline, which indicates that either there is a right side iliosacral inflare (if the right thumb moved during the standing flexion test), or there is a left side iliosacral outflare (if the left thumb moved during the standing flexion test).

The practitioner's eyes should be directly over the pelvis with the thumbs resting on the ASISs.

Rotations:

1. The side of the positive hip flexion test is the dysfunctional side, and if that is the side which appears inferior (compared to its pair) it is assumed that the ilium on the inferior side has rotated anteriorly on the sacrum on that side.
2. The side of the positive hip flexion test is the dysfunctional side, and if the ASIS appears superior to its pair on that side, then the ilium has rotated posteriorly on the sacrum on that side.

Flares While in the same position, to observe the ASIS positions, note is made as to the relative positions of these landmarks in relation to the midline of the patient's abdomen, using either the linea alba or the umbilicus as a guide:

- Is one thumb closer to the umbilicus than the other? It is necessary at this stage to once again refer to which side is dysfunctional.
- Is the ASIS on the side which is further from the umbilicus outflared or is the ASIS which is closer to the umbilicus indicative of that side being inflared?

The ASIS associated with the side on which the thumb travelled is the dysfunctional side, and the decision as to whether it is an inflare (closer to umbilicus) or outflare (further from umbilicus) is therefore obvious.

Flare dysfunctions are usually treated prior to rotation dysfunctions.

MET treatment of iliac inflare (Fig. 6.21A, B)

The patient is supine and the practitioner stands on the same side as the problem, with the cephalad hand stabilising the non-affected side ASIS and the caudad hand holding the ankle of the affected side (Fig. 6.21A).

The affected side hip is flexed and abducted while full external rotation is introduced to the hip. The practitioner's forearm aligns with the lower leg, elbow stabilising the medial aspect of the knee. The patient is asked to lightly adduct the hip against the resistance offered by the restraining arm for 10 seconds while holding the breath.

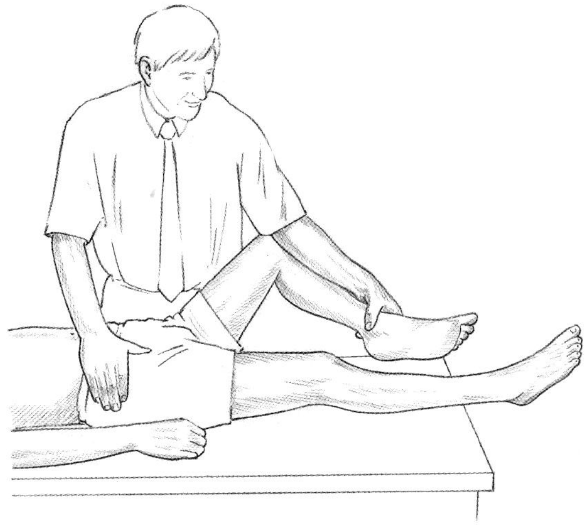

Figure 6.21A An MET treatment position for left side iliosacral inflare dysfunction. Note the stabilising hand on the right ASIS.

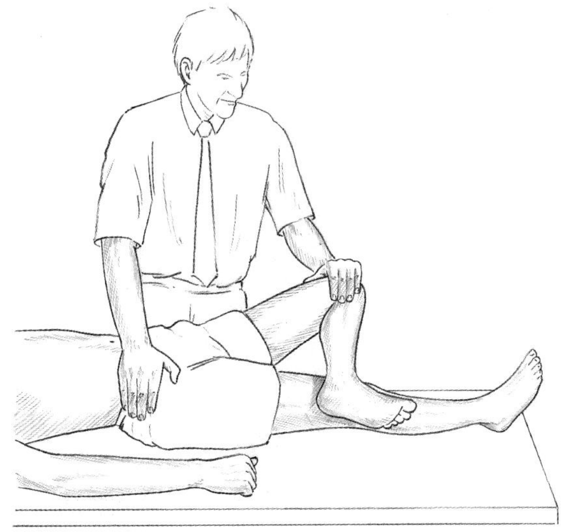

Figure 6.21B An alternative MET treatment position for left side iliosacral inflare dysfunction. Note the stabilising hand on the right ASIS.

On complete relaxation and on an exhalation, with the pelvis held stable by the cephalad hand, the flexed leg is taken into more abduction and external rotation, if new 'slack' is now available.

This process is repeated once or twice, at which time the leg is slowly straightened while abduction and external rotation of the hip are maintained. The leg is then returned to the table.

NOTE: Care should be taken not to use the powerful leverage available from the flexed and abducted leg; its own weight and gravity provide adequate leverage and the 'release' of tone achieved via isometric contractions will do the rest. It is very easy to turn an inflare into an outflare by overenthusiastic use of force. The degree of flare should be re-evaluated and any rotation then treated (see below).

MET treatment of iliac outflare (Fig. 6.22)

The patient is supine and the practitioner is on the same side as the dysfunctional ilium, supinated cephalad hand under the patient's buttocks with finger tips hooked into the sacral sulcus on the same side. The caudad hand holds the patient's foot on the treated side, with the forearm resting along the medial calf/shin area as the hand grasps the foot.

The hip on the treated side is fully flexed and adducted and internally rotated, at which time the patient is asked to abduct the hip against resistance, using up to 50% of strength, for 10 seconds while holding the breath.

Following this and complete relaxation, slack is taken out and the exercise repeated once or twice more.

As the leg is taken into greater adduction and internal rotation, to take advantage of the release of tone following the isometric contraction the fingers in the sacral sulcus exert a traction towards the practitioner, effectively guiding the ilium into a more inflared position.

After the final contraction, adduction and internal rotation are maintained as the leg is slowly returned to the table.

The evaluation for flare dysfunction is then repeated and if relative normality has been restored, any rotational dysfunction is then treated, as per the methods described below.

MET treatment of anterior iliac rotation (Fig. 6.23)

The patient is prone. The practitioner stands at the side to be treated, at waist level.

The affected leg and hip are flexed and brought over the edge of the table. The foot/ankle area is grasped between the practitioner's legs. The table-side hand stabilises the sacral area while the other hand supports the flexed knee and guides it into greater flexion, inducing posterior iliac rotation, until the restriction barrier is sensed:

- By the palpating 'sacral contact' hand
- By virtue of a sense of greater effort in guiding the flexed leg

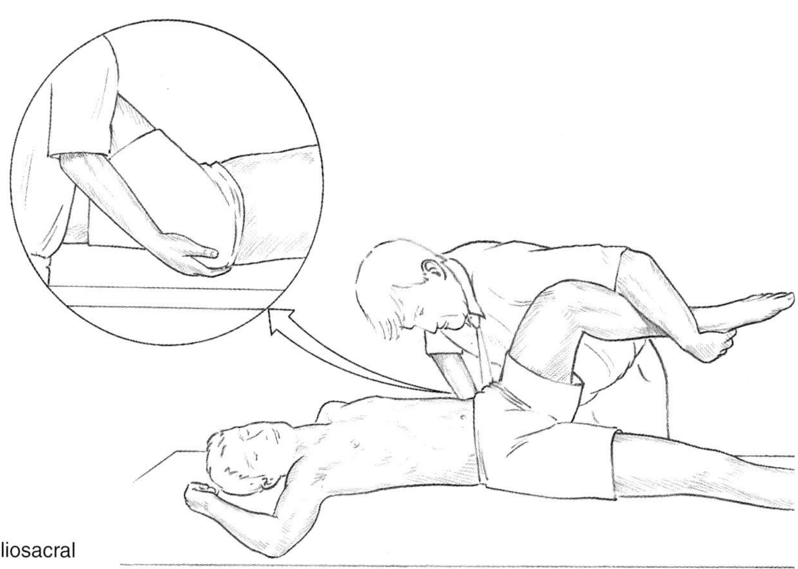

Figure 6.22 MET treatment of iliosacral outflare on the left.

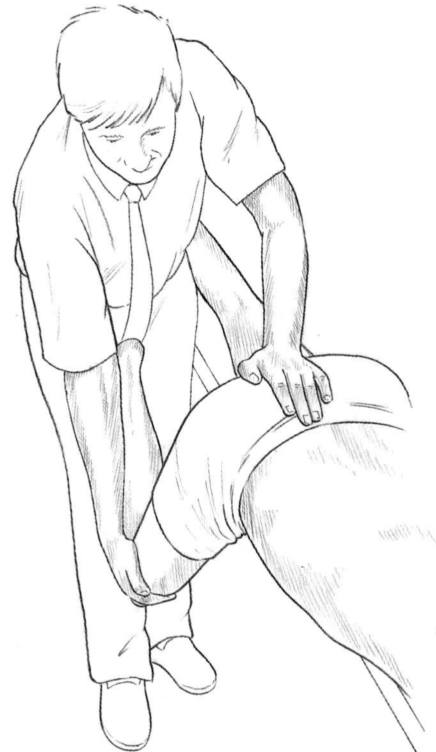

Figure 6.23 MET treatment of an anterior iliosacral restriction.

- By observation of pelvic movement as the barrier of resistance is passed.

The patient is asked to inhale, to hold the breath and to attempt to straighten the leg against unyielding resistance, for 10 seconds using no more than 20% of available strength.

On releasing the breath and the effort, and on complete relaxation and on an exhalation, the leg/innominate is guided to its new barrier.

Subsequent contractions can involve different directions of effort ('try to push your knee sideways', or 'try to bend your knee towards your shoulder', etc.) in order to bring into operation a variety of muscular factors to encourage release of the joint.[1]

[1] The same mechanics precisely can be incorporated into a side-lying position. The only disadvantage of this is the relative instability of the pelvic region compared to that achieved in the prone position described above.

The standing flexion test (see p. 186) should be performed again to establish whether the joint is now free.

MET for treatment of posterior iliac rotation (Fig. 6.24)

The patient is prone and the practitioner stands on the side opposite the dysfunctional iliosacral joint. The table-side hand supports the anterior aspect of the patient's knee while the other rests on the PSIS of the affected side to evaluate bind.

The affected leg is hyperextended until free movement ceases, as evidenced by the following observations:

- Bind is noted under the palpating hand
- Sacral and pelvic motion are observed as the barrier is passed
- A sense of effort is increased in the arm extending the leg.

With the practitioner holding the joint at its restriction barrier, the patient is asked, with no more than 20% of strength, to flex the hip against resistance for 10 seconds while holding the breath.

After cessation of the effort, releasing the breath and completely relaxing, on an exhalation, the leg is extended further to its new barrier. No force is used at all; the movement after the

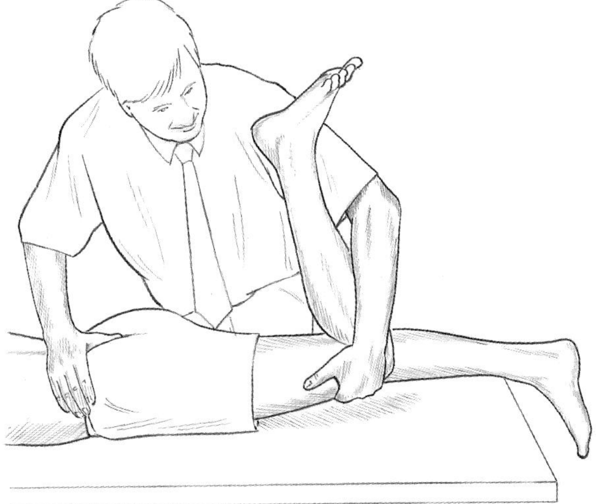

Figure 6.24 MET treatment of a posterior iliosacral restriction.

contraction simply takes advantage of whatever slack is now available.

Variations in the direction of the contraction (perhaps involving abduction or adduction or even attempted extension) are sometimes useful if no appreciable gain is achieved using hip and knee flexion.

The standing flexion test (p. 186) is performed again to establish whether iliosacral movement is now free, once a sense of 'release' has been noted following one of the contractions.

MET treatment for temporomandibular joint dysfunction

Dysfunction of the TMJ is a vast subject, and the implications of such problems have been related to a variety of other areas of dysfunction, ranging from cranial lesions to spinal and general somatic alterations and endocrine imbalance (Gelb 1977). The reader is referred to Janda's observations on postural influences on TMJ problems (Ch. 2).

Diagnosis of the particular pattern of dysfunction is, of course, essential before safe therapeutic intervention is possible. There are many possible causes of TMJ dysfunction, and a cooperative relationship with a skilled dentist is an advantage in such problems, since many aspects relate to the presence of faults in the bite of the patient.

A knowledge of cranial mechanics is useful, and a history of trauma should be sought in those patients presenting with TMJ involvement. One common source of injury is the equipment used in applying spinal traction, in which a head halter with a chinstrap is used. This can cause the mandible to be forced into the fossae, impacting the temporal bones into internal rotation. A strap causing pressure on the occipital region could jam the occipitomastoid and lambdoid sutures upwards and forwards, also resulting in internal rotation of the temporals. This can cause major dysfunction of cranial articulation and function which would be further exaggerated were there imbalances present in these structures prior to the trauma.

Inept manipulative measures can also traumatise the area, especially thrusting forces exerted onto the occiput while the head and neck are in extreme rotation. Any situation in which the patient is required to maintain the mouth opened for lengthy periods, such as during dental work, or when a laryngoscope is being used, may induce strain, especially if the neck is extended at the time.

All, or any, such patterns of injury should be sought when TMJ pain, or limitation of mouth opening is observed. Apart from correction of cranial dysfunction via skilled cranial osteopathic work, the muscular component invites attention, using MET methods and other appropriate measures. Gelb suggests a form of MET which he terms 'stretch against resistance' exercises.

MET TMJ method 1 (Fig. 6.25A) Reciprocal inhibition is the objective when the patient is asked to open the mouth against resistance applied by the practitioner's, or the patient's own, hand (patient places elbow on table, chin in hand, and attempts to open mouth against resistance for 10 seconds or so). The jaw would have been opened to its comfortable limit before attempting this, and after the attempt it would be taken to its new barrier before repeating. This MET method would have a relaxing effect on the muscles which are shortened or tight.

MET TMJ method 2 (Fig. 6.25B) To relax the short tight muscles using postisometric relax-

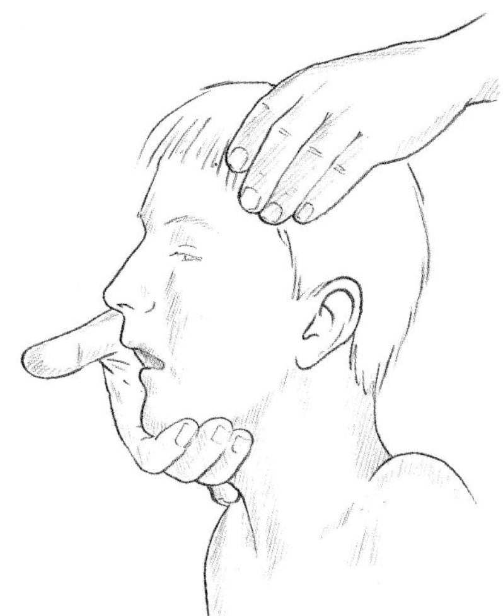

Figure 6.25A MET treatment of TMJ restriction, involving limited ability to open the mouth. The isometric contraction phase of treatment is illustrated as the patient attempts to open against resistance.

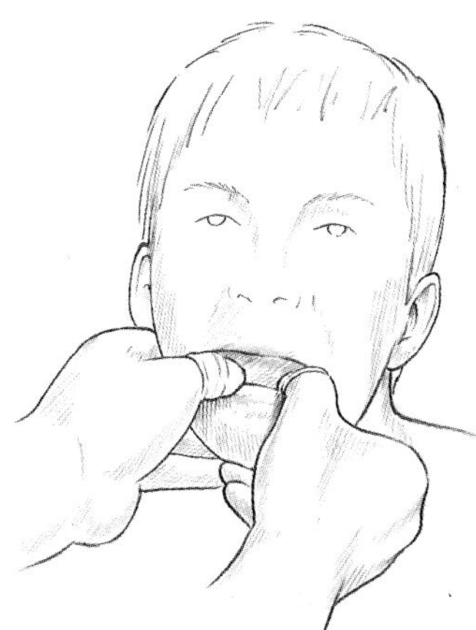

Figure 6.25B MET treatment of TMJ restriction, involving an isometric contraction in which the patient attempts to close the mouth against resistance.
Following both these procedures (A and B), the patient would be encouraged to gently stretch the muscles by opening the mouth widely. This can be assisted by the practitioner.

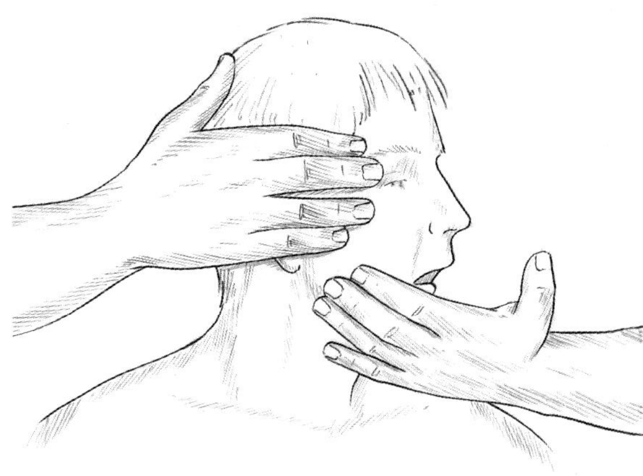

Figure 6.25C MET treatment of lateral restrictions of the TMJ. Following the isometric contraction as described, the lateral excursion is increased.

ation, counter-pressure would be required in order to prevent the open jaw from closing (using minimal force). This would require the thumbs (suitably protected) to be placed along the superior surface of the lower back teeth while an isometric contraction was performed by the patient. In this exercise the practitioner is directing force through the barrier (practitioner-direct method) rather than the patient (patient-direct) as in the first method (above).

MET TMJ method 3 (Fig. 6.25C) Lewit, maintaining that laterolateral movements are important, suggests the following method of treating TMJ problems using postisometric relaxation. The patient sits with the head turned to one side (say the left in this example). The practitioner stands behind him and stabilises the patient's head against his chest.

The patient opens his mouth, allowing the chin to drop, and the practitioner cradles the mandible with his left hand, so that the fingers are curled under the jaw, away from him. The practitioner draws the jaw gently towards his chest, and when the slack has been taken up, the patient offers a degree of resistance to its being taken further, laterally.

After a few seconds of gentle isometric contraction, the practitioner and patient relax simultaneously, and the jaw will usually have an increased lateral excursion.

This is repeated three times. This should be performed so that the lateral pull is away from the side to which the jaw deviates, on opening.

TMJ self-treatment exercise 1 Gelb suggests a retrusive exercise be used in conjunction with the above, both methods being useful in eliminating 'clicks' on opening the mouth. The patient curls the tongue upwards, placing the tip as far back on the roof of the mouth as possible. While this is maintained in position, the patient is asked to slowly open and close the mouth (gently), to reactivate the suprahyoid, posterior temporalis and posterior digastric muscles (the retrusive group).

TMJ self-treatment exercise 2 The patient places an elbow on a table, jaw resting on the clenched fist. This offers some resistance to the slow opening of the mouth. This is done five times with hand pressure, and then five times without, ensuring that the lower jaw does not come forward. The lower teeth should always remain behind the upper teeth on closing. A total of 25 such movements are performed, morning and evening.

JOINTS, END-FEEL AND MET

In the text thus far there have been descriptions of MET applications to spinal, pelvic, cervical, shoulder, acromioclavicular and sternoclavicular joints and TMJ, as well as to a multitude of muscles relating to most of the joints in the body.

In order to apply the principles embodied in MET methodology to joint dysfunction not specifically covered in the text, all that is required is an appreciation of restriction barriers, which in essence means having an awareness of what represents the norm in so far as range of movement and end-feel is concerned. What are the physiological and anatomical barriers which a particular joint should enjoy?

With that information and a keen sense of end-feel (what the end of a movement should feel like compared with what is actually presented) should come an appreciation of what is needed in order to position a joint for receipt of MET input, irrespective of which joint is involved.

If end-feel is sharp or sudden, it probably represents protective spasm of joint pathology, such as arthritis.

The benefits of MET to such joints will be limited to what the pathology will allow; however, even in arthritic settings, a release of soft tissues commonly produces benefits. Kaltenborn (1985) summarises normal end-feel variations as follows:

- Normal soft end-feel results from soft tissue approximation (as in flexing the knee) or soft tissue stretching (as in ankle dorsiflexion).
- Normal firm end-feel is the result of capsular or ligamentous stretching (internal rotation of the femur for example).
- Normal hard end-feel occurs when bone meets bone as in elbow extension.

He defines abnormal end-feel variations as follows:

- A firm, elastic feel is noted when scar tissue restricts movement or when shortened connective tissue is present.
- An elastic, less soft end-feel occurs when increased muscle tonus prevents free movement.
- An empty end-feel is noted when the patient stops the movement, or requests that it be stopped, before a true end-feel is reached, usually as a result of extreme pain such as might occur in active inflammation, or a fracture, or because of psychogenic factors.
- As noted above, a sudden, hard end-feel is commonly due to interosseous changes such as arthritis.

By engaging the barrier (*always* the barrier, never short of the barrier for joint conditions) and using appropriate degrees of isometric effort, the barriers can be pushed back by means of our two physiological tools, postisometric relaxation and reciprocal inhibition, as the soft tissues are encouraged to release. Remember also Ruddy's pulsed MET variation which is useful in joint problems (see Ch. 3).

Apart from those joints and areas already discussed in this chapter, no additional specific joint guidelines are described because it is assumed that the reader can employ the principles as explained, and the examples as given, to adapt and extrapolate the use of MET methods to any/most other joint conditions.

REFERENCES

Chaitow L 1996 Muscle energy techniques, 1st edn. Churchill Livingstone, Edinburgh

Evjenth O, Hamberg J 1984 Muscle stretching in manual therapy. Alfta Rehab, Alfta, Sweden

Fryette H 1954 Principals of osteopathic technique. American Academy of Osteopathy, Newark, Ohio

Gelb H 1977 Clinical management of head, neck and TMJ pain and dysfunction. W B Saunders, Philadelphia

Gibbons P, Tehan P 1998 Muscle energy concepts and coupled motion of the spine. Manual Therapy 3(2): 95–101

Goodridge J 1981 Muscle energy technique. Journal of the American Osteopathic Association 81: 249

Goodridge J, Kuchera W 1997 Muscle energy techniques for specific areas. In: Ward R (ed) Foundations of osteopathic medicine. Williams and Wilkins, Baltimore

Greenman P 1996 Principles of manual medicine, 2nd edn. Williams and Wilkins, Baltimore

Grieve G 1984 Mobilisation of the spine. Churchill Livingstone, Edinburgh

Harakal J 1975 An osteopathically integrated approach to whiplash complex. Journal of the American Osteopathic Association 74: 941–956

Hartman L 1985 Handbook of osteopathic technique. Hutchinson, London

Janda V 1988 In: Grant R (ed) Physical therapy of the cervical and thoracic spine. Churchill Livingstone, New York
Jones L 1981 Strain and counterstrain. Academy of Applied Osteopathy, Colorado Springs
Kaltenborn F 1985 Mobilisation of extremity joints. Olaf Norlis Boekhandel, Norway
Lewit K 1985 The muscular and articular factor in movement restriction. Manual Medicine 1: 83–85
McAtee R Charland J 1999 Faciltated stretching, 2nd edn. Human Kinetics, Champaign, Ilinois
Mitchell F 1995 The muscle energy manual. MET Press, East Lansing, Michigan
Patriquin D 1992 Evolution of osteopathic manipulative technique: the Spencer technique. Journal of the American Osteopathic Association 92: 1134–1146
Spencer H 1976 Shoulder technique. Journal of the American Osteopathic Association 15: 2118–2220
Steiner C 1994 Osteopathic manipulative treatment – what does it really do? Journal of the American Osteopathic Association 94(1): 85–87
Stiles E 1984a Manipulation – a tool for your practice? Patient Care 18: 16–42
Stiles E 1984b Manipulation – a tool for your practice. Patient Care 45: 699–704
Ward R (ed) 1997 Foundations of osteopathic medicine. Williams and Wilkins, Baltimore
Yates S 1991 Muscle energy techniques. In: DiGiovanna E (ed) Principles of osteopathic manipulative techniques. Lippincott, Philadelphia

CHAPTER CONTENTS

7

Integrated neuromuscular inhibition technique (INIT)

It is clear from the work of Travell and Simons in particular that myofascial trigger points are a primary cause of pain, dysfunction and distress of the sympathetic nervous system (Travell & Simons 1986). Melzack & Wall (1988), in their pain research, have shown that there are few chronic pain problems where myofascial trigger point activity is not a key feature maintaining or causing chronic pain.

As noted in Chapter 2, there are numerous causes for the production and maintenance of myofascial triggers, including postural imbalances (Barlow 1959, Goldthwaite 1949), congenital factors – warping of fascia via cranial distortions (Upledger 1983), short leg problems, small hemipelvis, etc. – occupational or leisure overuse patterns (Rolf 1977), emotional states reflecting into the soft tissues (Latey 1986), referred/reflex involvement of the viscera producing facilitated segments paraspinally (Beal 1983, Korr 1976), as well as trauma.

LOCAL FACILITATION

According to Korr, a trigger point is a localised area of somatic dysfunction which behaves in a facilitated manner, i.e. it will amplify and be affected by any form of stress imposed on the individual whether this is physical, chemical or emotional (Korr 1976).

A trigger point is palpable as an indurated, localised, painful entity with a reference (target) area to which pain or other symptoms are referred (Chaitow 1991a).

Muscles housing trigger points can frequently be identified as being unable to achieve their normal resting length using standard muscle evaluation procedures (Janda 1983), as described in Chapter 4. The trigger point itself always lies in hypertonic tissue, and not uncommonly in fibrotic tissue, which has evolved as the result of exposure of the tissues to diverse forms of stress.

TREATMENT METHODS

A wide variety of treatment methods have been advocated in treating trigger points, including inhibitory (ischaemic compression) pressure methods (Nimmo 1966, Lief 1982/1989), acupuncture and/or ultrasound (Kleyhans and Aarons 1974), chilling and stretching of the muscle in which the trigger lies (Travell & Simons 1986), procaine or Xylocaine injections (Slocumb 1984), active or passive stretching (Lewit 1992), and even surgical excision (Dittrich 1954).

Clinical experience has shown that while all or any of these methods can successfully inhibit trigger point activity short-term, in order to completely eliminate the noxious activity of the structure, more is often needed.

Travell and Simons have shown that whatever initial treatment is offered to inhibit the neurological overactivity of the trigger point, the muscle in which it lies has to be made capable of reaching its normal resting length following such treatment or else the trigger point will rapidly reactivate.

In treating trigger points the method of chilling the offending muscle (housing the trigger), while holding it at stretch in order to achieve this end, was advocated by Travell and Simons, while Lewit recommends muscle energy techniques in which a physiologically induced postisometric relaxation (or reciprocal inhibition) response is created, prior to passive stretching. Both methods are commonly successful, although a sufficient degree of failure occurs (trigger rapidly reactivates or fails to completely 'switch off') to require investigation of more successful approaches.

One reason for failure may relate to the possibility of the tissues which are being stretched not being the precise ones housing the trigger point.

Hypothesis

The author hypothesises that partial contraction (using no more than 20–30% of patient strength, as is the norm in MET procedures, see Ch. 3) may sometimes fail to achieve activation of the fibres housing the trigger point being treated, since the light contractions used in MET of this sort fail to recruit more than a percentage of the muscle's potential.

Subsequent stretching of the muscle may therefore only marginally involve the critical tissues surrounding and enveloping the myofascial trigger point.

Failure to actively stretch the muscle fibres in which the trigger is housed may account for the not infrequent recurrence of trigger point activity in the same site following treatment. Repetition of the same stress factors which produced it in the first place could undoubtedly also be a factor in such recurrence – which emphasises the need for re-education in rehabilitation.

A method which achieved precise targeting of these tissues (in terms of tonus release and subsequent stretching) would clearly be advantageous.

Selye's concepts

Selye has described the progression of changes in tissue which is being locally stressed (see Ch. 2 for more detail). There is an initial alarm (acute inflammatory) stage, followed by a stage of adaptation or resistance when stress factors are continuous or repetitive, at which time muscular tissue becomes progressively fibrotic, and as we have seen in earlier chapters (Ch. 2 in particular), if this change is taking place in muscle which has a predominantly postural rather than a phasic function, the entire muscle structure will shorten (Janda 1985, Selye 1984).

Such hypertonic and perhaps fibrotic tissue, lying in altered (shortened) muscle, may not be easily able to 'release' itself in order to allow the muscle to achieve its normal resting length (as we have seen, this is a prerequisite of normalisation of trigger point activity). Along with various forms of stretch (passive, active, MET, PNF, etc.), it has been noted above that inhibitory pressure is commonly employed in treatment of trigger points.

Such pressure technique methods (analogous to acupressure or shiatsu methodology) are often successful in achieving at least short-term reduction in trigger point activity and are variously dubbed 'neuromuscular techniques' (Chaitow 1991b).

Ischaemic compression validation

Researchers at the Department of Physical Medicine and Rehabilitation, University of California, Irvine, evaluated the immediate benefits of treating an active trigger point in the upper trapezius muscle by comparing four commonly used approaches as well as a placebo treatment (Hong et al 1993). The methods used included:

1. Ice spray and stretch (Travell & Simons approach)
2. Superficial heat applied by a hydrocolator pack (20–30 minutes)
3. Deep heat applied by ultrasound (1.2–1.5 watt/cm^2 for 5 minutes)
4. Dummy ultrasound (0.0 watt/cm^2)
5. Deep inhibitory pressure soft tissue massage (10–15 minutes of modified connective tissue massage and shiatsu/ischaemic compression).[1]

For the study 24 patients were selected who had active triggers in the upper trapezius which had been present for not less than 3 months and who had had no previous treatment for these for at least 1 month prior to the study (as well as no cervical radiculopathy or myelopathy, disc or degenerative disease). The following measurements were carried out:

- The pain threshold of the trigger point area was measured using a pressure algometer three times pre-treatment and within 2 minutes of treatment.
- The average was recorded on each occasion.
- A control group were similarly measured twice (30 minutes apart); this group received no treatment until after the second measurement.

The results showed that:

- All methods (but not the placebo ultrasound) produced a significant increase in pain threshold following treatment, with the greatest change being demonstrated by those receiving deep pressure treatment.
- The spray and stretch method was the next most efficient in achieving reduction in pain threshold.

Why is deep pressure technique more effective?

The researchers suggest that: 'Perhaps deep pressure massage, if done appropriately, can offer better stretching of the taut bands of muscle fibers than manual stretching because it applies stronger pressure to a relatively small area compared to the gross stretching of the whole muscle. Deep pressure may also offer ischemic compression which [has been shown to be] effective for myofascial pain therapy' (Simons 1989).

The use of algometrics in treating trigger points

An area of concern in trigger point evaluation lies in the non-standard degree of pressure being applied to tissues when they are being tested manually. In order to establish the 'type' and behaviour of trigger points, various researchers have evaluated the usefulness of an algometer in the process.

Belgian researchers Jonkheere & Pattyn (1998) explain that 'The purpose of algometrics is to define whether a trigger point is active, latent, falsely positive or absent'. In order to achieve this

---

[1] Application of inhibitory pressure may involve elbow, thumb, finger or mechanical pressure (a wooden rubber-tipped T-bar is commonly employed in the USA), or cross-fibre friction. Such methods are described in detail in a further text in this series (L Chaitow, *Modern Neuromuscular Techniques*, 1996).

objective, the 18 sites used in assessing for fibromyalgia are tested. Based on the results of this a 'myofascial pain index' (MPI) is calculated.

The purpose is to create an objective base (the MPI), which emerges initially from the patient's subjective pain reports, when pressure is applied to the test points. The calculation of the MPI determines the degree of pressure required to evoke pain in a trigger point, and helps to sift latent and 'false positive' from active points, with the latter receiving priority attention.

The Belgian researchers acknowledge that they have based their approach on earlier work by Hong et al (1994), who investigated pain pressure thresholds of trigger points and their surrounding soft tissues. Jonkheere and Pattyn define the various states of trigger points as follows:

- An active trigger point is sensitive to palpation and produces an identifiable pain which corresponds, completely or partially, with the known pattern of a trigger point located at that particular site.
- A latent trigger point is one which only produces localised pain on palpation.
- A 'false positive' trigger point is one which is sensitive to palpation, and which refers pain
  - — but which does not correspond with known patterns, or
  - — which produces a referral pattern which does correspond, completely or partially, with the known pattern of a trigger point located at that particular site, but only when the pressure required to evoke this response is greater than the myofascial pain index (MPI).

The 18 points tested are located in nine bilateral sites as defined by the American College of Rheumatology in 1990, as part of the diagnostic protocol for fibromyalgia syndrome (FMS) (American College of Rheumatology 1990). They are:

1. At the suboccipital muscle insertions (close to where rectus capitis posterior minor inserts)
2. At the anterolateral aspect of the intertransverse spaces between C5 and C7
3. At the midpoint of the upper border of upper trapezius muscle
4. At the origin of supraspinatus muscle above the scapula spine
5. At the second costochondral junctions, on the upper surface, just lateral to the junctions
6. 2 centimeters distal to the lateral epicondyles of the elbows
7. In the upper outer quadrant of the buttocks in the anterior fold of gluteus medius
8. Posterior to the prominence of the greater trochanter (piriformis attachment)
9. On the medial aspect of the knees, on the fatty pad, proximal to the joint line.

Using an algometer (the Belgian researchers used an Algoprobe®), pressure is applied to each of the points, sufficient to produce pain, with the measurement being taken when this is reported. The 18 values are recorded and then averaged, leaving a number which is the MPI. Once established, this amount of pressure is used to judge the nature (active, 'false positive', etc.) of all other potential trigger point sites.

A label of 'active' is assigned to any point where the referral pattern matches known referral distribution from that site, and which requires less than the MPI degree of pressure to produce this response. Those triggers which meet the definition of 'active trigger point' are therefore noted and treated first. If a greater degree of pressure than the MPI is required to evoke a pain response, the trigger point is not regarded as 'active' and its treatment is deferred.

Jonkheere & Pattyn (1998), utilising the basic research of Simons & Travell (1998), have also identified 'chains' of trigger points which seem to be functionally or structurally related to the patient's reported pain symptoms. Before treatment these are methodically tested using an algometer in the manner described above.

TARGETING WITH INTEGRATED NEUROMUSCULAR INHIBITION TECHNIQUE (INIT)

By combining the methods of direct inhibition (pressure mildly applied, continuously or in a make-and-break pattern), along with the concept of strain/counterstrain (see below) and MET, a specific targeting of dysfunctional soft tissues can be achieved (Chaitow 1994).

Strain/counterstrain (SCS) briefly explained

Jones (1981) has shown that particular painful 'points' relating to joint or muscular strain, chronic or acute, can be used as 'monitors' – pressure being applied to them as the body or body part is carefully positioned in such a way as to remove or reduce the pain felt in the palpated point.[2]

When the position of ease is attained (using what is known in SCS terminology as 'fine tuning') in which pain vanishes from the palpated monitoring tender point, the stressed tissues are felt to be at their most relaxed – and clinical experience indicates that this is so, since they palpate as 'easy' rather than having a sense of being 'bound' or tense (see Ch. 3, p. 66, for more detailed discussion of this phenomenon).

SCS is thought to achieve its benefits by means of an automatic resetting of muscle spindles which help to dictate the length and tone in the tissues. This resetting apparently occurs only when the muscle housing the spindle is at ease and usually results in a reduction in excessive tone and release of spasm. When positioning the body (part) in strain/counterstrain methodology, a sense of 'ease' is noted as the tissues reach the position in which pain vanishes from the palpated point.

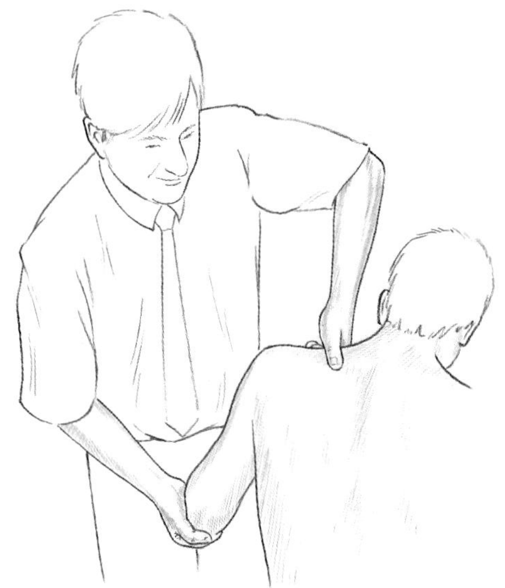

Figure 7.1A First stage of INIT in which a tender/pain/trigger point in supraspinatus is located and ischaemically compressed, either intermittently or persistently.

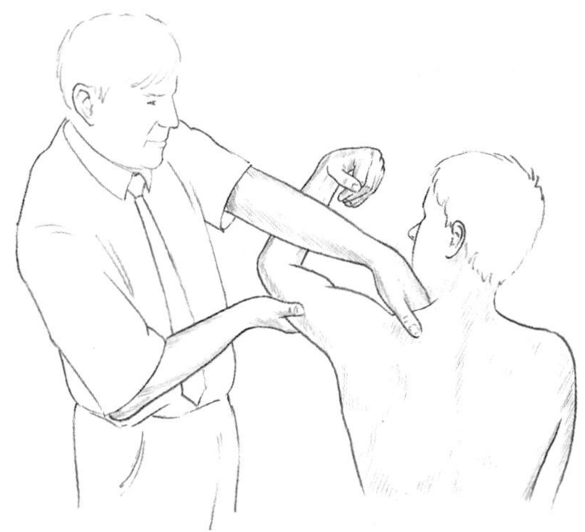

Figure 7.1B The pain is removed from the tender/pain/trigger point by finding a position of ease which is held for at least 20 seconds, following which an isometric contraction is achieved involving the tissues which house the tender/pain/trigger point.

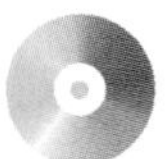

INIT method 1 (Fig. 7.1A, B, C)

It is reasonable to assume, and palpation confirms, that when a trigger point is being palpated by direct finger or thumb pressure, and when the very tissues in which the trigger point lies are positioned in such a way as to take away the pain (entirely or at least to a great extent), that the most (dis)stressed fibres in which the trigger point is housed are in a position of relative ease.

The trigger point would then be receiving direct inhibitory pressure (mild or perhaps intermittent) and (using SCS methods) would have

[2] These tender points, as described by Jones, are found in tissues which were short rather than being stretched at the time of injury (acute or chronic) and are usually areas in which the patient was unaware of pain previous to their being palpated. They seem to equate in most particulars with 'Ah shi' points in traditional Chinese medicine.

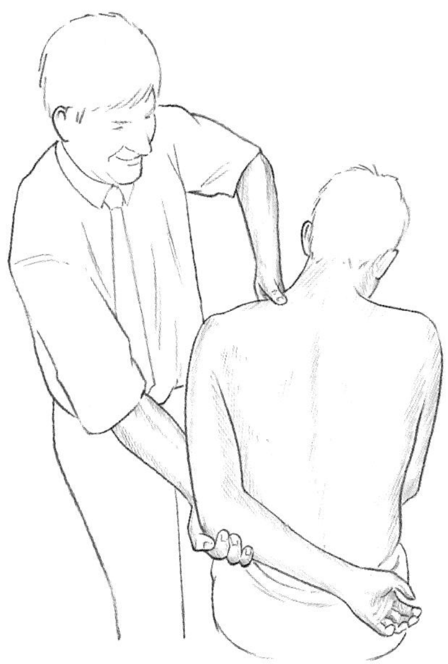

Figure 7.1C Following the holding of the isometric contraction for an appropriate period, the muscle housing the point of local soft tissue dysfunction is stretched. This completes the INIT sequence.

been positioned so that the tissues housing it are relaxed (relatively or completely).

Following a period of 20–30 seconds in this 'position of ease' – accompanied by inhibitory pressure – the patient would be asked to introduce an isometric contraction into the tissues housing the trigger (and currently 'at ease') and to hold this for 7–10 seconds, so involving the very fibres which had been repositioned to obtain the strain/counterstrain release.

Following the isometric contraction there would be a reduction in tone in these tissues (postisometric relaxation). These could then be gently stretched as in any muscle energy procedure (as described previously), with the strong likelihood that specifically involved fibres would be stretched (see Fig. 7.1C).

INIT method 2

There is another choice – a variation in which, instead of an isometric contraction followed by stretch being commenced following the period of ease (strain/counterstrain position), an isolytic approach could be used.

The muscle receiving attention would be actively contracted by the patient at the same time that a stretch was being introduced, resulting in mild trauma to the muscle and the breakdown of fibrous adhesions between it and its interface and within its structures (Mitchell et al 1979).

To introduce this method into trigger point treatment, following the application of inhibitory pressure and SCS release, the patient would be asked to contract the muscles around the palpating thumb or finger (lying on the now inhibited pain point) with the request that the contraction should not be a full strength effort, since the operator intends to gently stretch the tissues while the contraction is taking place.

This isotonic eccentric effort – designed to reduce contractions and break down fibrotic tissue – should target precisely the tissues in which the trigger point being treated lies buried.

Following the isolytic stretch, the tissues could benefit from effleurage and/or hot and cold applications to ease local congestion. An instruction should be given to avoid active use of the area for a day or so.

To complete the sequence

Ruddy's pulsed MET can be used to facilitate weak antagonists to finish the INIT sequence. The methods of pulsed MET as developed by Ruddy (1961) were illustrated in earlier chapters (see Ch. 4 for examples). To complete the INIT sequence, pulsating contractions of the weak antagonists to muscles housing trigger points would further inhibit these muscles, as well as helping to tone and proprioceptively re-educate the antagonists.

SUMMARY

The integrated use of inhibitory pressure, strain/counterstrain and one or other form of muscle energy technique, applied to a trigger point or other area of soft tissue dysfunction involving pain or restriction of range of motion (of soft tissue origin), is a logical approach since it has the advantage of allowing precise targeting of the culprit tissues.

Clearly, the use of an isolytic approach as part of this sequence will be more easily achieved in some regions than others, upper trapezius, for example, posing less of a problem in terms of positioning and application than might quadratus lumborum.

REFERENCES

American College of Rheumatology 1990 Criteria for the classification of fibromyalgia. Arthritis and Rheumatism 33: 160–172

Barlow W 1959 Anxiety and muscle tension pain. British Journal of Clinical Practice 13: 5

Beal M 1983 Journal of the American Osteopathic Association (July)

Chaitow 1991a Palpatory literacy. Harper Collins, London

Chaitow L 1991b Soft tissue manipulation. Healing Arts Press, Rochester, Vermont

Chaitow L 1994 INIT in treatment of pain and trigger points. British Journal of Osteopathy 13: 17–21

Dittrich R 1954 Somatic pain and autonomic concomitants. American Journal of Surgery

Goldthwaite J 1949 Essentials of body mechanics. Lippincott, Philadelphia

Hong C-Z, Chen Y-C, Pon C, Yu J 1993 Immediate effects of various physical medicine modalities on pain threshold of an active myofascial trigger point. Journal of Musculoskeletal Pain 1(2)

Hong C-Z, Chen Y-N, Twehouse D, Hong D 1994 Pressure threshold for referred pain by compression on trigger point and adjacent area. Journal of Musculoskeletal Pain

Janda V 1983 Muscle function testing. Butterworths, London

Janda V 1985 Pain in the locomotor system. In: Glasgow E (ed) Aspects of manipulative therapy. Churchill Livingstone, London

Jones L 1981 Strain/counterstrain. Academy of Applied Osteopathy, Colorado Springs

Jonkheere P, Pattyn J 1998 Myofascial muscle chains. Trigger vzw, Brugge, Belgium

Kleyhans, Aarons 1974 Digest of Chiropractic Economics (September)

Korr I 1976 Spinal cord as organiser of the disease process. Yearbook of the Academy of Applied Osteopathy, Newark, Ohio

Latey P 1986 Muscular manifesto. Latey, London

Lewit K 1992 Manipulation in rehabilitation of the locomotor system. Butterworths, London

Lief S 1982/9 Described in: Chaitow L Neuromuscular technique, 1982, revised as Soft tissue manipulation, 1989 (further revised in 1991). Thorsons, Wellingborough

Melzack R, Wall P 1988 The challenge of pain. Penguin, New York

Mitchell F, Moran P, Pruzzo N 1979 Evaluation of osteopathic muscle energy procedure. Valley Park, Missouri

Nimmo R 1966 Receptor tonus technique. Lecture notes

Rolf I 1977 The integration of human structures. Harper and Row, New York

Ruddy T 1961 Osteopathic rhythmic resistive duction therapy. Yearbook of Academy of Applied Osteopathy 1961, Indianapolis

Selye H 1984 The stress of life. McGraw Hill, New York

Simons D 1989 Myofascial pain syndromes. Current therapy of pain. pp 251–266, B C Decker

Simons D, Travell J 1998 Trigger point manual, 2nd edn. Williams and Wilkins, Baltimore

Slocumb J 1984 Neurological factors in chronic pelvic pain. American Journal of Obstetrics and Gynaecology 49: 536

Travell J, Simons D 1986 Trigger point manual, 1st edn. Williams and Wilkins, Baltimore

Upledger J 1983 Craniosacral therapy. Eastland Press, Seattle

CHAPTER CONTENTS

8

Results of MET

The research examples given in this chapter relate to the application of MET in very different situations: chronic muscle pain, fibromyalgia, low back problems and acute joint problems following internal bleeding, as well as self-applied MET for unstable pelvic problems.

The sources are all derived from peer-reviewed literature relating to work carried out in settings as diverse as Polish, Swedish and Czech medical hospitals as well as a southside Chicago osteopathic hospital.

The diverse spectrum of dysfunction involved mirrors much that is faced on a daily basis by therapists and practitioners, and it is hoped that review of these reports will encourage the wider use of the variety of MET possibilities as outlined in this and earlier chapters.

MET RESULTS IN TREATMENT OF MYOFASCIAL PAIN

(Lewit & Simons 1984)

David Simons, co-researcher with Janet Travell into trigger points, and Karel Lewit, the Czech developer of gentler MET, have fairly conclusively demonstrated the efficiency of MET in a study involving assessment and treatment of severe muscular pain using MET. The study involved 244 patients with pain diagnosed as musculoskeletal in nature. These patients were examined and found to have between them 351 muscle groups requiring attention, based on their having:

1. Trigger points in the muscle and/or its insertion

2. Increased muscular tension during stretch
3. Muscular tension shortening which was not secondary to movement restriction caused by joint dysfunction.

These were muscular/soft tissue restrictions and not joint problems.

The method used in treating these muscles involved Lewit's postisometric relaxation approach (as described in Chs 3 and 4) in which prolonged but mild isometric contractions against resistance were carried out for 10 seconds before releasing. Following complete 'letting go' by the patient, and on a subsequent exhalation, any additional slack was taken up and the muscle moved to its new barrier ('stretch was stopped at the slightest resistance').

From the new position, the process was repeated, although if no release was apparent, contractions, which remained mild, were extended for up to 30 seconds. It was often noted that it was only after the second or third contraction that a release was obtained, and three to five repetitions were usually able to provide as much progress as was likely at one session.

When release was noted the operator was careful not to move too quickly: 'At this time the operator was careful not to interfere with the process and waited until the muscle relaxed completely. When the muscle reached a full range of motion the tension and the tender (trigger) points in the muscle were gone.'

The results were impressive, with 330 (94%) of the 351 muscles or muscle groups treated demonstrating immediate relief of pain and/or tenderness.

The technique was required to be precise concerning the direction of forces, which needed to be aligned to stretch the fibres demonstrating greatest tension. The patient's effort therefore needed to involve contraction in the direction which precisely affected these fibres. This was most important in triangular muscles such as pectoralis major and trapezius.

At a 3 month follow-up, lasting relief of pain was found to have been obtained in 63% (referring to the pain originally complained of) and lasting relief of tenderness (relating to relief of tenderness in the treated muscles) in a further 23% of muscles. Among the muscles treated in this study, those which were found to respond most successfully are given in Table 8.1.

The authors of the study point out that 'The technique not only abolished trigger points in muscles, but also relieved painful ligaments and periosteum in the region of attachment. The fact that increasing the length of shortened muscles relieved tenderness and pain, supports a muscu-

Table 8.1 Results of use of MET in myofascial pain study

Muscle	Number treated	Pain relief	Tenderness relief	No relief
Upper trapezius	7	7		
Wrist and finger flexors	5	5		
Lateral epicondyle of arm involving supinator, wrist and finger extensors and/or biceps brachii	20	19	1	
Suboccipital	23	21	2	
Soleus (Achilles tendon)	6	5	1	
Sternomastoid	9	7	2	
Hamstrings	8	5	2	1
Pelvic muscles/ligaments	29	22	4	3
Gluteus maximus (coccyx attachment)	27	15	9	3
Levator scapulae	19	10	7	2
Piriformis	21	11	6	4
Erector spinae	28	13	12	3
Deep paraspinal	15	7	5	3
Upper pectorals	22	10	5	7
Biceps femoris (fibula head)	18	8	6	4
Biceps femoris (long head)	7	2	0	5

lar origin of the pain.' They further point out that those patients achieving the greatest degree of long-term relief were those who carried out home treatment using MET stretches under instruction.

MET RESULTS IN TREATMENT OF FIBROMYALGIA

Drs Stotz and Kappler of the Chicago College of Osteopathic Medicine have treated patients with fibromyalgia (Stotz & Kappler 1992) utilising a variety of osteopathic approaches including MET. The results given below were achieved by incorporating MET alongside positional release methods and a limited degree of more active manipulation (personal communication to the author, 1994).

Fibromyalgia is notoriously unresponsive to standard methods of treatment and continues to be treated, in the main, by resort to mild antidepressant medication, despite many of the primary researchers' insistence that in most instances depression is a result, rather than a cause of the condition (Block 1993, Duna & Wilke 1993).

The Chicago physicians measured the effects of osteopathic manipulative therapy (OMT – which includes MET as a major element) on the intensity of pain reported from tender points in 18 patients who met all the criteria for fibromyalgia syndrome (FMS) (Goldenberg 1993).

Each patient had six visits/treatments and it was found over a 1 year period that 12 of the patients responded well in that their tender points became less sensitive (14% reduction against a 34% increase in the six patients who did not respond well). Activities of daily living were significantly improved and general pain symptoms decreased.

In another study, 19 patients with all the criteria of FMS were treated once a week for 4 weeks at Kirksville, Missouri, College of Osteopathic Medicine, using OMT which included MET as a major component. 84.2% showed improved sleep patterns, 94.7% reported less pain and most patients had fewer tender points on palpation (Rubin et al 1990).

MET RESULTS IN TREATMENT OF LOW BACK PAIN

Harald Brodin, of the Karolinska Hospital in Stockholm, describes the effects of using MET in a group of long-term, low back pain (lumbar area only) sufferers, specifically excluding patients with signs of disc compression, spondylitis or sacroiliac lesions, but not those with radiographic evidence of common degenerative signs – spondylosis deformans (Brodin 1987).

The group comprised 41 patients (24 female, 17 male) who had suffered pain in one or two lumbar segments, with reduced mobility, for a duration of at least 2 months. The patients were randomly assigned to two groups, one receiving no treatment and the other receiving MET treatment three times weekly for 3 weeks (see details below of the approach, which is described as 'a modification of the technique described by Lewit ... a variation of Mitchell's MET').

Both groups of patients recorded their pain level at rest and during activity according to a 9-graded scale each week.

Results

After 3 weeks, the group receiving treatment showed pain reduction statistically greater than in the non-treated group, as well as an increase in mobility of the lumbar spine:

- Of the treated group, four remained the same or were worse, while 17 were improved, of whom seven became totally pain free.
- Only one in the non-treated group became totally pain free, while 16 remained the same or were worse. A total of four of this group, including the one who was totally improved, showed some improvement.

What was the treatment offered in this study?

This was divided into two phases, inhibition and facilitation, as follows:

1. Inhibition

- The patient was side-lying, with the lumbar spine rotated by moving the upper shoulder backwards, with the table-side shoulder drawn forwards until the restricted segment of the spine was engaged.

- The practitioner stabilised the patient's pelvis as they pushed their shoulder forwards with a very small amount of effort, against resistance from the practitioner, for 7 seconds.
- During relaxation, the practitioner increased the degree of lumbar rotation to the new barrier, and repeated the isometric resistance phase again, until no further gain was made, usually four or five times in all.

2. Facilitation

- Active, rhythmic, small rotatory movements against the resistance barrier were carried out (see notes in Ch. 4 on Ruddy's approach).
- The patient held a deep breath and turned the head and looked in the direction of the rotation (towards the barrier).
- There was an isometric attempt, against the barrier, to reduce this, to increase rotation.

Additional information given by the author of this study includes the fact that sometimes rotation away from the barrier was the starting point for treatment, with rotation towards the pain-free direction of motion. It is not noted when this decision (to move away from the barrier at the outset) was made but it is logical to assume that it was adopted when engagement of the restriction barrier was painful.

Patients were advised to use pain-free movements and positions during everyday life.

The author states, 'From this study we can conclude that in preselected cases, muscle energy technique is an effective treatment for lower back pain.'

Direct attention to soft tissue imbalances might therefore be seen to be a means of helping to normalise painful spinal joints in many instances, especially if 'mobility is decreased, or its end-feel abnormally distinct' (Brodin 1982).

MET SELF-TREATMENT OF PELVIC INSTABILITY

Broadhurst (1997) describes a long-term Australian based study in which, over a 5–6 year period, he gathered evidence relating to 88 patients (64 female, 24 male) with deep-seated low back pain which proved to be of non-visceral origin. The most common characteristics (in no particular order of importance) were:

- A history of trauma, mainly twisting and compression type accidents causing pelvic torque (summarised as five after pregnancy; 16 following nursing injury; 11 as a result of motor vehicle accident; 56 following a forceful twist)
- Very low back pain
- Favoured one buttock when sitting
- Straight leg raise 70° without pain
- Constant diffuse pelvic discomfort
- Difficulty in weight-bearing on affected side
- No pain referral beyond pelvis
- Pain noted on inclines and stairs.

None of the patients were found to have thoracolumbar functional syndrome, or pelvic rotational or upslip dysfunction. All had been investigated with MRI or CT and all were found to be 'normal'.

Broadhurst notes that the combination of favouring one buttock on sitting, inability to weight-bear on the affected side, and the exacerbation of symptoms when going down stairs or inclines should alert to the possibility of an unstable SI joint. Further examination in these cases involved provocation to reproduce symptoms, rectal examination to stress the sacrospinous ligament on the ipsilateral side, and evaluation of tenderness at the symphysis pubis.

All 88 patients who entered the study were given pelvic support belts, and were asked to perform regular pelvic floor exercises. At 6 week follow-up most (63%) reported benefit from the pelvic support. Most had not complied with the exercises. A choice of additional therapy was offered to those still in pain, including trigger point injections, cortisone injections and sclerosing (dextrose) injections, as well as MET in the form of postisometric exercises (five repetitions twice daily) directed at psoas and piriformis.

Results were not statistically reliable because of the small numbers; however, what emerges from the MET self-care exercises was that 37% of those doing these exercises attributed their subsequent relief from pain to them.

Comment: This population represents a very difficult set of patients, as all bodyworkers will recognise. The choice of psoas and piriformis exercises seems arbitrary (based, it is reported, on the work of Lewit (1991) and Fishman & Zybert (1992)). Identification of specific shortness in other associated muscles (possibly hamstrings or quadratus lumborum) would have been straightforward, as would the prescribing of MET self-treatment as appropriate. The fact that, despite this, almost two out of five patients benefited attests to the possibilities inherent in this approach.

MET TREATMENT OF JOINTS DAMAGED BY HAEMOPHILIA

Just how useful MET can be in treating joint problems in even severely ill patients is illustrated by a Polish study of the effects of use of MET in a group of haemophiliac patients in whom bleeding had occurred into the joints. There had also been bleeding into muscles such as iliopsoas, quadriceps and gastrocnemius (Kwolek 1989).

The study notes that 'As a result of haemorrhage into the joints and muscles the typical signs and symptoms of inflammation develop; if they are untreated or treated incorrectly or rehabilitation is neglected, motion restriction, deformation, athrodesis, muscle atrophy, scarring and muscular contractures may occur.'

Standard medical treatment used included electromagnetic field applications, heat, paraffin baths and massage as well – where appropriate – as the use of casts for limbs and other medical and surgical procedures.

All patients received instruction as to self-application of breathing, relaxation and general fitness exercise as well as rehabilitation methods for the affected joints using postisometric relaxation methods (MET). These were performed twice daily, for a total of 60 minutes.

Range of movement was assessed, and it was found that those patients using PIR (MET) methods achieved an improvement in range of movement of between 5° and 50° in 87% of the 49 joints treated – mainly involving ankles, knees and elbows (there was a reduction in motion range of 5–10° in just six joints). These undoubtedly impressive results for MET in a group of severely ill and vulnerable patients further highlights the safety of the method, since anything approaching aggressive intervention in treating such patients would be contraindicated.

The researchers, having pointed to frequent complications arising in the course of more traditional approaches, concluded: 'The 87% improvement in movement range of 5° to 50° and the lack of complications when rehabilitating articulations with haemophiliac arthropathy speaks in favour of routine application of the post isometric relaxation methods for patients with haemophilia.'

REFERENCES

Block S 1993 Fibromyalgia and the rheumatisms. Controversies in Rheumatology 119(1): 61–78

Broadhurst N 1997 Deep-seated low back pain – a triad of symptoms for pelvic instability. In: Vleeming A, Mooney V, Dorman T, Snijders C, Stoeckart R (eds) Movement stability and low back pain. Churchill Livingstone, Edinburgh

Brodin H 1982 Lumbar treatment using MET. Osteopathic Annals 10: 23–24

Brodin H 1987 Inhibition-facilitation technique for lumbar pain treatment. Manual Medicine 3: 24–26

Duna G, Wilke W 1993 Diagnosis, etiology and therapy of fibromyalgia. Comprehensive Therapy 19(2): 60–63

Fishman L, Zybert P 1992 Electrophysiologic evidence of piriformis syndrome. Archives of Physical Medicine and Rehabilitation 73: 359–364

Goldenberg D 1993 Fibromyalgia, chronic fatigue syndrome and myofascial pain syndrome. Current Opinion in Rheumatology 5: 199–208

Kwolek A 1989 Rehabilitation treatment with post-isometric muscle relaxation for haemophilia patients. Journal of Manual Medicine 4: 55–57

Lewit K, Simons D 1984 Myofascial pain: relief by post-isometric relaxation. Archives of Physical Medicine and Rehabilitation 65: 452–456

Lewit K 1991 Manipulative therapy in rehabilitation of the motor system. Butterworths, London

Rubin B et al 1990 Treatment options in fibromyalgia syndrome. Journal of the American Osteopathic Association 90(9): 844–845

Stotz A, Kappler R 1992 Effects of osteopathic manipulative treatment on tender points associated with fibromyalgia. Journal of the American Osteopathic Association 92(9): 1183–1184

Index

Page numbers in **bold** *type refer to illustrations and tables*

A

B

C

D

E